Interstitium, Connective Tissue and Lymphatics

Animal Experimentation and the Future of Medical
  Research

Embryonic Development and Manipulation in Animal
  Production

Immunotechnology

Nitric Oxide: Brain and Immune System

Proteolysis and Protein Turnover

Temperature Adaptation of Biological Membranes

The Biology of Nitric Oxide
  Parts 1–4, including
  Enzymology, Biochemistry and Immunology
  Physiological and Clinical Aspects

Interstitium, Connective Tissue and Lymphatics

Proceedings of the XXXII
Congress of the International
Union of Physiological
Sciences, Glasgow, U.K.

Editors

R. K. Reed
N. G. McHale
J. L. Bert
C. P. Winlove
G. A. Laine

PORTLAND PRESS

Published by Portland Press, 59 Portland Place, London WIN 3AJ, U.K.
In North America orders should be sent to Ashgate Publishing Co.,
Old Post Road, Brookfield, VT 05036-9704, U.S.A.

© 1995 Portland Press Ltd, London

ISBN 1 85578 073 9   ISSN 0966-4068

British Library Cataloguing in Publication Data
A catalogue record for this book is available from the British Library

Typeset by Unicus Graphics Ltd, Horsham, Sussex and
Printed in Great Britain by Whitstable Litho Printers Ltd

Front cover shows illustration of morpho-functional arrangement of the
pleural structures (D. Negrini, Milan, Italy).

K. Åhlén
Department of Medical and Physiological Chemistry, University of Uppsala, BMC, Box 575, S-751 23 Uppsala, Sweden

S.J. Allen
Department of Veterinary Physiology and Pharmacology, College of Veterinary Medicine, Texas A&M University, TX 77843-4466, U.S.A.

K. Aukland
Department of Physiology, University of Bergen, Årstadveien 19, 5009 Bergen, Norway

G.T. Belz
Department of Anatomical Sciences, University of Queensland, Brisbane, Qld. 4072, Australia

E. Benaim
Julius Silver Institute of Biomedical Engineering Sciences, Department of Biomedical Engineering, Technion, Israel Institute of Technology, Haifa 32000, Israel

J.L. Bert
Department of Chemical Engineering, University of British Columbia, 2216 Main Mall, Vancouver, Canada V6T 1Z4

M.J. Crowe
The Neuroscience Group, Discipline of Human Physiology, Faculty of Medicine and Health Sciences, University of Newcastle, Callaghan, NSW 2308, Australia

K.L. Davis
Department of Veterinary Physiology and Pharmacology, College of Veterinary Medicine, Texas A&M University, TX 77843-4466, U.S.A.

J. Dudhia
Kennedy Institute of Rheumatology, Bute Gardens, Hammersmith, London W6 7DW, U.K.

A.J. Fosang
Orthopaedic Molecular Biology Research Unit, Royal Children's Hospital, Melbourne, Victoria, Australia

S.T. Greiner
Department of Medical Physiology, Texas A&M University Health Science Center, College Station, TX 77843-1114, U.S.A.

A.J. Grodzinsky
Department of Electrical Engineering and Computer Science, Department of Mechanical Engineering, Massachusetts Institute of Technology, Cambridge, MA 02139, U.S.A.

A.C. Guyton
University of Mississippi Medical Center, Department of Physiology and Biophysics, 2500 N. State Street, Jackson, MS 39216-4505, U.S.A.

T.E. Hardingham
Kennedy Institute of Rheumatology, Bute Gardens, Hammersmith, London W6 7DW, U.K.

J.B. Hay
Trauma Research Program, Sunnybrook Health Science Centre, 2075 Bayview Avenue, North York, Ontario M4N 3M5, Canada

T.J. Heath
Department of Anatomical Sciences, University of Queensland, Brisbane, Qld. 4072, Australia

M.G. Johnston
Trauma Research Program, Sunnybrook Health Science Centre, 2075 Bayview Avenue, North York, Ontario, Canada M4N 3M5

P.L. Khimenko
Department of Physiology, University of South Alabama, College of Medicine, Mobile, AL 36688-0002, U.S.A.

G.A. Laine
Department of Veterinary Physiology and Pharmacology, College of Veterinary Medicine, Texas A&M University, TX 77843-4466, U.S.A.

T.C. Laurent
Department of Medical and Physiological Chemistry, Biomedical Center, Box 575, S-751 23 Uppsala, Sweden

J.R. Levick
Department of Physiology, St George's Hospital Medical School, London SW17 0RE, U.K.

C.S. Lowden
Department of Anatomical Sciences, University of Queensland, Brisbane, Qld. 4072, Australia

A. Maroudas
Julius Silver Institute of Biomedical Engineering Sciences, Department of Biomedical Engineering, Technion, Israel Institute of Technology, Haifa 32000, Israel

M. Martinez
Department of Chemical Engineering, University of British Columbia, 2216 Main Mall, Vancouver, Canada V6T 1Z4

J.N. McDonald
Department of Physiology, St George's Hospital Medical School, London SW17 0RE, U.K.

N.G. McHale
Department of Physiology, School of Biomedical Science, The Queen's University of Belfast, 97 Lisburn Road, Belfast BT9 7BL, Northern Ireland, U.K.

U. Mehlhorn
Department of Veterinary Physiology and Pharmacology, College of Veterinary Medicine, Texas A&M University, TX 77843-4466, U.S.A.

J. Mizrahi
Julius Silver Institute of Biomedical Engineering Sciences, Department of Biomedical Engineering, Technion, Israel Institute of Technology, Haifa 32000, Israel

T.M. Moore
Department of Physiology, University of South Alabama, College of Medicine, Mobile, AL 36688-0002, U.S.A.

D. Negrini
Istituto di Fisiologia Umana, Via Mangiagalli 32, 20133 Milano, Italy

K.H. Parker
Physiological Flow Studies Group, Centre for Biological and Medical Systems, Imperial College of Science, Technology and Medicine, London SW7 2BY, U.K.

R.K. Reed
Department of Physiology, University of Bergen, Årstadveien 19, N-5009 Bergen, Norway

E.M. Renkin
Department of Human Physiology, University of California, Davis, CA 95616, U.S.A.

A. Rizzo
Department of Surgery, University of South Alabama, College of Medicine, Mobile, AL 36688-0002, U.S.A.

K. Rubin
Department of Medical and Physiological Chemistry, University of Uppsala, BMC, Box 575, S-751 23 Uppsala, Sweden

C. Sundberg
Department of Medical and Physiological Chemistry, University of Uppsala, BMC, Box 575, S-751 23 Uppsala, Sweden

A.E. Taylor
Department of Physiology, University of South Alabama, College of Medicine, Mobile, AL 36688-0002, U.S.A.

D.G. Taylor
Department of Chemical Engineering, University of Ottawa, 161 Louis Pasteur, Ottawa, Canada K1N 6N5

O. Tenstad
Department of Physiology, University of Bergen, Årstadveien 19, 5009 Bergen, Norway

V.L. Tucker
Department of Human Physiology, University of California, Davis, CA 95616, U.S.A.

J.P.G. Urban
University Laboratory of Physiology, Oxford University, Oxford OX1 3PT, U.K.

D.F. van Helden
The Neuroscience Group, Discipline of Human Physiology, Faculty of Medicine and Health Sciences, University of Newcastle, Callaghan, NSW 2308, Australia

P.-Y. von der Weid
The Neuroscience Group, Discipline of Human Physiology, Faculty of Medicine and Health Sciences, University of Newcastle, Callaghan, NSW 2308, Australia

C.P. Winlove
Physiological Flow Studies Group, Centre for Biological and Medical Systems, Imperial College of Science, Technology and Medicine, London SW7 2BY, U.K.

A.J. Young
Department of Immunology and Pathology, University of Toronto, Toronto, Canada

D.C. Zawieja
Department of Medical Physiology, Texas A&M University Health Science Center, College Station, TX 77843-1114, U.S.A.

A-II	Angiotensin II
AA	Atrial-appendectomized
ALDO	Aldosterone
ANP	Atrial natriuretic peptide
CHO	Chinese hamster ovary
COP	Colloid osmotic pressure
CS	Chondroitin sulphate
CVP	Central venous pressure
ECF	Extracellular fluid
ECM	Extracellular matrix
EDRF	Endothelium-derived relaxing factor
EF	Extrafibrillar
EGF	Epidermal growth factor
EJF	Ejection fraction
EJP	Excitatory junction potential
ELG	Electrolymphangiogram
F	Lymphatic contraction frequency
FCD	Fixed charge density
GAG	Glycosaminoglycan
HA$_6$	Hyaluronan hexasaccharide
HA$_{12}$	Hyaluronan dodecasaccharide
HPH	High concentration of H_2O_2
HPL	Low concentration of H_2O_2
5-HT	5-Hydroxytryptamine
IAP	Intra-articular pressure
IF	Intrafibrillar
IFNγ	Interferon γ
IGD	Interglobular domain
IL	Interleukin
IL-I	Interleukin I
IP$_3$	Inositol 1,4,5-trisphosphate
ISF	Interstitial fluid
ISFV	Interstitial fluid volume
KS	Keratan sulphate
LDL	Low-density lipoprotein
LPF	Lymph pump flow index
NO	Nitric oxide
NPY	Neuropeptide Y
P$_{if}$	Interstitial fluid pressure
P$_{int}$	Myocardial interstitial pressure
PDGF	Platelet-derived growth factor
PG	Proteoglycan
PKC	Protein kinase C
pp125^{FAK}	Focal adhesion protein tyrosine kinase
SH	High generation rate of superoxide anions
SL	Low generation rate of superoxide anions
SOD	Superoxide dismutase
STD	Spontaneous transient depolarization
SV	Stroke volume

TEA	Tetraethylammonium ion
TGF-β	Transforming growth factor β
TNF-α	Tumour necrosis factor α
VA	Albumin distribution volume
VLDL	Very-low-density lipoprotein

Structure of the extracellular matrix and the biology of hyaluronan

Torvard C. Laurent
Department of Medical and Physiological Chemistry, University of Uppsala, Uppsala, Sweden

Introduction

This contribution is divided into three separate parts. Being asked to give the first paper at the symposium, I thought that it would be appropriate to start with a short review of the history of the interstitium and the extracellular matrix. My own main interest during the last 45 years has been the interstitial polysaccharide hyaluronan. In the second section I have therefore given an overview of research on this compound, especially after 1980. Finally in the third section I have dealt with a recent experiment on hyaluronan which may have interesting physiological implications.

In order not to overload the article with references I have, whenever possible, cited review articles rather than original work. For this I apologize to all those who have made the primary observations.

History of matrix research

The interstitium

The birth of the interstitium must be the discovery of blood circulation by William Harvey in 1628 and the discoveries in the early 1650s of the lymph vessels by Thomas Bartholin, Olaus Rudbeckius and Jean Pecquet.

The interstitium (although I doubt that the word was used at that time) could then be defined as the 'black box' in which fluid flowed between the blood circulation and the lymph vessels. Marcello Malpighi's discovery of the capillaries, also in the 17th century, gave a closer anatomical location of the black box.

The next step came during the 19th century. Although Malpighi had already discovered cells in plant material, it would take 200 years before it was shown by Theodore Schwann that the animal organism was also formed by a large number of cells. After that the interstitium could, in principle, be defined as the space between the cells. The French physiologist Claude Bernard coined, in 1857, the term 'milieu interieur' for the composition of the intercellular phase.

Correspondence address: Department of Medical and Physiological Chemistry, University of Uppsala, Box 575, S-75123 Uppsala, Sweden.

The extracellular material (the matrix)
We now know that the space between the cells is filled with macro-molecular material which forms the matrix. Important prerequisites for the discovery of these components were the dyes produced in the German chemical industry during the 19th century. It was with the aid of these dyes that one could, before the turn of the century, distinguish between striated fibres, that we now know as collagen, and an amor-phous ground substance in the connective tissue. For some historical data on the matrix see Schubert and Hamerman [1] and Mathews [2].

The presence of collagen, however, was known much earlier. It was used for industrial purposes to generate glue, and Berzelius described in 1810 that heating cartilage as well as bone yielded similar glues. Although the leather-industry chemists were interested in the nature of collagen, due to the insolubility of its fibres its molecular structure was not defined until the second half of the present century. Since then there has been rapid progress in the collagen field and we now know of a large number of different types of collagens. We also know of other fibres in the matrix, e.g. elastic fibres.

The history of the ground substance started in 1838 when Mulder was able to show the presence of sulphate in material isolated from cartilage. Through the work of Krukenberg, Mörner and Schmiedeberg in the 1880s carbohydrate-containing material was isolated from cartilage, i.e. chondroitin sulphate and cartilage proteoglycans. However, the chemical structures of the various connective-tissue polysaccharides were not determined until the 1950s, especially by Karl Meyer and his collaborators (see e.g. Brimacombe and Webber [3]). We have now defined a number of polysaccharides: hyaluronan, chondroitin sulphates, dermatan sulphate, heparan sulphate and keratan sulphate, and also the covalent complexes formed between polysaccharides and proteins, the proteoglycans. The final determination of the structures of the latter was not accomplished until the development of modern molecular biology.

A third group of matrix substances was ill-defined for a long time and usually called insoluble-tissue glycoproteins. We now know that this group embraces a number of proteins with very specific properties, functions and tissue distributions, such as fibronectin, laminin, tenascin, bone-specific sialoprotein, osteopontin, etc. The elucidation of their structures and interactions in the last few decades has given a completely new insight into the biology of the matrix. We know that many of these proteins bind specifically to 'receptors' on the cell surface; in most instances to members of the integrin family.

The function of the matrix
Our concept of the function of the matrix has gradually changed. When I started to work on connective tissue at the end of the 1940s the general concept was that collagen gave strength and stability to the tissues and the ground substance was an undefined colloid which filled the space between the fibres.

Gersh and Catchpole [4] summarized, in 1960, the hypothetical functions of the ground substance, as shown in Table 1. The first point is identical with the 'milieu interieur' of Claude Bernard and the second is in essence the function as a filling material. The barrier function against bacterial invasion was discovered by Duran-Reynals in 1928 when

	Proposed function	Table I
1	The actual homoeostatic environment of most cells and a sink for their metabolites	
2	Stabilizer of the spatial and functional relations between cells	
3	The mother liquor from which come connective-tissue fibres	
4	A barrier to bacterial invasion	
5	Site of changes in growth, differentiation, regeneration and ageing	
6	A target of hormonal action	
7	A site of changes in inflammation, oedema, rickets, periodontosis, scurvy, arteriosclerosis and collagen diseases	
8	A site of normal and pathological calcification	

Suggested functions of the ground substance proposed by Gersh and Catchpole in 1960 [4]

he showed that particles were spreading more rapidly in skin after injection of a 'spreading factor' which turned out to be hyaluronidase. The evidence for the last four functions in Table 1 was collected essentially from histological observations and none had a solid molecular basis.

Through work mainly in the 1960s and 1970s a new insight into the possible functions of the polysaccharides developed [5,6] (Table 2). Physicochemical studies on semi-dilute solutions of the polysaccharides showed that they behaved as entangled networks with remarkable properties that could be connected with defined physiological roles. The rheological properties of hyaluronan solutions indicated that they could act as lubricants in joints and tissues. The non-ideal osmotic properties of polysaccharide solutions made them ideal osmotic buffers. This, and a high flow resistance in polymer networks, gave the polysaccharides a role in water homoeostasis. The discovery of exclusion of other macromolecules from polysaccharide compartments was taken to suggest a role for the polysaccharides in regulating various reactions, such as the physiological partitioning of proteins between different compartments or the pathological precipitation of immune complexes and lipoproteins. Finally, the network of chains could act as a barrier for, or a carrier of, macromolecules and particles, and could play a role in regulating transport through the connective tissue.

The organization of the matrix

The next step in the development came in 1972, when Hardingham and Muir discovered that proteoglycans from cartilage could aggregate with hyaluronan (see Hardingham [7]). It was the first example of a specific interaction between two extracellular matrix components. Since then we have obtained knowledge of a large number of specific interactions between various matrix components, as well as between matrix components and the cell surface. Our concept of the amorphous ground substance has now developed into the recognition of a highly ordered supra-macromolecular structure. This is illustrated in Figure 1, reproduced from Heinegård and Oldberg [8].

Table 2

	Function	Property
1	Lubrication	Viscoelasticity Non-Newtonian flow
2	Water homoeostasis	
	Flow barriers	High flow resistance
	Osmotic buffers	Non-ideal osmotic pressure
3	Partition of plasma proteins	Exclusion of macromolecules from
	Formation of precipitates	polysaccharide compartments
	Stabilization of structures	
4	Regulation of macromolecular	Molecular sieving
	transport through the	Ordered convective transport
	interstitium	

Functions of connective-tissue polysaccharides related to their physical and chemical properties (see e.g. [5,6])

Figure 1

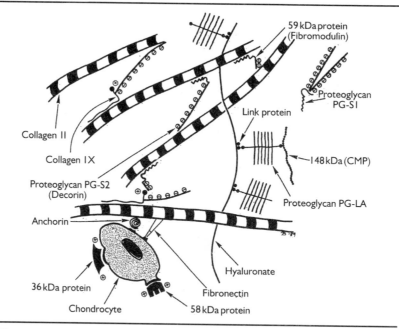

Illustration of the highly complex supramolecular structure of the matrix in cartilage

A number of specific interactions occur between the various matrix components and between matrix components and the cell surface. Reproduced from Heinegård and Oldberg [8] with permission.

What is especially interesting in the new concept is that the cells themselves are part of the structures. Via cell-surface binding proteins the cells are directly bound to collagen fibres, polysaccharide chains, fibronectin, laminin, basal membranes, etc. This means that the properties and functions of the matrix components are not static and independent of cellular reactions but are under the constant influence of cellular activities. The cells influence the matrix both by synthesis and degradation of the extracellular material and by direct interaction with the organized matrix.

We have, to my knowledge, at present two examples of how interplay between cells and matrix determines a physiological process for which we previously thought the properties of the matrix components alone were responsible. One of them concerns the influence of cellular activity on the interstitial pressure [9]. The other has been published by Tay et al. [10] and concerns the interplay between endothelial cells and the basal membranes in regulating the glomerular permeability of the kidney.

We have thus come a long way from the black box and the inert amorphous ground substance to a highly structured and cellularly regulated matrix.

Hyaluronan research

Hyaluronan [11,12] — previously called hyaluronic acid — was described, in 1934, by Karl Meyer and it was also Meyer and co-workers who determined the structure of the polymer to be a linear chain of D-glucuronic acid and N-acetyl-D-glucosamine linked by β1-3 and β1-4 glycosidic linkages. The chain is relatively stiff, presumably due to stabilizing hydrogen bonds between the sugar residues.

Hyaluronan from most sources has a relative molecular mass of several million. In solution the molecule behaves as a very extended coil which immobilizes a large amount of solvent. Already at concentrations of 1 mg/ml the coils start to entangle and at higher concentrations they form a more or less continuous network in solution. As mentioned above, the physical properties of these networks have been associated with various physiological functions in the matrix.

A turning point for hyaluronan research occurred in 1980. The clinical and commercial interest in the compound had increased after its introduction as an aid in eye surgery but there were also methodological breakthroughs which made biological and medical experiments feasible. Some of the techniques developed at that time are listed in Table 3. Most important of all of them were the new assays to measure hyaluronan specifically in nanogram quantities. The first one was introduced by Anders Tengblad and made it possible to determine hyaluronan concentrations routinely in blood. Some aspects of hyaluronan research, which have been prominent in the last decade, are discussed below:

Biosynthesis of hyaluronan
Mainly through work by Peter Prehm [13] it has been clarified that hyaluronan is synthesized in the plasma membrane by addition of sugars to the reducing end of the chain. The chain is translocated from the cytoplasmic side to the pericellular space where it forms a thick coat on the cell surface. A number of inflammatory mediators and growth factors activate the synthesis [14] and several laboratories are working on the mechanism of regulation of the biosynthesis.

Table 3

	Technique
1	New specific assays for hyaluronan which can quantify nanogram amounts directly in body fluids
2	New gel chromatographic techniques which can determine M_r distributions on a microgram scale
3	Histochemical techniques to visualize hyaluronan specifically using affinity probes
4	Availability of biosynthetically labelled radioactive hyaluronan for turnover studies
5	Hyaluronan coupled with ligands which could be used to pinpoint the site of degradation of the polysaccharide
6	New techniques to separate liver cells

New techniques introduced during the 1980s which promoted the progress of hyaluronan research

Figure 2

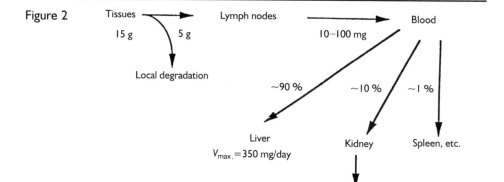

An overview of the turnover of hyaluronan in the adult human
Reproduced from [16] with permission.

Catabolic pathways
The discovery that hyaluronan is present in blood, although at very low concentrations, started an investigation of the turnover of hyaluronan [15–17]. It was shown that the serum hyaluronan originates in the tissues and is carried to the blood by the lymph. It is rapidly cleared from the circulation. Figure 2 describes our present concept of the turnover of hyaluronan; the data are based not only on studies on humans but are also extrapolated from experiments on animals.

From measurements in rats we expect that the adult human body should contain about 15 g of hyaluronan, more than half of which will be in the skin. Approximately one-third is turning over each day, which is a surprisingly high figure. We now know that part of it is degraded locally but part is carried by the lymph to the lymph nodes, where the major portion is taken up and degraded, and part is carried to the bloodstream. About 30–40 mg is turning over in the circulation every day in the adult. The concentration of hyaluronan in serum is in the order of 30–40 ng/ml in a middle-aged man. The half-life of hyaluronan in blood is 2–5 min and at least 90% is taken up by the liver. Special hyaluronan receptors on the endothelial cells in the liver sinusoids mediate the internalization, and the polysaccharide is finally degraded in the lysosomes. The degradation products appear in blood 20 min after uptake. A minor amount of the circulating hyaluronan is apparently metabolized in the kidney and spleen. A very small amount of low-molecular-mass hyaluronan appears in urine.

The fraction of hyaluronan in the tissues which is carried by the lymph to the circulation varies [17]. Hyaluronan in the intestine seems to be very mobile and can, to a large extent, be washed out by an increased lymph flow. However, only a small fraction of the hyaluronan in skin and lung is removed under similar conditions.

Hyaladherins

One of the most interesting aspects of hyaluronan research in recent years deals with proteins which specifically recognize hyaluronan. Many of them are anchored to cell surfaces and are often called receptors. Toole has suggested a collective name for these proteins, hyaladherins [18]. The first proteins described in this family were the aggregating proteoglycan and the link proteins, which are extracellular proteins. The first indication that cell-surface proteins bind hyaluronan came from studies showing that hyaluronan aggregates certain cells. Later, Underhill and Toole isolated a hyaluronan-binding protein from SW3T3 cells which now seems to be identical to the lymphocyte homing receptor CD44. Smedsröd et al. showed the presence of the liver endothelial receptor for hyaluronan and Eva Turley isolated a protein that she termed RHAMM (receptor for hyaluronan mediating motility). There are also a number of other proteins described such as hyaluronectin (Delpech et al., see [11]) and a 68000-M_r protein from rat tissues (Datta et al., see [11]).

The cell–matrix interactions mediated by hyaladherins have presumably important biological implications in development, formation of structured extracellular matrix, cellular behaviour, metastasis of tumours, etc. [19]. We are only beginning to understand the cell-biological role of hyaluronan.

Pathology of hyaluronan metabolism

One of the practical consequences of the metabolic studies on hyaluronan has been the discovery that the polysaccharide can be used to monitor pathological processes and probably also be the cause of certain pathological phenomena.

When it became possible to measure blood hyaluronan, its level was recorded in a number of patients [20]. It became immediately apparent that in liver disease the level was often highly elevated (up to 100-fold). High serum hyaluronan correlated to liver cirrhosis documented by liver biopsies. Although the most apparent cause for the increased level seems to be impaired function of the liver endothelial cells, there are alternative explanations, such as an increased production of hyaluronan by the liver, a decreased blood flow through the liver, or an increased amount of hyaluronan carried by the lymph from the splanchnic region to the circulation in portal hypertension. Another condition in which serum hyaluronan has been an important diagnostic sign is the rejection of a liver graft.

In several diseases a high serum hyaluronan level is a sign of an increased synthesis of the polysaccharide. Many of these conditions are inflammatory, e.g. rheumatoid arthritis. As mentioned above, a large number of inflammatory mediators [14] (growth factors, interleukins, prostaglandins, etc.) activate hyaluronan synthesis in the tissues and therefore more is carried to the circulation. In rheumatoid arthritis the highest serum levels are found after the patients first get out of bed in the morning. The reason is that hyaluronan accumulates in the inflamed joints overnight and is then pumped out into the circulation by the muscular activity. The observation also gives an explanation for the symptom of morning stiffness in these patients — the hyaluronan accumulated in the joints attracts water and causes an oedema.

Other diseases where high serum levels of hyaluronan have been noticed include sepsis, certain tumours, such as Wilms' tumour and mesothelioma, and some rare hereditary diseases such as Werner's syndrome.

The observation that accumulation of hyaluronan impairs the normal activity of the joint has been followed by other discoveries in which a hyaluronan-induced oedema damages organ functions. Alveolitis in the lung activates hyaluronan synthesis, and gas exchange becomes reduced [20]. Also, organ transplants which are rejected contain large amounts of hyaluronan. This could be a cause of the oedema seen in rejected kidneys [21]. Hyaluronan accumulation has also been observed after ischaemic heart disease [22].

Clinical use of hyaluronan

As mentioned above, one of the reasons for the growing interest in hyaluronan has been its introduction in clinical practice. The person mainly responsible for this development has been Endre Balazs [23]. Although hyaluronan was tried at an early stage in the treatment of joint disease, the first actual success came in ophthalmic surgery in about 1980 [24]. Hyaluronan is especially used to protect the delicate structures of the anterior chamber during cataract surgery. Since then the use in joint treatment has increased and the possibility of using the polysaccharide in improving wound healing, preventing adhesions and as a drug carrier is being actively pursued.

The above examples indicate how, for at least one matrix component (hyaluronan), interest has changed in the last decade from studies on the chemical and macromolecular properties of the poly-saccharide towards its metabolism, specific interactions with proteins and cell-biological role. The results have generated interesting conse-quences for physiology, pathology and clinical medicine.

On the nature of the pericellular coat

Clarris and Fraser [25] discovered 25 years ago 'clouds' or 'coats' around fibroblasts in cell cultures. These cannot be seen by histological fixation and staining but can be visualized if particles such as red blood cells are added to the cultures. The particles are excluded from a large volume around the fibroblasts by some invisible structure (Figure 3). The structure disappears when hyaluronidase is added to the cultures. This pericellular layer has received increasing attention in recent years. There are at least two possible means of anchoring the hyaluronan coat to the cell. One is via hyaluronan synthase, which continuously translocates the hyaluronan molecule into the pericellular space. The other is by binding of an exogenous hyaluronan molecule to a hyaluronan receptor on the cell surface. Both mechanisms probably exist.

The extension of the pericellular layer is of the same order as the diameter of the cell and the total length of the elongated hyaluronan molecule. This is paradoxical as the hyaluronan molecule appears in solution in a coiled form. It is also difficult to envisage free elongated hyaluronan molecules being able to withstand the mechanical pressure of erythrocytes. There must therefore be some stabilizing forces in the coat. One possible stabilizing factor could be the binding of proteoglycans along the hyaluronan chains.

Heldin and Pertoft [26] in my laboratory have studied the properties of the pericellular coat around mesothelial cells with image analysis. When followed in culture a coat of maximal size is formed in about 5 h. The investigators also added exogenous compounds to the cultures in order to influence the coat formation. The addition of neither high-M_r hyaluronan nor aggregating proteoglycans had any visible effect on the size of the coat. This argued against the possibility that the coat originated from exogenous macromolecules. However, the addition of a hyaluronan dodecasaccharide (HA_{12}) prevented the coat formation.

Figure 3

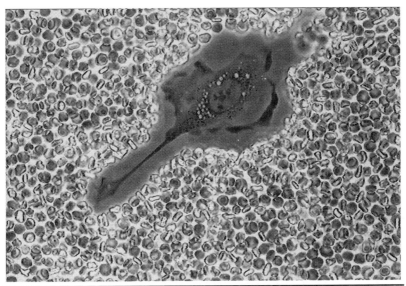

A human mesothelial cell grown *in vitro*
The hyaluronan-containing coats visualized by the exclusion of erythrocytes.
Reproduced from Heldin and Pertoft [26] with permission.

It was first ascertained, by incorporation of radioactive precursors, that HA_{12} did not inhibit the synthesis of hyaluronan by the cells. This conclusion was also verified when it was found that HA_{12}, when added to cells which already had developed coats, dissolved these within 15 min. Secondly, it was tested whether the oligosaccharide did compete with the binding of hyaluronan to a hyaladherin on the cell surface. Such a protein should recognize a hexasaccharide (HA_6), but HA_6 had no effect on the cloud formation. Neither could hyaladherins on the cell surface be detected by binding of radioactive hyaluronan or by immunological techniques. Another possible action of HA_{12} was also found to be improbable, i.e. the competition with the endogenous hyaluronan for aggregating proteoglycans and link proteins. As mentioned, addition of aggrecan to the cultures had no effect on the coat formation; nor had the addition of exogenous hyaluronan which could, as well as HA_{12}, compete for endogenous aggrecans.

A possible explanation came from studies on oligosaccharides of increasing length. HA_6 had no effect on the coat, HA_{10} had a medium effect and HA_{12} had a maximal effect but with further increased length of the oligosaccharide the activity decreased and a polymer with a relative molecular mass of 40000 stabilized rather than destabilized the coat. This behaviour could fit with a role for the oligosaccharides as competitors to chain–chain interaction between hyaluronan molecules. John Scott and colleagues [27] have shown that there is a possibility for chain–chain interactions based on the conformation of the hyaluronan chain and they also have evidence from electron microscopy that hyaluronan forms networks stabilized by chain interactions.

Short oligosaccharides could compete with such interactions while longer hyaluronan chains would stabilize the network by binding to two or more chains. This is consistent with the work of Rees and collaborators [28] whose rheological studies on hyaluronan provided evidence for transient chain–chain interactions which disappeared when hyaluronan molecules with 60 disaccharides were added.

It is not probable that intermediate oligosaccharides are formed *in vivo* in such concentrations that they will interfere with the normal formation of a hyaluronate network. However, oligosaccharides could be an interesting tool with which to study the role of the hyaluronan matrix. It is noteworthy in this context that West and Kumar [29] observed that intermediate oligosaccharides can induce angiogenesis. For the matrix researcher, whether physiologist or cell biologist, hyaluronan oligosaccharide-induced matrix 'collapse' should be a new and powerful experimental tool.

Summary

The aim of this chapter has been threefold. As an introduction to a book on the interstitium I have tried to provide a short historical description of how our view of the matrix has changed from that of a black box to a highly organized structure integrated with the cell surface. The new concepts developed by the biochemists should influence profoundly the thinking of physiologists. In the second part I have outlined research on hyaluronan during the last decade. This molecule is turning over remarkably quickly and its metabolism may be of consequence for both physiological and pathological phenomena in the interstitium. Finally, I have described recent experiments, which indicate that the hyaluronan matrix can be broken down by addition of hyaluronan oligosaccharides, probably due to interference with chain–chain interactions in the hyaluronan network.

I am grateful to all my co-workers over the years. This contribution was supported by grants from the Swedish Medical Research Council (3X-4).

References

1. Schubert, M. and Hamerman, D. (1968) *A Primer on Connective Tissue Biochemistry*, Lea & Febiger, Philadelphia
2. Mathews, M.B. (1975) *Connective Tissue: Macromolecular Structure and Evolution*, Springer-Verlag, Berlin
3. Brimacombe, J.S. and Webber, J.M. (1969) *Mucopolysaccharides*, Elsevier, Amsterdam
4. Gersh, I. and Catchpole, H.R. (1960) The nature of ground substance of connective tissue. *Perspect. Biol. Med.* **3**, 282–319
5. Laurent, T.C. (1970) The structure and function of the intercellular polysaccharides in connective tissue. In *Capillary Permeability* (Crone, V. and Lassen, N.A., eds.), pp. 261–277, Munksgaard, Copenhagen
6. Comper, W.D. and Laurent, T.C. (1978) Physiological function of connective tissue poly-saccharides. *Physiol. Rev.* **58**, 255–315
7. Hardingham, T. (1981) Proteoglycans: their structure, interactions and molecular organizations in cartilage. *Biochem. Soc. Trans.* **9**, 489–497
8. Heinegård, D. and Oldberg, Å. (1989) Structure and biology of cartilage and bone matrix noncollagenous macromolecules. *FASEB J.* **3**, 2042–2051
9. Reed, R.K., Rubin, K., Wiig, H. and Rodt, S.Å. (1992) Blockade of β_1-integrins in skin causes edema through lowering of interstitial fluid pressure. *Circ. Res.* **71**, 978–983
10. Tay, M., Comper, W.D. and Singh, A.K. (1991) Charge selectivity in kidney filtration is associated with glomerular uptake of transport probes. *Am. J. Physiol.* **260**, F549–F554
11. Evered, D. and Whelan, J. (eds.) (1989) *The Biology of Hyaluronan*, Wiley, Chichester
12. Laurent, T.C. and Fraser, J.R.E. (1992) Hyaluronan. *FASEB J.* **6**, 2397–2404
13. Prehm, P. (1984) Hyaluronate is synthesized at plasma membranes. *Biochem. J.* **220**, 597–600
14. Laurent, T.C. and Fraser, J.R.E. (1986) The properties and turnover of hyaluronan. In *Functions of the Proteoglycans* (Evered, D. and Whelan, J., eds.), pp. 9–29, Wiley, Chichester
15. Fraser, J.R.E. and Laurent, T.C. (1989) Turnover and metabolism of hyaluronan. In *The Biology of Hyaluronan* (Evered, D. and Whelan, J., eds.), pp. 41–59, Wiley, Chichester
16. Laurent, T.C. and Fraser, J.R.E. (1991) Catabolism of hyaluronan. In *Degradation of Bioactive Substances: Physiology and Pathophysiology* (Henriksen, J.H., ed.), pp. 249–265, CRC Press, Boca Raton, FL
17. Laurent, U.B.G. and Reed, R.K. (1991) Turnover of hyaluronan in the tissues. *Advanced Drug Delivery Rev.* **7**, 237–256
18. Toole, B.P. (1990) Hyaluronan and its binding proteins, the hyaladherins. *Curr. Opin. Cell Biol.* **2**, 839–844
19. Knudson, C.B. and Knudson, W. (1993) Hyaluronan-binding proteins in development, tissue homeostasis, and disease. *FASEB J.* **7**, 1233–1241
20. Engström-Laurent, A. and Laurent, T.C. (1989) Hyaluronan as a clinical marker. In *Clinical Impact of Bone and Connective Tissue Markers* (Lindh, E. and Thorell, J.I., eds.), pp. 235–252, Academic Press, London
21. Tufveson, G., Gerdin, B., Larsson, E., Laurent, T.C., Wallander, J., Wells, A. and Hällgren, R. (1992) Hyaluronic acid accumulation; the mechanism behind graft rejection edema. *Transplant. Int.* **5** (Suppl. 1), 688–689
22. Waldenström, A., Martinussen, H.J., Gerdin, B. and Hällgren, R. (1991) Accumulation of hyaluronan and tissue edema in experimental myocardial infarction. *J. Clin. Invest.* **88**, 1622–1628
23. Balazs, E.A., Band, P.A., Denlinger, J.L., Goldman, A.I., Larsen, N.E., Leshchiner, E.A., Leshchiner, A. and Morales, B. (1991) Matrix Engineering. *Blood Coagulation and Fibrinolysis* **2**, 173–178
24. Miller, D. and Stegmann, R. (eds.) (1983) *Healon (Sodium Hyaluronate): A Guide to its Use in Ophthalmic Surgery*, Wiley, New York
25. Clarris, B.J. and Fraser, J.R.E. (1968) On the pericellular zone of some mammalian cells *in vitro*. *Exp. Cell Res.* **49**, 181–193
26. Heldin, P. and Pertoft, H. (1993) Synthesis and assembly of the hyaluronan-containing coats around normal human mesothelial cells. *Exp. Cell Res.* **208**, 422–429

27. Scott, J.E., Cummings, C., Brass, A. and Chen, Y. (1991) Secondary and tertiary structures of hyaluronan in aqueous solution, investigated by rotary shadowing-electron microscopy and computer simulation. *Biochem. J.* **274**, 699–705

28. Welsh, E.J., Rees, D.A., Morris, E.R. and Madden, J.K. (1980) Competitive inhibition evidence for specific intermolecular interactions in hyaluronate solutions. *J. Mol. Biol.* **138**, 375–382

29. West, D.C. and Kumar, S. (1989) Hyaluronan and angiogenesis. In *The Biology of Hyaluronan* (Evered, D. and Whelan, J., eds.), pp. 187–207, Wiley, Chichester

2

Proteoglycans in connective tissues: structure and function of aggrecan in cartilage

Timothy E. Hardingham*, Amanda J. Fosang† and Jayesh Dudhia‡
*School of Biological Sciences, University of Manchester, Manchester, U.K.,
‡Kennedy Institute of Rheumatology, Hammersmith, London, U.K. and
†Orthopaedic Molecular Biology Research Unit, Royal Children's Hospital,
Melbourne, Australia

Summary

Aggrecan, the large aggregating proteoglycan from cartilage, contains
chondroitin sulphate and keratan sulphate chains attached to a
multidomain protein core. It aggregates by binding to hyaluronan and
this is further stabilized by a separate globular link protein. There are
two structurally related N-terminal globular domains, G1 and G2, of
which only G1 and not G2 is involved in aggregation. The interglobular
domain joining G1 and G2 contains proteinase-sensitive sequences which
appear to be the key site for cleavage during aggrecan turnover. Much of
the keratan sulphate and all of the chondroitin sulphate is attached to
the long extended glycosaminoglycan attachment region. The function
of the C-terminal G3 domain is unknown. It contains a mammalian
type-C lectin and complement regulatory protein motifs. These may
have interactive properties that contribute to matrix organization. The
carbohydrate composition of aggrecan varies with cartilage source,
development and age, and is heterogeneous in each sample. There is
evidence of a close control of chondroitin sulphate synthesis that
determines chain length and disaccharide composition and which
changes during development and in pathology. Monoclonal antibodies
that recognize specific sequences within chondroitin sulphate chains
enable some of these changes in fine structure to be detected.
Progressive digestion of chains with chondroitinase ACII has provided
evidence of a pattern of sulphation with 6-sulphated disaccharides more
abundant towards the protein core, although the disaccharide next to the
linkage region is predominantly non-sulphated.

Proteoglycans in solution at high concentration, similar to that in
cartilage, have complex viscoelastic properties due to network formation.
The concentration of aggrecan, the formation of aggregates, the size of
aggregates and their stabilization by link protein all contribute separately
to these network properties. These intermolecular interactions of
aggrecan are sensitive to shear disruption and they do not provide the
shear stiffness of cartilage, but they help to organize and immobilize the
collagen fibres in an extended state so that they bear tensile forces

---

*To whom correspondence should be addressed.

during shear deformation. It is the combined properties of aggrecan and collagen that together give cartilage its load-bearing properties.

General biology of aggrecan

Articular cartilage has a high content of proteoglycan, which is mainly aggrecan, the large aggregating proteoglycan. Aggrecan has several features that contribute to the specialized biomechanical properties of cartilage [1] (Figure 1). Its structure consists of an extended protein core to which many chondroitin sulphate and keratan sulphate chains are attached. This forms a densely substituted branched or 'bottle brush' structure, which provides a highly focused concentration of polyanion. This structure is fully hydrated and space-filling, but of much lower viscosity and with a smaller excluded volume than a long-chain, unbranched polyanion of comparable relative molecular mass, such as hyaluronan. Aggrecan is thus able to diffuse within the cartilage matrix when newly secreted by the chondrocyte. However, it forms aggregates by specifically binding to hyaluronan [1,2] and this provides an extracellular mechanism for helping to immobilize it within the matrix. This is assisted by a separate globular link protein, which binds to both aggrecan and hyaluronan [3,4]. Although the main components of the aggregate, aggrecan and hyaluronan, are both synthesized by the chondrocytes within cartilage, they do not become mixed within intracellular compartments. Whereas proteoglycan and link protein follow the pathways of biosynthesis of other secretory proteins through compartments of the rough and smooth (Golgi) endoplasmic reticulum, there is evidence that hyaluronan is synthesized at the plasma membrane [5]. This would also explain the observation that hyaluronan synthesis by chondrocytes was unaffected by the Na^+/K^+ ionophore monensin at a concentration where the late stages of proteoglycan synthesis in the Golgi were completely blocked [6]. Aggrecan and link protein thus only have the opportunity to interact with hyaluronan after their secretion from the chondrocyte. Aggrecan also appears to undergo a slow

Figure 1

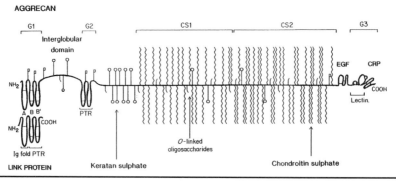

Schematic of the protein and carbohydrate structures of aggrecan and link protein
Abbreviations used: CRP, complement regulatory protein-like domain; EGF, epidermal growth factor-like domain; PTR, proteoglycan tandem repeat.

Figure 2

1. Increasing the
   proportion
   aggregated

2. Increasing the
   size (M_r) of
   hyaluronan

3. Increasing the
   proportion of
   aggrecan per
   hyaluronan
   (packing density)

4. Decreasing the
   size (M_r) of
   aggrecan by
   C-terminal cleavage

5. Variable length
   of CS/KS chains
   on aggrecan

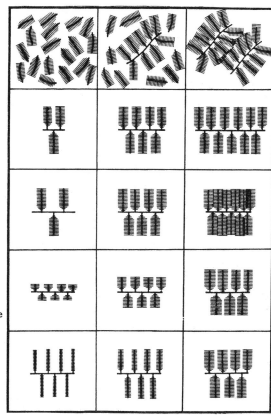

Factors affecting the supramolecular structure of aggregates formed from aggrecan and hyaluronan
Abbreviations: KS, keratan sulphate; CS, chondroitin sulphate.

maturation process whereby its full avidity for hyaluronan only develops over 1–2 days following secretion from the chondrocyte [7,8]. This may further facilitate the diffusion of aggrecan away from the cells that produce it.

For 'mature' aggrecan extracted from cartilage the affinity for hyaluronan has a K_d value of approx. 2×10^{-8} M [9], but in the presence of link protein, the dissociation of aggrecan from a link-stabilized aggregate is not experimentally detected [4]. The dissociation constant must therefore be below 1×10^{-11} M. The size of proteoglycan aggregates is determined by a number of parameters (Figure 2). Hyaluronan chains can be of very great length, up to an M_r of $(5–6) \times 10^6$ and 10 μm long, but most chains in articular cartilage are in the range M_r 3×10^5–6×10^5 [10] (although newly synthesized chains are considerably larger). The length of the hyaluronan chain determines the number of aggrecan molecules than can bind to it, and this is also limited by the proximity of adjacent molecules. There appear to be steric restrictions which space proteoglycans, such that each occupies a length of hyaluronan of M_r 7000 at maximum packing density [11]. This is only seen when there is an excess of aggrecan. However, in most tissues there is sufficient hyaluronan to bind all the aggrecan, and lower packing densities, with more space between each aggrecan molecule, are commonly seen in most aggregate preparations reformed from tissue extracts. The size of proteoglycan aggregates thus varies from being very small (2–5 aggrecan molecules), when there is a large excess of hyaluronan and/or it is of short chain length, up to exceedingly large aggregates (400–800 aggrecans), when the hyaluronan is of particularly long chain length and there is an excess of aggrecan. These aggregates, by some criteria, such as gel chromatography on Sepharose 2B, would all appear to be excluded from the column and therefore similar. It would require a technique such as rate zonal sedimentation or quasi-elastic light scattering (photon correlation spectroscopy) to distinguish them [12,13]. They can also be distinguished as they have very different rheological flow properties and viscoelastic behaviour [14].

Aggrecan protein structure

Investigation of the protein core has shown it to be the product of a single gene copy. It has an interesting multidomain structure (Figure 1) which, by rotary shadowing electron microscopy, appears as three globular and two extended segments [15]. The complete sequences from several species (human, rat, mouse, and chicken [16–18]) have been determined and partial sequences from several other species are known. The N-terminal region of the protein core contains two globular domains, G1 and G2, separated by a 21 nm extended segment. The major extended region, containing much of the keratan sulphate and all of the chondroitin sulphate, appears to be about 260 nm long by rotary shadowing and joins G2 to the C-terminal globular domain G3 [15]. The G1 and G3 domains are structural motifs that are common to a family of hyaluronan-binding proteoglycans. Versican is a large chondroitin sulphate proteoglycan produced by fibroblasts and smooth muscle cells [19], and neurocan and brevican are found in brain tissue [20,21]. All three contain G1 and G3 domains which are related to those of aggrecan, although their chondroitin sulphate attachment regions are of entirely unrelated sequence structure.

G1 and G2 domains

The N-terminal globular G1 and G2 domains have been prepared from pig laryngeal cartilage aggrecan by proteolytic digestion [22,23]. Extensive tryptic digestion of proteoglycan aggregate leaves the G1 domain and link protein largely intact and still bound to hyaluronan. Both the G1 domain and link protein retain their functional properties when prepared in this way [22], although link protein loses a short N-terminal peptide under these conditions. The G1 fragment isolated in this way contains about 25% carbohydrate, some keratan sulphate as well as oligosaccharides, and migrates on SDS/PAGE with an M_r of 65 000. However, it still appears as a simple globular domain by rotary shadowing and binds non-cooperatively to hyaluronan and also interacts with link protein [24].

When proteoglycan aggregates were digested with trypsin under more gentle conditions a larger fragment was isolated which contained both G1 and G2 domains [23]. This appeared as a double-globe structure by rotary shadowing electron microscopy and interaction experiments showed that only one domain (G1) was active in binding to hyaluronan and to link protein [24]. The G2 domain was isolated from the G1–G2 preparation by digestion with V8 proteinase under non-denaturing conditions [23]. It contained even more keratan sulphate than the G1 domain and migrated on SDS/PAGE as a broad band of M_r 110000 which is sharpened to M_r 70000 after keratanase digestion. Removal of a major part of the keratan sulphate was also necessary for the detection of a protein epitope by monoclonal antibody 1-C-6 [25]. The isolated G2 domain also showed no properties of interaction with hyaluronan, link protein or other soluble matrix proteins [23].

Investigation of the protein structures of the G1 and G2 domains and link protein has shown them to be closely related [26,27]. Both the G1 domain and link protein contain two structural motifs, an N-terminal immunoglobulin-fold (Ig-fold) and a tandem repeat sequence (a disulphide-bonded double loop structure; Figure 1). The G2 domain was also shown to contain a similar tandem repeat sequence, but no Ig-fold.

Comparison of the Ig-fold motifs of G1 domain and link protein using consensus sequence methods and structure prediction identified the pattern of β-sheet structure found in variable Ig-folds for which the crystal structure was known [27]. This established that both contained the basic structural framework of an Ig-fold and formed part of a broad family of proteins containing related Ig-fold motifs, the immunoglobulin superfamily. The analysis also identified the regions in which the Ig-folds of G1 domain and link protein showed the greatest differences from each other which was in sequences comparable with the hyper-

Domain	Motifs	Protein		Table 1
		M_r ($\times 10^{-3}$)	Function	
G1	Ig-fold	38	Binding link protein	
	Tandem repeat		Binding hyaluronan	
E1	Extended segment	12	Proteinase sites	
G2	Tandem repeat	25	Unknown	
E2	KS-attachment	5–15	KS attachment	
	CS-attachment	~55	CS (and some KS) attachment	
G3	EGF, mammalian type C lectin	25	Gal/Fuc lectin binding?	
	Complement regulatory protein (CRP)		Protein binding?	

Domain structure of aggrecan

Abbreviations: KS, keratan sulphate; CS, chondroitin sulphate; EGF, epidermal growth factor; Gal, galactose; Fuc, fucose.

Figure 3

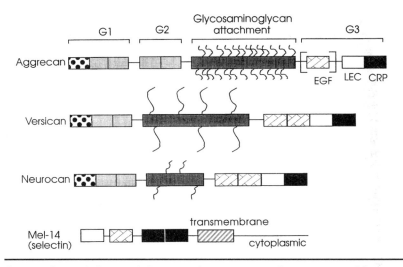

Comparison of the modular protein structure of aggrecan, with other related proteoglycans, versican and neurocan, and the cell-surface molecule E-selectin (Mel-14)

Abbreviations used: CRP, complement regulatory protein-like domain; EGF, epidermal growth factor-like domain; LEC, lectin-like domain.

variable loop regions. These form part of the Ig-fold motif that may be involved in protein–protein interactions and thus might provide the site for binding between G1 domain and link protein (Table 1).

No comparable crystal structures are available for the tandem repeat structure. However, a related sequence has been identified in a lymphocyte homing receptor CD-44 and this has been identified as a cell-surface receptor for hyaluronan [28] (Figure 3). The observations support the results from experiments which showed that hyaluronan binding of link protein was associated with the C-terminal tandem repeat region [29]. The sequence in CD-44 contains only a single loop structure and has specificity for a hexasaccharide of hyaluronan, whereas G1 domain and link protein both have specificity for a decasaccharide. The double loop structure found in G1 domain and link protein may thus be necessary to provide a site for binding to a longer segment of hyaluronan. This may offer greater stability or greater specificity of binding.

The G1 domain of aggrecan is a 'tough' structure [11,30]; it is generally resistant to proteinase attack, is resistant to thermal denaturation ($t_{1/2}$ at $80°C = 120$ min) and survives exposure to most solvents (ethanol, acetone, ether) and chaotropic agents (guanidine hydrochloride, KSCN and urea). Even after reduction of its disulphide bonds it renatures under oxidizing conditions with considerable efficiency. The native state of the G1 domain is thus very stable and thermodynamically preferred and these are perhaps appropriate properties for a matrix protein with a lifetime that may extend to several years within the cartilage matrix.

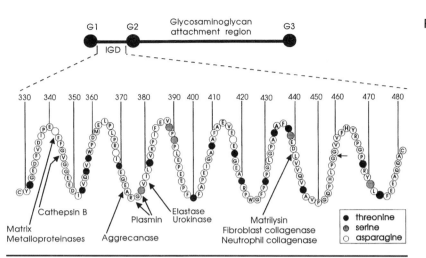

Figure 4

Proteinase cleavage sites within the interglobular domain of aggrecan

Interglobular domain

The interglobular domain (IGD) that links the G1 and G2 domains has attracted considerable recent interest, as it provides the site for proteolytic attack on aggrecan during extracellular turnover and matrix degradation (Figure 4). This is a key site for cleavage because it separates the major glycosaminoglycan-bearing proteoglycan from the G1 domain that anchors it in the matrix. A major and predominant cleavage site within the IGD was identified in natural and interleukin-1 (IL-1)-stimulated turnover [31–35], but all attempts to purify the proteinase responsible for cleavage from cartilage or chondrocyte extracts, have failed. The proteinases that form the major candidates for matrix degradation, the neutral metalloproteinases, comprising stromelysins, gelatinases and collagenases, all appeared to cleave aggrecan at a common site N↓FF (residues 341–342) which is 32 amino acids N-terminal of the 'aggrecanase' cleavage site E↓AR (residues 373–374) [36–38] (Figure 4). Other proteinases, such as cathepsin B, cathepsin L and elastase, also cleaved within the IGD, but not at the 'aggrecanase' site. However, in a recent report [39] it has been shown that natural and recombinant neutrophil collagenase (MMP-8) will cleave at the E↓AR site *in vitro*. Under these conditions it also cleaves initially at the N↓FF site. This is an important observation, as it establishes that a metalloproteinase is able to cleave at the 'aggrecanase' site. Although it is unclear whether neutrophil collagenase is expressed by chondrocytes, other metalloproteinases, including stromelysin (MMP-3) and collagenase (MMP-1), are expressed and it remains to be determined if they contain 'aggrecanase' activity under the special conditions that occur within the cartilage matrix. These special conditions include a very high concentration of aggrecan, which has important volume exclusion effects, and in recent experiments it has been shown that when polyethylene glycol (with similar volume exclusion effects) is added to digests, concentrations of MMP-8 as low as 10 μg/ml will cleave at the aggrecan-ase site [39]. The high concentration of aggrecan in cartilage may therefore have a direct influence on the action of the proteinases.

G3 domain

The C-terminal G3 domain of aggrecan (Figure 1, Table 1) was identified when the first cDNA sequences were determined for the protein core [40] and independently at the same time by the use of rotary shadowing electron microscopy to visualize proteoglycans [15]. The failure to detect it prior to these investigations largely resulted from the difficulty of detecting small differences in protein core size/composition among the heterogeneous population of aggrecan extracted from cartilage, and also, probably more importantly, because only a fraction of the molecules extracted from cartilage appear to retain an intact G3 domain [41]. Many aggrecan molecules in the tissue appear to have lost some part of their C-terminal structure including the G3 domain, together with varying proportions of the chondroitin sulphate attachment region, presumably as a result of proteolytic action in the matrix. Accurate figures have not yet been published on the content of G3 in purified aggrecan from different sources, but estimates from rotary shadowing electron microscopy suggest that only 10–50% of aggrecan in cartilage extracts has an intact G3 domain [42].

The amino acid sequence of the G3 domain has been determined in several species. It is entirely unrelated to the G1 and G2 domains, but contains elements with sequence similarities with two other protein families (Figure 3). The first of these is a family of cell-surface carbohydrate-binding proteins, the mammalian type-C lectin, a notable member of which is the hepatic asialoglycoprotein receptor. The second family is related to complement B component, although it is reported that for human aggrecan there is an alternatively spliced form lacking the complement B component [43]. There are 10 cysteine residues in the G3 domain and the amino acid sequence is highly conserved (>90%) among aggrecans from different species [41]. There is also considerable simi-larity in sequence ($\sim$65%) with the corresponding C-terminal domain of the fibroblast proteoglycan versican [19] and the brain proteoglycan neurocan [20] (Figure 3). The G3 domain has been expressed from cDNA, and weak carbohydrate binding with some specificity for fucose and galactose has been detected [44]. Lectin binding was also detected in an expressed G3 construct from PG-M (a chicken versican-related proteoglycan) [45] and deletion of the complement sequence from the lectin protein abolished its lectin-like properties [46]. The G3 domain may thus have some binding specificity itself, with a role in matrix organization; although, alternatively, it may be important during the intracellular synthesis, translocation, glycosylation and secretion of proteoglycan [47], rather than during its lifetime in the matrix.

The sequence similarity to complement B components is low and was established by consensus sequence methods [48]. There is a large family of other proteins, many of which contain repetitive copies of this sequence, such as complement proteins, other serum proteins and cell-surface molecules, including the cell adhesion molecules the selectins [1] (Figure 3). This is particularly interesting as the selectins also contains a lectin-like region and an epidermal growth factor (EGF)-like sequence. The cDNA for human aggrecan G3 has been shown to have a splicing variant with one or two EGF-like sequences next to its lectin-like region [43,49]. The structural elements in G3 can thus be similar to those in a selectin, although lacking transmembrane and cytoplasmic domains. Any specific functions of EGF-like sequences have not been separately tested.

Chondroitin sulphate- and keratan sulphate-rich regions

The substitution of chondroitin sulphate on the protein core is entirely restricted to the regions between the G2 and G3 domains, whereas keratan sulphate is found much closer to the N-terminus of the protein core including on the IGD domain, as well as in a more specific keratan sulphate-rich region on the C-terminal side of the G2 domain (Figure 1, Table 1). This keratan sulphate-rich region was absent from the cDNA of rat chondrosarcoma aggrecan, but was present in different lengths in bovine and human sequences [50]. The bovine keratan sulphate-rich region contained 23 consecutive six-amino-acid repeats, of similar but not identical sequence, whereas the human molecule had only 13 repeats and the rat only four [51]. The long chondroitin sulphate attachment region was interesting in that it consisted of two regions each with distinct repeating sequence patterns within them, but these were part of the same large single exon in the DNA sequence. The human sequence also contained a long repeating string (19 repeats) of 19 amino acids in the first part of the chondroitin sulphate attachment region. This was longer than in the rat sequence, such that it contained 77 Ser-Gly sequences compared with 49 in the rat [41]. The second region of chondroitin sulphate attachment was more similar in the two species.

The available sequences from different species so far show that these structures of the globular protein domains are highly conserved, whereas the extended highly glycosylated regions are more variable. The chondroitin sulphate-attachment regions all contain a high content of Ser–Gly residues, but there is considerable variation in their number and in their spatial distribution. The conserved sequences in globular domains may be associated with the greater constraints placed upon amino acid side chains in globular structures compared with extended sequences. However, it is clear that the lack of conservation of the detailed distribution of chondroitin sulphate chains suggests that this is unlikely to be of crucial importance in determining their function on proteoglycans in the matrix.

Variations in glycosaminoglycan structure

Cartilage proteoglycans of the aggrecan type show great variation in carbohydrate composition and this was a severe handicap in the elucidation of their structure [11]. Cartilage aggrecan contains chondroitin sulphate, keratan sulphate and O-linked and N-linked oligosaccharides. The number, size, sulphation pattern, and charge density of these substituents are known to change with development and ageing, and vary from site to site, but in no preparation has the full range of structural variation been studied in any precise molecular detail. Some of the changes apparent in aggrecan extracted from cartilage may reflect matrix degradation processes, which, for example, can create protein-rich, keratan sulphate-rich proteoglycan fragments that are of relatively small size. Some changes in biosynthetic glycosylation may thus be obscured by structural changes within the extracellular matrix and few details of the changes in the pattern of glycosylation during biosynthesis have been investigated. The factors that influence and control glyco-sylation of aggrecan are poorly understood.

Some aspects of chondroitin sulphate biosynthesis can be modulated *in vitro*. The addition to chondrocytes of β-xyloside, which acts as an acceptor for chondroitin sulphate synthesis, stimulates the synthesis of more chains, most of which are on the free xyloside and are of shorter average length. At the same time fewer, but similarly shortened chains, are made on the proteoglycan [52]. In contrast, if the supply of protein core is limited by inhibiting protein synthesis, there is less net synthesis, but the chains are much longer. This also occurs if the temperature is dropped from 37°C to 25°C or lower; a smaller number of longer chains are synthesized. In relatively short experiments it is thus possible to show that the rate of chain synthesis is inversely correlated with chain length [52]. However, if chain synthesis is perturbed by more physiological methods, such as by stimulating it with growth factors (in fetal calf serum) or inhibiting it with cytokines, such as IL-1, the rate of synthesis is changed, but there is no change in chain length [53]. Under these circumstances it appears that the enzymes and mechanism of chain synthesis are all up-regulated or down-regulated co-ordinately with protein core synthesis, such that chain characteristics are maintained despite changes in the rate of synthesis.

Several factors now suggest that many details of chondroitin sulphate structure are in fact closely controlled during biosynthesis [1]. Comparison of the chondroitin sulphate chains on aggrecan and on decorin (small chondroitin sulphate-proteoglycan) in pig laryngeal cartilage showed the chains to differ in size and also in disaccharide composition [54]. Since they were apparently made by the same cells within the same tissue, this implies that the chondroitin sulphate synthesized on aggrecan was made differently to that synthesized on decorin. This suggests that the protein core was able to influence glycosylation and sulphation, even on these long, extended glyco-saminoglycan chains. This comparison of chondroitin sulphate chains on different proteoglycans in human articular cartilage was even more revealing [54], as not only were there differences in chain length and disaccharide composition for aggrecan and decorin, but those attached to aggrecan were chondroitin sulphate whereas those attached to decorin were dermatan sulphate, with considerable epimerization of glucuronate to iduronate. This provided further evidence of differential chain synthesis distinguishing one proteoglycan from another and apparently being made within the same cellular biosynthetic system.

Further details of chondroitin sulphate chain structure and its biological modulation have been investigated in two different ways. First, a series of monoclonal antibodies have been prepared that recognize specific epitopes within chondroitin sulphate chain structure [55,56]. They are therefore able to provide techniques that distinguish between chondroitin sulphate with a low or high epitope content. The epitopes involve chain terminal structures or particular patterns of sulphation within the chains. Application of these monoclonals has been used to show developmentally regulated changes in chondroitin sulphate structure associated with cell differentiation and morphogenesis of cartilaginous and non-cartilaginous tissues [55,56]. Furthermore, in mature articular cartilage they have been shown to detect changes in chondroitin sulphate structure associated with a canine experimentally induced model of osteoarthritis [56]. Chondroitin sulphate chain synthesis was therefore being modulated by chondrocytes in response to the early changes associated with articular cartilage pathology.

A second and complementary approach to investigating chondroitin sulphate chain structure has focused on determining the changes in the pattern of disaccharide sulphation from the non-reducing terminus of a chondroitin sulphate chain to its linkage with the protein core. This was carried out by analysing partial chondroitinase AC and ABC digests of cartilage proteoglycans [57]. By determining the disaccharide composition of the released digest products at each stage of digestion, and comparing them with the disaccharide composition of the shortened chondroitin sulphate chain remaining attached to the proteoglycan, the results reveal the average composition of chains as their length is shortened. For a pig laryngeal proteoglycan preparation some characteristics of the chain were revealed by this technique. The proportion of 6-sulphated (relative to 4-sulphated) disaccharides increased as the chains were shortened, except in the region immediately adjacent to the neutral sugar linkage to protein where a non-sulphated disaccharide was most abundant. Further experiments are necessary to determine whether there are general patterns common to aggrecan in all cartilages, or if they vary with anatomical site (and 4/6-sulphate ratio), and also how the pattern of chain structure is modulated in chondrocytes in response to growth factors or cytokines. Changes in chain structure may be part of the mechanisms by which the chondrocyte can control the properties of the cartilage extracellular matrix that surrounds it.

Rheological properties of aggrecan

Aggrecan in articular cartilage is present at 50–80 mg/ml, but what physical form does it have? At this concentration its hydrodynamic domains would be predicted to overlap greatly [58]. Overlapping would imply that there is considerable interdigitation of the chains of adjacent molecules, but another possibility is that the domains contract. Evidence for the contraction of aggrecan domains at high concentrations has come from other physical measurements [59]. The determination of the limiting viscosity number of aggrecan in various concentrations of dextran or chondroitin sulphate showed that it decreased as the total concentration of polymer increased and, in the determination of the hydrodynamic volume of aggrecan by gel chromatography, the elution of aggrecan was much later in the presence of dextran. Both of these results suggested that the aggrecan was behaving as though it was of smaller size.

The study of the rheological properties of aggrecan at high concentrations has also given some insight into the nature and extent of intermolecular interactions [14,60].

Solutions of aggrecan show complex viscoelastic properties that are highly non-linearly concentration-dependent. Measurement of the dynamic shear modulus at concentrations up to 55 mg/ml in a cone-on-plate viscometer using small amplitude sinusoidal shear oscillations showed that solutions of aggregates formed stronger intermolecular networks in solution which could store more energy than monomers. Measurements of viscosity made at different shear rates showed that aggrecan solutions exhibited shear-thinning, and this was most pronounced with the aggregates. Extrapolation of the data to zero shear predicted that intermolecular interactions were maximal in unperturbed solutions and that the network was sensitive to disruption at low shear rates [14]. This was also shown in experiments investigating the time-dependent growth in stress at the onset of steady shear (Figure 5). There was a significant stress overshoot, which reflected the force required to disrupt the intermolecular network formed in the absence of shear and was found to be much greater for solutions of aggregates than for monomers [60].

Figure 5

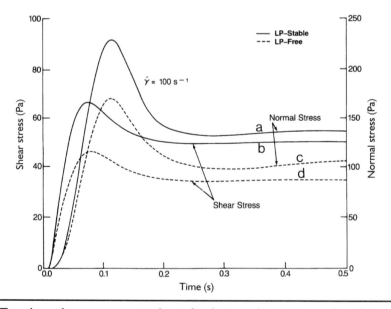

Transient shear stress overshoot (and normal stress overshoot) in link protein-free and link protein-stable aggregate solutions
Aggrecan solutions (40 mg/ml in PBS) containing link protein-free and link protein-stable aggregates were subject to a sudden application of shear at $100 \, s^{-1}$. Curves (a) and (b) measure normal stress (force pushing the viscometer plates apart) and curves (c) and (d) measure the shear stress from the start of rotation in a cone-on-plate viscometer [60].

The contribution of link protein to the rheological properties of the aggregate was also evident. It might be envisaged that at 50 mg/ml the equilibrium of aggrecan–hyaluronan binding would be strongly in favour of the bound form and that link protein may therefore have little additional effect. However, the presence of link protein was found to increase the dynamic modulus of aggregates and to show a larger stress overshoot effect (Figure 5), reflecting the presence of a stronger intermolecular network [60]. The more tightly bound aggregate formed in the presence of link protein was thus shown to form stronger networks that were more resistant to shear disruption than aggregates formed from aggrecan and hyaluronan alone. These results show that there is considerable intermolecular interaction among aggrecan molecules at high concentration, and they appear most consistent with an interpretation where, although there is some contraction of aggrecan domains, there is also some overlap. The investigation of different preparations showed that the concentration of aggrecan, the formation of aggregates, the size of aggregates and their stabilization by link protein all contribute separately and additively to the network properties present in solution. It is clear that the function of aggrecan in cartilage is not to provide shear stiffness itself, but to organize and immobilize the collagen framework in an extended state so that the collagen fibrils are tensed during shear deformation [61]. It is the combined properties of the fibrillar collagen and the proteoglycan that give cartilage its essential load-bearing properties.

This work was carried out with the support of the Arthritis and Rheumatism Council and the Medical Research Council (U.K.), and the Arthritis Foundation and NH and MRC (Australia).

References

1. Hardingham, T.E. and Fosang, A.J. (1992) Proteoglycans: many forms, many functions. *FASEB J.* **6**, 861–870
2. Hardingham, T.E. and Muir, H. (1972) The specific interaction of hyaluronic acid with cartilage proteoglycans. *Biochim. Biophys. Acta* **279**, 401–405
3. Heinegård, D. and Hascall, V.C. (1974) Aggregation of cartilage proteoglycans. III. Characterisation of the proteins isolated from trypsin digests of aggregates. *J. Biol. Chem.* **249**, 4250–4256
4. Hardingham, T.E. (1979) The role of link protein in the structure of cartilage proteoglycan aggregates. *Biochem. J.* **177**, 237–247
5. Prehm, P. (1983) Synthesis of hyaluronate in differentiated teratocarcinoma cells. Characterisation of the synthase. *Biochem. J.* **211**, 181–189
6. Mitchell, D. and Hardingham, T. (1982) Monensin inhibits synthesis of proteoglycan, but not hyaluronate, in chondrocytes. *Biochem. J.* **202**, 249–254
7. Bayliss, M.T., Ridgeway, G.D. and Ali, S.Y. (1984) Delayed aggregation of proteoglycans in adult human articular cartilage. *Biosci. Rep.* **4**, 827–833
8. Sandy, J.D., O'Neill, J.R. and Ratzlaff, L.C. (1989) Acquisition of hyaluronate-binding affinity in vivo by newly synthesised proteoglycans. *Biochem. J.* **258**, 875–880
9. Nieduszynski, I.A., Sheehan, J.K., Phelps, C.F., Hardingham, T.E. and Muir, H. (1980) Equilibrium binding studies of pig laryngeal proteoglycans with hyaluronate oligosaccharide fractions. *Biochem. J.* **185**, 104–114
10. Holmes, M.W.A., Bayliss, M.T. and Muir, H. (1988) Hyaluronic acid in human articular cartilage. *Biochem. J.* **250**, 435–441
11. Hardingham, T.E. (1981) Proteoglycans: Their structure, interactions and molecular organisation in cartilage. *Biochem. Soc. Trans.* **9**, 489–497
12. Pita, J., Muller, F., Morales, S. and Alarcon, E. (1979) Ultracentrifugal characterisation of proteoglycans from rat growth cartilage. *J. Biol. Chem.* **254**, 10313–10320
13. Ohno, H., Blackwell, J., Jamieson, A.M., Carrino, D.A. and Caplan, A.I. (1986) Calibration of the relative molecular mass of proteoglycan subunit by column chromatography on Sepharose CL-2B. *Biochem. J.* **235**, 553–557

14. Hardingham, T.E., Muir, H., Kwan, M.K., Lai, W.M. and Mow, V.C. (1987) Viscoelastic properties of proteoglycan solutions with varying properties present as aggregates. *J. Orthop. Res.* **5**, 36–46

15. Paulsson, M., Mörgelin, M., Wiedemann, H., Beardmore-Gray, M., Dunham, D., Hardingham, T.E., Heinegård, D., Timpl, R. and Engel, J. (1987) Extended and globular protein domains in cartilage proteoglycans. *Biochem. J.* **245**, 763–772

16. Doege, K.J., Sasaki, M., Horigan, E., Hassell, J.R. and Yamada, Y. (1987) Complete primary structure of the rat cartilage proteoglycan core protein deduced from cDNA clones. *J. Biol. Chem.* **262**, 17757–17767

17. Doege, K.J., Sasaki, M., Kimura, T. and Yamada, Y. (1991) Complete coding sequence deduced primary structure of the human cartilage large aggregating proteoglycan, aggrecan. *J. Biol. Chem.* **266**, 894–902

18a. Walez, E., Deak, F., Erhardt, P., Coulter, S.N., Fulop, C., Horrath, P., Doege, K.J. and Glant, T.T. (1994) Complete coding sequence deduced primary structure, chromosomal localization and structural analysis of murine aggrecan. *Genomics* **22**, 364–371

18. Chandrasekeran, L. and Tanzer, M.L. (1992) Molecular cloning of chicken aggrecan. *Biochem. J.* **288**, 903–910

19. Zimmerman, D.R. and Rouslahti, E. (1989) Multiple domains of the large fibroblast proteoglycan, versican. *EMBO J.* **8**, 2975–2981

20. Rauch, V., Karthikeyan, L., Maurel, P., Margolis, R.U. and Margolis, R.K. (1992) Cloning and primary structure of neurocan, a developmentally regulated aggregating chondroitin sulfate proteoglycan of brain. *J. Biol. Chem.* **267**, 19536–19547

21. Yamada, H., Watanabe, K., Shimonaki, M. and Yamaguchi, M. (1994) Molecular cloning of brevican, a novel brain proteoglycan of the aggrecan/versican family. *J. Biol. Chem.* **269**, 10119–10126

22. Bonnet, F., Dunham, D. and Hardingham, T.E. (1985) Structure and interactions of cartilage proteoglycan binding region and link protein. *Biochem. J.* **228**, 77–85

23. Fosang, A.J. and Hardingham, T.E. (1989) Isolation of the N-terminal globular domains from cartilage proteoglycans. *Biochem. J.* **261**, 801–809

24. Mörgelin, M., Paulsson, M., Hardingham, T.E., Heinegård, D. and Engel, J. (1988) Cartilage proteoglycans: assembly with hyaluronate and link protein as studied by electron microscopy. *Biochem. J.* **253**, 175–185

25. Fosang, A.J. and Hardingham, T.E. (1991) 1-C-6 epitope in cartilage proteoglycan G2 domain is masked by keratan sulphate. *Biochem. J.* **273**, 369–373

26. Neame, P.J., Christner, J.E. and Baker, J.R. (1987) Cartilage proteoglycan aggregates. The link protein and proteoglycan amino-terminal globular domains have similar structure. *J. Biol. Chem.* **262**, 17768–17778

27. Perkins, S.J., Nealis, A.S., Dudhia, J. and Hardingham, T.E. (1989) Immunoglobulin fold tandem repeat structures in proteoglycan N-terminal domains and link protein. *J. Mol. Biol.* **206**, 737–753

28. Aruffo, A., Stamenkovic, I., Melnick, M., Underhill, C.B. and Seed, B. (1990) CD44 is the principle cell surface receptor for hyaluronate. *Cell* **61**, 1303–1313

29. Goetinck, P.F., Stirpe, N.S., Tsonis, P.A. and Carlone, D. (1987) The tandemly repeated sequence of cartilage link protein contains the site for interaction with hyaluronic acid. *Cell* **105**, 2403–2408

30. Hardingham, T.E., Ewins, R.J.F. and Muir, H. (1976) Cartilage proteoglycans. Structure and heterogeneity of the protein core and the effects of specific protein modifications on the binding to hyaluronate. *Biochem. J.* **157**, 127–143

31. Sandy, J.D., Neame, P.J., Boynton, R.E. and Flannery, C.R. (1991) Catabolism of aggrecan in cartilage explants: identification of a major cleavage site within the interglobular domain. *J. Biol. Chem.* **266**, 8683–8685

32. Ilic, M.Z., Handley, C.J., Robinson, H.C. and Mok, M.T. (1992) Mechanism of catabolism of aggrecan by articular cartilage. *Arch. Biochem. Biophys.* **294**, 115–122

33. Sandy, J.D., Flannery, C.R., Neame, P.J. and Lohmander, L.S. (1992) The structure of aggrecan fragments in human synovial fluid. *J. Clin. Invest.* **89**, 1512–1516

34. Loulakis, P., Shrikhande, A., Davis, G. and Maniglia, C.A. (1992) N-terminal sequence of proteoglycan fragments isolated from medium of interleukin-1 treated articular cartilage cultures. *Biochem. J.* **284**, 589–593

35. Lohmander, L.S., Neame, P.J. and Sandy, J.D. (1993) The structure of aggrecan fragments in human synovial fluid: evidence that aggrecanase mediates cartilage degradation in inflammatory joint disease, joint injury and osteoarthritis. *Arthritis Rheum.* **36**, 1214–1222

36. Fosang, A.J., Neame, P.J., Hardingham, T.E., Murphy, G. and Hamilton, J.A. (1991) Cleavage of cartilage proteoglycan between G1 and G2 domains by stromelysins. *J. Biol. Chem.* **266**, 15579–15582

37. Fosang, A.J., Neame, P.J., Last, K., Hardingham, T.E., Murphy, G. and Hamilton, J.A. (1992) The interglobular domain of cartilage aggrecan is cleaved by PUMP, gelatinases and cathepsin B. *J. Biol. Chem.* **267**, 19470–19474

38. Fosang, A.J., Last, K., Neame, P.J., Murphy, G., Hardingham, T.E., Tschesche, H. and Hamilton, J.A. (1993) Fibroblast and neutrophil collagenase cleave at two sites in the cartilage aggrecan interglobular domain. *Biochem. J.* **295**, 273–276

39. Fosang, A.J., Last, K., Neame, P.J., Murphy, G., Knauper, V., Tschesche, H., Hughes, C.E., Caterson, B. and Hardingham, T.E. (1994) Neutrophil collagenase (MMP-8) cleaves at the aggrecanase site E^{373}–A^{374} in the interglobular domain of cartilage aggrecan. *Biochem. J.* **304**, 347–351

40. Sai, S., Tanaka, T., Kosher, R.A. and Tanzer, M.L. (1986) Cloning and sequence analysis of a partial cDNA for chicken cartilage proteoglycan core protein. *Proc. Natl. Acad. Sci. U.S.A.* **83**, 5081–5085

41. Hardingham, T.E., Fosang, A.J. and Dudhia, J. (1990) Domain structure in aggregating proteoglycans from cartilage. *Biochem. Soc. Trans.* **18**, 794–796

42. Flannery, C., Stanescu, V., Mörgelin, M., Boynton, R., Gordy, J. and Sandy, J. (1992) Variability in the G3 domain content of bovine aggrecan from cartilage extracts and chondrocyte cultures. *Arch. Biochem. Biophys.* **297**, 52–58

43. Baldwin, C.T., Reginato, A.M. and Prockop, D.J. (1989) A new epidermal growth factor-like domain in the human core protein for the large cartilage specific proteoglycan. *J. Biol. Chem.* **264**, 15747–15750

44. Halberg, D.H., Proulx, G., Doege, K., Yamada, Y. and Drickamer, K. (1988) A segment of the cartilage proteoglycan core protein has lectin-like activity. *J. Biol. Chem.* **263**, 9486–9490

45. Shinomura, T., Nishida, Y., Ito, K. and Kimata, K. (1993) cDNA cloning of PG-M a large chondroitin sulfate proteoglycan expressed during chondrogenesis in chick limb buds. *J. Biol. Chem.* **268**, 14461–14469

46. Ujita, M., Shinomura, T., Ito, K., Kitagawa, Y. and Kimata, Y. (1994) Expression and binding activity of the carboxy-terminal portion of the core protein of PG-M, a large chondroitin sulfate glycoprotein. *J. Biol. Chem.* **269**, 27603–27609

47. Vertel, B.M., Walters, L.M., Grier, B., Maine, N. and Goetinck, P.F. (1993) Nanomelic chondrocytes synthesize but fail to translocate a truncated aggrecan precursor. *J. Cell Sci.* **104**, 939–948

48. Patthy, L. (1987) Detecting homology of distantly related proteins with consensus sequences. *J. Mol. Biol.* **198**, 567–577

49. Fülöp, C., Walcz, E., Valym, M. and Glant, T.T. (1993) Expression of alternatively spliced epidermal growth factor-like domains in aggrecans of different species. *J. Biol. Chem.* **268**, 17377–17383

50. Antonsson, P., Heinegård, D. and Oldberg, A. (1989) The keratan sulfate-enriched region of bovine cartilage proteoglycan consists of consecutively repeated hexapeptide motifs. *J. Biol. Chem.* **264**, 16170–16173

51. Barry, F.P., Neame, P.J., Sasse, J. and Pearson, D. (1994) Length variation in the keratan sulfate domain of mammalian aggrecan. *Matrix Biol.* **14**, 323–328

52. Mitchell, D.C. and Hardingham, T.E. (1982) The control of chondroitin sulphate biosynthesis and its influence on the structure of cartilage proteoglycans. *Biochem. J.* **202**, 387–395

53. Mitchell, D. and Hardingham, T.E. (1981) The effects of cycloheximide on the biosynthesis and secretion by chondrocytes in culture. *Biochem. J.* **196**, 521–529

54. Sampaio, L., Bayliss, M.T. and Hardingham, T.E. (1988) Dermatan sulphate proteoglycan from human articular cartilage. *Biochem. J.* **254**, 757–764

55. Sorrell, J.M., Mahmoodian, F., Schafer, I.A., Davis, B. and Caterson, B. (1990) Identification of monoclonal antibodies that recognise novel epitopes in native chondroitin/dermatan sulphate glycosaminoglycan chains: their use in mapping functionally distinct domains of human skin. *J. Histochem. Cytochem.* **38**, 8393–8402

56. Caterson, B., Mahmoodian, F., Sorrell, J.M., Hardingham, T.E., Bayliss, M.T., Carney, S.L., Ratcliffe, A. and Muir, H. (1990) Modulation of native chondroitin sulphate structure in tissue development and in disease. *J. Cell Sci.* **97**, 411–417

57. Hardingham, T., Fosang, A., Hey, N., Hazell, P., Kee, W.-J. and Ewins, R. (1994) Modulation of native chondroitin sulphate structure in tissue development and in disease. *Carbohydr. Res.* **255**, 241–254

58. Hascall, V.C. and Hascall, G.K. (1981) Proteoglycans. In *Cell Biology of Extracellular Matrix* (Hay, E.D., ed.), pp. 39–63, Plenum Press, New York

59. Harper, G.S. and Preston, B.N. (1987) Molecular shrinkage of proteoglycans. *J. Biol. Chem.* **262**, 8088–8095

60. Mow, V.C., Zhu, W., Lai, W.M., Hardingham, T.E., Hughes, C. and Muir, H. (1989) The influence of link protein stabilisation on the viscometric properties of proteoglycan aggregate solutions. *Biochim. Biophys. Acta* **992**, 201–208

61. Hardingham, T.E., Hughes, C., Mow, V.C. and Lai, W.M. (1989) Flow properties of proteoglycan solutions. In *Dynamic Properties of Biomolecular Assemblies* (Harding, S.E. and Rowe, A.J., eds.), pp. 246–255, Royal Society of Chemistry, Cambridge, U.K.

3

Integrins: transmembrane links between the extracellular matrix and the cell interior

Kristofer Rubin*‡, Christian Sundberg*, Karina Åhlén* and Rolf K. Reed†
*Department of Medical and Physiological Chemistry, University of Uppsala, BMC, Box 575, S-751 23 Uppsala, Sweden and †Department of Physiology, University of Bergen, Årstadsveien 19, N-5009 Bergen, Norway

Integrins: a growing family of adhesion receptors that mediate dynamic adhesive interactions

Integrins [1–3] comprise a large family of membrane-spanning glycoproteins that mediate cell adhesion to extracellular matrix (ECM) proteins, as well as to other cells (for recent reviews see [4–8]). A complete primary structure of an integrin β-subunit was determined for the first time in 1986 by Tamkun *et al.* [9]; these authors also introduced the name integrin.

Integrins do not merely mediate cellular adhesion, but also function as signalling molecules conveying information from the outside to the cell interior, the so called outside-in signalling by integrins [8]. Integrins regulate a plethora of cell physiological processes *in vitro* including regulation of cellular growth, motility and gene expression [10–14]. Clustering of certain integrins at the cell surface with anti-integrin antibodies or ligand binding leads to a rapid increase in intracellular free Ca^{2+}, alkalinization of the cytosol and phosphorylation of intracellular proteins [8,13,14]. Less information is available concerning *in vivo* functions of integrins. Integrins have, however, been shown to be involved in such diverse processes as normal embryonic development, inflammatory processes and malignancies [4–8]. As will be discussed later in this chapter, and also in Chapter 7 by Reed in this volume, evidence for a role of integrins in the control of dermal interstitial fluid pressure (P_{if}) has been presented [15].

Integrins are non-covalently associated heterodimers built from one α- and one β-subunit. At present, eight β- and 15 α-subunits have been characterized; these integrin subunits associate to form the 20 or so different integrin heterodimers described to date [4–8,16]. Isolated α- or β-subunits do not appear on cell surfaces; α/β heterodimers are assembled intracellularly and transported to the cell surface during synthesis. Both subunits contribute to the ligand-binding domain of the heterodimeric receptors; isolated integrin subunits possess no ligand-binding capacity. Integrins are dependent on bivalent cations for their functions and α-subunits possess three or four repeats of aspartic acid-rich sequences that are likely to participate in bivalent cation binding. Molecular characteristics shared by all integrin β-subunits are

‡To whom correspondence should be addressed.

the presence of cysteine-containing repeats close to the transmembrane segment and also several disulphide-bonded intramolecular loops in the molecule. Both the α and β-subunits have short cytoplasmic domains, containing 50 or fewer amino acids. One reported exception is the $\sim$1000-amino-acid large cytoplasmic domain of the β_4-subunit.

Integrins have been grouped in subfamilies based on the particular β-subunit that is shared by members within each subfamily. The β_1 integrins act as receptors for several ECM glycoproteins such as collagens, laminins and fibronectins. In addition, some β_1 integrins mediate cell–cell adhesion. The integrin β_2 subfamily encompasses leucocyte adhesion receptors that mediate intercellular adhesion. The platelet fibrinogen receptor, gpIIb/β_3, and the classical vitronectin receptor, $\alpha_V\beta_3$, constitute the β_3 subfamily. Some α-subunits can associate with more than one β-subunit, a prominent example being the α_V-subunit that can associate with the β_1-, β_3-, β_5- and β_6-subunits. The $\alpha_6\beta_4$ integrin acts as a laminin receptor in cultured cells. In tissues, $\alpha_6\beta_4$ is localized to hemidesmosomes of epithelia and is present in endothelia.

The β_1 integrin subfamily encompasses ten integrins, $\alpha_1\beta_1$ to $\alpha_9\beta_1$ and $\alpha_V\beta_1$. One feature common to several of these integrins is their ability to bind to more than one ligand. This can be illustrated by the $\alpha_1\beta_1$ and $\alpha_2\beta_1$ integrins. These have affinity for collagen, and are of major importance for the primary adhesion of different types of cells to immobilized collagen [8,17,18]. In some cells $\alpha_3\beta_1$ can also act as a collagen receptor [19,20]. All three integrins function as laminin receptors, and $\alpha_3\beta_1$ is a fibronectin receptor as well [19,21,22]. In addition, evidence that $\alpha_2\beta_1$ and $\alpha_3\beta_1$ mediate intercellular adhesion has been presented [23–26]. Thus, many integrins exhibit a broad binding specificity and recognize several ligands. It is not known whether these diverse ligands contain a common three-dimensional structure that is recognized by all three integrins. In the case of $\alpha_1\beta_1$ and $\alpha_2\beta_1$ data have been presented which suggest that these integrins recognize distinct sites in collagen [18,27]. Other β_1 integrins include the laminin receptors $\alpha_6\beta_1$ and $\alpha_7\beta_1$, and the fibronectin receptors $\alpha_4\beta_1$ and $\alpha_5\beta_1$. Many β_1 integrins, such as the fibronectin-binding integrins $\alpha_5\beta_1$ and $\alpha_V\beta_1$, recognize the amino acid sequence Arg-Gly-Asp [28]. The functions of others, such as the collagen-binding integrins $\alpha_1\beta_1$ and $\alpha_2\beta_1$, are not inhibited by Arg-Gly-Asp-containing peptides. The fact that several integrins can act as receptors for one particular ECM glycoprotein indicates that ligand occupation of different integrins may give different functional consequences. In fact, a recent study demonstrated that the cytoplasmic domains of the α_2-, α_4- and α_5-subunits mediate distinct and different functions with regard to migration and contraction [29].

An additional level of complexity results from the fact that many integrin subunit precursor mRNAs are alternatively spliced, leading to the presence of integrin isoforms. Among α-subunits, α_3, α_6 and α_7 are known to occur in isoforms differing in the primary structure of the cytoplasmic domains (for a review see [30]). The presence of three different β_1 integrin isoforms has been demonstrated [31,32], and these different isoforms seem to have different functions [33].

The expression of integrins in various tissues has been investigated by immunolocalization techniques [34–41]. Most normal tissues express a restricted number of integrins that are most easily detected in epithelial, smooth muscle and endothelial cells, i.e. cells which are in intimate contact with basement membranes. Dermal fibroblasts express the collagen-binding integrin $\alpha_2\beta_1$ *in situ* [19,42].

Integrins link intracellular fibres with the extracellular matrix at focal adhesions

Focal adhesions are sites of close contact between the cell membrane and the underlying substrate. At these sites integrins are concentrated and co-localize with several cytoskeletal components [14,43–45]. Examples of the latter include talin and α-actinin, both of which interact directly with the integrin β_1-subunit [46,47]. The recently described focal adhesion protein tyrosine kinase, pp125^{FAK} [48–50], protein kinase C (PKC) [51] and, in transformed cells, p60^{v-src} [52] have been found to be concentrated in focal adhesions. Other intracellular proteins that localize to focal adhesions include vinculin, paxillin, zyxin and tensin.

Several lines of evidence point to the importance of protein phosphorylation events in the regulation of adhesion of cells to ECM glycoproteins and for the formation of focal adhesions. The focal adhesion proteins pp125^{FAK} and paxillin become phosphorylated on tyrosine residues during attachment and spreading of cells [48,49,53,54]. Treatment of fibroblasts with the tyrosine kinase inhibitor herbimycin A blocks formation of focal adhesions and stress fibres [54]. Similarly, inhibitors of PKC inhibit the formation of focal adhesions [55]. Furthermore, membrane-bound PKC becomes activated when Chinese hamster ovary (CHO) cells spread on immobilized fibronectin. Phorbol esters enhance both processes, whereas an inhibitor of PKC activity abolishes the spreading reaction [56]. It has furthermore been shown that members of the rho-subfamily of GTP-binding, ras-related proteins are important for growth factor-induced assembly of focal adhesions [57]. Some growth factors, e.g. platelet-derived growth factor (PDGF), are able to affect the integrity of focal adhesions. Thus PDGF stimulation leads to a transient translocation of vinculin from focal adhesions in fibroblasts [58] and to phosphorylation and/or re-distribution of other focal adhesion proteins, including pp125^{FAK} [59,60]. Studies in our own laboratory have revealed that PDGF stimulation also leads to a transient redistribution of β_1 integrins from focal adhesions to the cell circumference in fibroblasts (K. Åhlén and K. Rubin, unpublished work).

Integrins exhibit functional specificity in that they organize into focal adhesions only after having bound to their proper ligands. Thus, $\alpha_5\beta_1$ will only assemble in focal adhesions in cells cultured on fibronectin and $\alpha_1\beta_1$ in cells cultured on collagen. The structural information necessary to assemble β_1 integrins into focal adhesions seems to reside in the β_1-subunit. This is demonstrated by the observation that chimeric proteins containing only the β_1 cytoplasmic domain will assemble in focal adhesions spontaneously [61]. It is further suggested that the α-subunit masks the site in the β-subunit which possesses a default affinity for focal adhesion components, as removal of the cytoplasmic domain from the α_1-subunit leads to the formation of an $\alpha_1\beta_1$ which also assembles into focal adhesions on cells cultured on fibronectin [62].

It is likely that the supramolecular organization at focal adhesions does not merely serve as a mechanical link between ECM structures and the cytoskeleton, but also forms a framework facilitating the spatial organization of regulatory intracellular proteins. Such organizations are probably needed for proper signal transduction evoked by either integrin or growth factor stimulation. It has been shown that integrin-mediated adhesion, for example, is necessary for a PDGF-induced increase in free cytoplasmic Ca^{2+} [63]. In this context it is interesting to note that integrins transduce different intracellular signals depending on the three-dimensional structure of the ligand [64].

Regulation of integrin activity

Many integrin-mediated adhesion reactions are dynamic and rapidly regulated. Well-recognized examples are the adhesive properties of platelets and leucocytes. Activated platelets acquire a high affinity for fibrinogen, leading to platelet aggregation, and chemo-attractant-stimulated leucocytes acquire a high affinity for activated endothelium, leading to diapedesis. These reactions are dependent on the integrin gpIIb/β_3 and the β_2 integrins respectively. These integrins have the ability to undergo intramolecular affinity modulation [65–67]. Integrins have relatively low affinities with K_d values in the micromolar range. Determinations of K_d values for $\alpha_L\beta_2$ (LFA-1) present on T cells revealed a 200-fold increase in affinity after T-cell activation, although only a portion of the LFA-1 molecules acquired the high-affinity state [68]. The molecular background to this activation is not completely understood, but available data favour the hypothesis that transitions between the two affinity states result from changes in conformation of the integrin heterodimers [69–72]. It has been shown that gpIIb/β_3 heterodimers, in which the cytoplasmic domains of the gpIIb-subunit have been removed by recombinant DNA methods, are constitutively in the high-affinity state [73,74]. A tentative schematic description, based on available data, of the high- and low-affinity transition states of integrins is presented in Figure 1.

Bivalent cations can affect the affinity of soluble $\alpha_5\beta_1$; Mn^{2+} increases the affinity to fibronectin [75]. Evidence that β_1 integrins may exist in low- and high-affinity states is provided by the observation that certain monoclonal anti-(β_1 integrin) antibodies are able to increase the affinity of avian [76] and human [77–80] β_1 integrins. Stimulation of CHO cells with phorbol esters increases attachment of these cells to fibronectin [81]. In contrast, phosphorylation of integrins by pp60[src] reduces their affinity for both talin and fibronectin [82]. Thus the available data strongly suggest that β_1 integrins exist in high- and low-affinity states, and also indicate that intracellular phosphorylation events can regulate β_1 integrin activity.

The intrinsic property of integrins of being able to undergo intramolecular affinity modulation makes these adhesion receptors ideal mediators of tensile force in processes where swift changes of contractile tension are needed. β_1 integrins have been shown to function as mechanoreceptors which can increase cytoskeletal stiffness in cells [83].

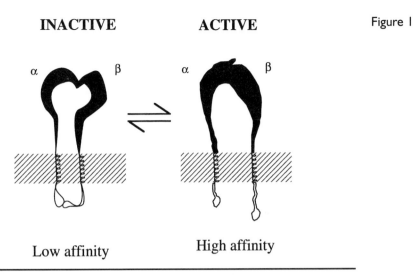

INACTIVE   ACTIVE   Figure I

α   β   α   β

Low affinity   High affinity

Tentative schematic illustration of the two affinity states of integrin heterodimers
The figure is based on studies referenced in the text. The two states differ with respect to conformation; the high-affinity state exposes binding sites for cytoskeletal proteins present on the β-subunit cytoplasmic domain.

Regulation of integrin expression *in vitro*

Stimulation of cultured cells with a number of growth factors or cytokines leads to changes in integrin expression. Transforming growth factor-β (TGF-β), interleukin-1 (IL-1) and tumour necrosis factor-α (TNF-α) have all been shown to stimulate integrin expression in cultured fibroblasts. TGF-β increases steady-state levels of β_1-subunit mRNA, as well as synthesis and post-translational processing [84,85]. Furthermore, in WI-38 fibroblasts, TGF-β increases the synthesis of several α-subunits, including the α_1-, α_2- and α_3-subunits. IL-1 and TNF-α stimulate the expression of $\alpha_1\beta_1$ on fibroblasts but not the synthesis of $\alpha_2\beta_1$ and $\alpha_3\beta_1$ [86]. In contrast, studies in our own laboratory have shown that PDGF-BB stimulates the synthesis of α_2, but not α_1 or α_3 [87a].

Integrins in other types of cells have also been shown to be regulated by soluble factors. Fibroblast growth factor increases the expression of several integrins on microvascular endothelial cells [87,88]. In a comparison of the effects of TGF-β and PDGF-BB on integrin expression it was found that these factors differ in which of the integrin heterodimers they stimulate [89]. Finally, epidermal growth factor (EGF) stimulates the expression of $\alpha_2\beta_1$ on human keratinocytes [90]. This effect is likely to be of importance for EGF-promoted keratinocyte locomotion on collagen.

Contraction of three-dimensional collagen lattices *in vitro*

Fibroblasts cultured in three-dimensional lattices of reconstituted collagen fibres compact the collagen fibres leading to a decrease in lattice volume, the so called fibroblast-mediated collagen gel contraction [91–95]. A visible decrease in lattice volume can usually be observed within hours after the initiation of the contraction process. This process has been suggested to result from fibroblast migration through the lattice and the subsequent arrangement of collagen fibres into bundles. Fibroblasts which are cultured in a contracting collagen gel will change their morphology, as well as alter other phenotypic characteristics, such as collagen synthesis, and come more closely to resemble cells *in vivo* [91,96,97]. Culture in collagen gels also leads to a decreased cellular sensitivity for growth factor stimulation [98] and PDGF β-receptors at the cell surface decrease in number or become refractory [99,100].

The contraction process depends on cytoskeletal integrity. Reagents disrupting cytoskeletal fibres, such as cytochalasin A, effectively block collagen gel contraction [101]. A role for β_1 integrins has been implicated in fibroblast-mediated collagen gel contraction [102]. The collagen-binding integrin $\alpha_2\beta_1$ seems to play a particularly important role [12,103,104]. Increases in intracellular cyclic AMP inhibit collagen gel contraction [105,106], probably mediated by changes in phosphorylation of myosin light chain kinase [107]. A direct role of PKC in collagen gel contraction has also been demonstrated [108].

Growth factors and cytokines influence the ability of fibroblasts to contract collagen gels. TGF-β [109], PDGF [102,110] and endothelins [111] stimulate collagen gel contraction. A direct comparison of the effects of TGF-β and PDGF, using the same assay system, revealed that the effects of PDGF are evident after a few hours, whereas the stimulatory effect of TGF-β had a slower onset [99]. These findings indicate that TGF-β and PDGF exert their stimulatory effects via different intracellular signalling pathways. The inhibitory effects of anti-(β_1 integrin) antibodies on fibroblast-mediated collagen gel contraction could be overcome by increasing the concentration of PDGF-BB in the medium [102], suggesting that PDGF-BB induces an increase in collagen-binding β_1 integrin expression and/or activity. In contrast, certain inflammatory cytokines are able to inhibit collagen gel contraction, including IL-1 and TNF-α [99,112], as well as prostaglandin E_2 [105]. The inhibitory activity of at least some of the latter factors may be due to changes in intracellular levels of cyclic AMP.

It is interesting to note that contraction of fibroblast-populated collagen gels is regulated by a number of growth factors and cytokines that are produced locally during wound healing. Collagen gel contraction has in fact been suggested to be a suitable *in vitro* model for wound contraction [92,113]. The strong and rapid modulation of collagen gel contraction *in vitro*, by inflammatory factors such as PDGF and prostaglandin E_2, suggests that the *in vivo* counterpart to collagen gel contraction is of importance also in some aspects of inflammatory reactions.

Control of interstitial fluid pressure (P_{if}) in dermis: the possible role of β_1 integrins in contraction of the ECM *in vivo*

P_{if} constitutes a major driving force in the formation of acute inflammatory oedema. For a more extensive discussion of P_{if} and control of interstitial fluid balance see Chapter 7 by Reed in this volume. In a recent report we presented data demonstrating a role for β_1 integrins in the control of dermal P_{if} [15]. Furthermore, injection of polyclonal

FLUID

Figure 2

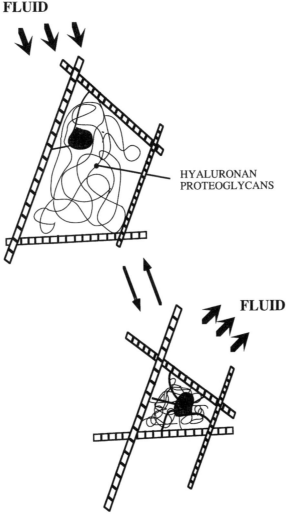

HYALURONAN
PROTEOGLYCANS

FLUID

Hypothetical role of integrin-mediated fibroblast tension on collagen fibres in the control of tissue fluid content
Fibroblasts are able to modulate their tension on the collagen network by regulating the activity of cell-surface β_1 integrins. These integrins function as adhesion receptors, linking cells to the surrounding network of ECM collagen fibres.

anti-(β_1 integrin) IgG in rat dermis leads to the formation of oedema. In later studies we have found that certain agents modulating P_{if} *in vivo* also modulate contraction of fibroblast-populated collagen gels. Examples are anti-(β_1 integrin) antibodies (both IgG and monovalent Fab fragments) and cyclic AMP which inhibit collagen gel contraction *in vitro*, and decrease P_{if} *in vivo* [114].

On the basis of the available data we propose a model in which fibroblasts regulate P_{if} in dermis by exerting a tensile force on a collagen network which restrains a hyaluronan–proteoglycan gel from swelling (Figure 2; see also Chapter 10 by Winlove and Parker in this book). According to this hypothesis, the tensile force on the collagen fibre network is generated by the cytoskeletal contractile apparatus that acts on the collagen fibres via collagen-binding β_1 integrins. The activity of these integrins can be modulated by cytokines, growth factors and prostaglandins, allowing for rapid changes in the balance between grip and release. This will lead to the compaction or swelling of the hyaluronan–proteoglycan gel, in turn affecting P_{if} and the water content of the tissue.

We wish to acknowledge financial support from The Swedish Cancer Foundation, Konung Gustaf V:s 80-Ürsfond, and The Norwegian Council for Science and The Humanities.

References

1. Ruoslahti, E. and Pierschbacher, M.D. (1987) New perspectives in cell adhesion: RGD and integrins. *Science* **238**, 491–497
2. Hynes, R.O. (1987) Integrins: a family of cell surface receptors. *Cell* **48**, 549–554
3. Buck, C.A. and Horwitz, A.F. (1987) Integrin, a transmembrane glycoprotein complex mediating cell-substratum adhesion. *J. Cell Sci.* **8** (Suppl.), 231–250
4. Albelda, S.M. and Buck, C.A. (1990) Integrins and other cell adhesion molecules. *FASEB J.* **4**, 2868–2880
5. Hemler, M.E. (1990) VLA proteins in the integrin family: structures, functions, and their role on leukocytes. *Annu. Rev. Immunol.* **8**, 365–400
6. Springer, T.A. (1990) Adhesion receptors of the immune system. *Nature (London)* **346**, 425–434
7. Ruoslahti, E. (1991) Integrins. *J. Clin. Invest.* **87**, 1–5
8. Hynes, R.O. (1992) Integrins: versatility, modulation, and signaling in cell adhesion. *Cell* **69**, 11–25
9. Tamkun, J.W., DeSimone, D.W., Fonda, D., Patel, R.S., Buck, C., Horwitz, A.F. and Hynes, R.O. (1986) Structure of integrin, a glycoprotein involved in the transmembrane linkage between fibronectin and actin. *Cell* **46**, 271–282
10. Damsky, C.H. and Werb, Z. (1992) Signal transduction by integrin receptors for extracellular matrix: cooperative processing of extracellular information. *Curr. Opin. Cell Biol.* **4**, 772–781
11. Leavesley, D.I., Schwartz, M.A., Rosenfeld, M. and Cheresh, D.A. (1993) Integrin β1- and β3-mediated endothelial cell migration is triggered through distinct signaling mechanisms. *J. Cell Biol.* **121**, 163–170
12. Schiro, J.A., Chan, B.M., Roswit, W.T., Kassner, P.D., Pentland, A.P., Hemler, M.E., Eisen, A.Z. and Kupper, T.S. (1991) Integrin $\alpha_2\beta_1$ (VLA-2) mediates reorganization and contraction of collagen matrices by human cells. *Cell* **67**, 403–410
13. Juliano, R.L. and Haskill, S. (1993) Signal transduction from the extracellular matrix. *J. Cell Biol.* **120**, 577–585
14. Schwartz, M.A. (1992) Transmembrane signalling by integrins. *Trends Cell Biol.* **2**, 304–308
15. Reed, R.K., Rubin, K., Wiig, H. and Rodt, S.A. (1992) Blockade of β_1-integrins in skin causes edema through lowering of interstitial fluid pressure. *Circ. Res.* **71**, 978–983
16. Palmer, E.L., Ruegg, C., Ferrando, R., Pytela, R. and Sheppard, D. (1993) Sequence and tissue distribution of the integrin α9 subunit, a novel partner of β1 that is widely distributed in epithelia and muscle. *J. Cell Biol.* **123**, 1289–1297
17. Kunicki, T.J., Nugent, D.J., Staats, S.J., Orchekowski, R.P., Wayner, E.A. and Carter, W.G. (1988) The human fibroblast class II extracellular matrix receptor mediates platelet adhesion to collagen and is identical to the platelet glycoprotein Ia-IIa complex. *J. Biol. Chem.* **263**, 4516–4519
18. Gullberg, D., Gehlsen, K.R., Turner, D.C., Ahlen, K., Zijenah, L.S., Barnes, M.J. and Rubin, K. (1992) Analysis of $\alpha_1\beta_1$, $\alpha_2\beta_1$ and $\alpha_3\beta_1$ integrins in cell–collagen interactions: identification of

conformation dependent $\alpha_1\beta_1$ binding sites in collagen type I. EMBO J. **11**, 3865–3873

19. Wayner, E.A., Carter, W.G., Piotrowicz, R.S. and Kunicki, T.J. (1988) The function of multiple extracellular matrix receptors in mediating cell adhesion to extracellular matrix: preparation of monoclonal antibodies to the fibronectin receptor that specifically inhibit cell adhesion to fibronectin and react with platelet glycoproteins Ic-IIa. *J. Cell Biol.* **107**, 1881–1891

20. Elices, M.J., Urry, L.A. and Hemler, M.E. (1991) Receptor functions for the integrin VLA-3: fibronectin, collagen, and laminin binding are differentially influenced by Arg-Gly-Asp peptide and by divalent cations. *J. Cell Biol.* **112**, 169–181

21. Elices, M.J. and Hemler, M.E. (1989) The human integrin VLA-2 is a collagen receptor on some cells and a collagen/laminin receptor on others. *Proc. Natl. Acad. Sci. U.S.A.* **86**, 9906–9910

22. Languino, L.R., Gehlsen, K.R., Wayner, E., Carter, W.G., Engvall, E. and Ruoslahti, E. (1989) Endothelial cells use $\alpha_2\beta_1$ integrin as a laminin receptor. *J. Cell Biol.* **109**, 2455–2462

23. Carter, W.G., Wayner, E.A., Bouchard, T.S. and Kaur, P. (1990) The role of integrins $\alpha_2\beta_1$ and $\alpha_3\beta_1$ in cell-cell and cell-substrate adhesion of human epidermal cells. *J. Cell Biol.* **110**, 1387–1404

24. Larjava, H., Peltonen, J., Akiyama, S.K., Yamada, S.S., Gralnick, H.R., Uitto, J. and Yamada, K.M. (1990) Novel function for β1 integrins in keratinocyte cell-cell interactions. *J. Cell Biol.* **110**, 803–815

25. Symington, B.E., Takada, Y. and Carter, W.G. (1993) Interaction of integrins $\alpha 3$ $\beta 1$ and $\alpha 2\beta 1$: potential role in keratinocyte intercellular adhesion. *J. Cell Biol.* **120**, 523-535

26. Sriramarao, P., Steffner, P. and Gehlsen, K.R. (1993) Biochemical evidence for a homophilic interaction of the $\alpha 3 \beta 1$ integrin. *J. Biol. Chem.* **268**, 22036–22041

27. Kern, A., Eble, J., Golbik, R. and Kuhn, K. (1993) Interaction of type IV collagen with the isolated integrins $\alpha 1\beta 1$ and $\alpha 2\beta 1$. *Eur. J. Biochem.* **215**, 151–159

28. Pierschbacher, M., Hayman, E.G. and Ruoslahti, E. (1983) Synthetic peptide with cell attachment activity of fibronectin. *Proc. Natl. Acad. Sci. U.S.A.* **80**, 1224–1227

29. Chan, B.M., Kassner, P.D., Schiro, J.A., Byers, H.R., Kupper, T.S. and Hemler, M.E. (1992) Distinct cellular functions mediated by different VLA integrin α subunit cytoplasmic domains. *Cell* **68**, 1051–1060

30. Sastry, S.K. and Horwitz, A.F. (1993) Integrin cytoplasmic domains: mediators of cytoskeletal linkages and extra- and intracellular initiated transmembrane signaling. *Curr. Opin. Cell Biol.* **5**, 819–831

31. Altruda, F., Cervella, P., Tarone, G., Botta, C., Balzac, F., Stefanuto, G. and Silengo, L. (1990) A human integrin β1 subunit with a unique cytoplasmic domain generated by alternative mRNA processing. *Gene* **95**, 261–266

32. Languino, L.R. and Ruoslahti, E. (1992) An alternative form of the integrin β_1 subunit with a variant cytoplasmic domain. *J. Biol. Chem.* **267**, 7116–7120

33. Balzac, F., Belkin, A.M., Koteliansky, V.E., Balabanov, Y.V., Altruda, F., Silengo, L. and Tarone, G. (1993) Expression and functional analysis of a cytoplasmic domain variant of the β_1 integrin subunit *J. Cell Biol.* **121**, 171–178

34. Buck, C., Albelda, S., Damjanovich, L., Edelman, J., Shih, D.T. and Solowska, J. (1990) Immunohistochemical and molecular analysis of β_1 and β_3 integrins. *Cell. Differ. Dev.* **32**, 189–202

35. Defilippi, P., van Hinsbergh, V., Bertolotto, A., Rossino, P., Silengo, L. and Tarone, G. (1991) Differential distribution and modulation of expression of alpha1/beta1 integrin on human endothelial cells. *J. Cell Biol.* **114**, 855–863

36. Albelda, S.M. (1992) Differential expression of integrin cell-substratum adhesion receptors on endothelium. *Experientia* **61**, 188–192

37. Stallmach, A., von Lampe, B., Matthes, H., Bornhoft, G. and Riecken, E.O. (1992) Diminished expression of integrin adhesion molecules on human colonic epithelial cells during the benign to malign tumour transformation. *Gut* **33**, 342–346

38. Damjanovich, L., Albelda, S.M., Mette, S.A. and Buck, C.A. (1992) Distribution of integrin cell adhesion receptors in normal and malignant lung tissue. *Am. J. Respir. Cell Mol. Biol.* **6**, 197–206

39. van den Berg, T.K., van der Ende, M., Dopp, E.A., Kraal, G. and Dijkstra, C.D. (1993) Localization of β_1 integrins and their extracellular ligands in human lymphoid tissues. *Am. J. Pathol.* **143**, 1098–1110

40. Mette, S.A., Pilewski, J., Buck, C.A. and Albelda, S.M. (1993) Distribution of integrin cell adhesion receptors on normal bronchial epithelial cells and lung cancer cells in vitro and in vivo. *Am. J. Respir. Cell Mol. Biol.* **8**, 562–572

41. Johnson, B.A., Haines, G.K., Harlow, L.A. and Koch, A.E. (1993) Adhesion molecule expression in human synovial tissue. *Arthritis Rheum.* **36**, 137–146

42. Zutter, M.M. and Santoro, S.A. (1990) Widespread histologic distribution of the $\alpha_2\beta_1$ integrin cell-surface collagen receptor. *Am. J. Pathol.* **137**, 113–120

43. Burridge, K., Fath, K., Kelly, T., Nuckolls, G. and Turner, C. (1988) Focal adhesions: transmembrane junctions between the extracellular matrix and the cytoskeleton. *Annu. Rev. Cell Biol.* **4**, 487–525

44. Turner, C.E. and Burridge, K. (1991) Transmembrane molecular assemblies in cell-extracellular matrix interactions. *Curr. Opin. Cell Biol.* **3**, 849–853

45. Turner, C.E. (1994) Paxillin: a cytoskeletal target for tyrosine kinases *BioEssays* **16**, 47–52

46. Otey, C.A., Pavalko, F.M. and Burridge, K. (1990) An interaction between α-actinin and the β_1 integrin subunit *in vitro*. *J. Cell Biol.* **111**, 721–729

47. Horwitz, A., Duggan, K., Buck, C., Beckerle, M.C. and Burridge, K. (1986) Interaction of plasma

membrane fibronectin receptor with talin–a transmembrane linkage. *Nature (London)* **320**, 531–533

48. Hanks, S.K., Calalb, M.B., Harper, M.C. and Patel, S.K. (1992) Focal adhesion protein-tyrosine kinase phosphorylated in response to cell attachment to fibronectin. *Proc. Natl. Acad. Sci. U.S.A.* **89**, 8487–8491

49. Kornberg, L., Earp, H.S., Parsons, J.T., Schaller, M. and Juliano, R.L. (1992) Cell adhesion or integrin clustering increases phosphorylation of a focal adhesion-associated tyrosine kinase. *J. Biol. Chem.* **267**, 23439–23442

50. Schaller, M.D., Hildebrand, J.D., Shannon, J.D., Fox, J.W., Vines, R.R. and Parsons, J.T. (1994) Autophosphorylation of the focal adhesion kinase, pp125FAK, directs SH2-dependent binding of pp60src. *Mol. Cell. Biol.* **14**, 1680–1688

51. Jaken, S., Leach, K. and Klauck, T. (1989) Association of type 3 protein kinase C with focal contacts in rat embryo fibroblasts. *J. Cell Biol.* **109**, 697–704

52. Rohrschneider, L.R. (1980) Adhesion plaques of Rous sarcoma virus transformed cells contain the src gene product. *Proc. Natl. Acad. Sci. U.S.A.* **77**, 3514–3518

53. Guan, J.L. and Shalloway, D. (1992) Regulation of focal adhesion-associated protein tyrosine kinase by both cellular adhesion and oncogenic transformation. *Nature (London)* **358**, 690–692

54. Burridge, K., Turner, C.E. and Romer, L.H. (1992) Tyrosine phosphorylation of paxillin and pp125FAK accompanies cell adhesion to extracellular matrix: a role in cytoskeletal assembly. *J. Cell Biol.* **119**, 893–903

55. Woods, A. and Couchman, J.R. (1992) Protein kinase C involvement in focal adhesion formation. *J. Cell Sci.* **101**, 277–290

56. Vuori, K. and Ruoslahti, E. (1993) Activation of protein kinase C precedes $\alpha_5\beta_1$ integrin-mediated cell spreading on fibronectin. *J. Biol. Chem.* **268**, 21459–21462

57. Ridley, A.J. and Hall, A. (1992) The small GTP-binding protein rho regulates the assembly of focal adhesions and actin stress fibers in response to growth factors. *Cell* **70**, 389–399

58. Herman, B. and Pledger, W.J. (1985) Platelet-derived growth factor-induced alterations in vinculin and actin distribution in BALB/c-3T3 cells. *J. Cell Biol.* **100**, 1031–1040

59. Tidball, J.G. and Spencer, M.J. (1993) PDGF stimulation induces phosphorylation of talin and cytoskeletal reorganization in skeletal muscle. *J. Cell Biol.* **123**, 627–635

60. Rankin, S. and Rozengurt, E. (1994) Platelet-derived growth factor modulation of focal adhesion kinase (p125FAK) and paxillin tyrosine phosphorylation in Swiss 3T3 cells. Bell-shaped dose response and cross-talk with bombesin. *J. Biol. Chem.* **269**, 704–710

61. Geiger, B., Salomon, D., Takeichi, M. and Hynes, R.O. (1992) A chimeric N-cadherin/β_1-integrin receptor which localizes to both cell- cell and cell-matrix adhesions. *J. Cell Sci.* **103**, 943–951

62. Briesewitz, R., Kern, A. and Marcantonio, E.E. (1993) Ligand-dependent and -independent integrin focal contact localization: the role of the α chain cytoplasmic domain. *Mol. Biol. Cell* **4**, 593–604

63. McNamee, H.P., Ingber, D.E. and Schwartz, M.A. (1993) Adhesion to fibronectin stimulates inositol lipid synthesis and enhances PDGF-induced inositol lipid breakdown. *J. Cell Biol.* **121**, 673–678

64. Schwartz, M.A. and Ingber, D.E. (1994) Integrating with integrins. *Mol. Biol. Cell* **5**, 389–393

65. Shattil, S.J., Hoxie, J.A., Cunningham, M. and Brass, L.F. (1985) Changes in the platelet membrane glycoprotein IIb.IIIa complex during platelet activation. *J. Biol. Chem.* **260**, 11107–11114

66. Du, X.P., Plow, E.F., Frelinger, A., O'Toole, T.E., Loftus, J.C. and Ginsberg, M.H. (1991) Ligands 'activate' integrin $\alpha_{IIb}\beta_3$ (platelet GPIIb-IIIa). *Cell* **65**, 409–416

67. Dustin, M.L. and Springer, T.A. (1989) T-cell receptor cross-linking transiently stimulates adhesiveness through LFA-1. *Nature (London)* **341**, 619–624

68. Lollo, B.A., Chan, K.W.H., Hanson, E.M., Moy, V.T. and Brian, A.A. (1993) Direct evidence for two affinity states for lymphocyte function-associated antigen 1 on activated T cells. *J. Biol. Chem.* **268**, 21693–21700

69. Sims, P.J., Ginsberg, M.H., Plow, E.F. and Shattil, S.J. (1991) Effect of platelet activation on the conformation of the plasma membrane glycoprotein IIb-IIIa complex. *J. Biol. Chem.* **266**, 7345–7352

70. Calvete, J.J., Mann, K., Schafer, W., Fernandez-Lafuente, R. and Guisan, J.M. (1994) Proteolytic degradation of the RGD-binding and non-RGD-binding conformers of human platelet integrin glycoprotein IIb/IIIa: clues for identification of regions involved in the receptor's activation. *Biochem. J.* **298**, 1–7

71. Humphries, M.J., Mould, A.P. and Tuckwell, D.S. (1993) Dynamic aspects of adhesion receptor function–integrins both twist and shout. *BioEssays* **15**, 391–397

72. Williams, J.M., Hughes, P.E., O'Toole, T.E. and Ginsberg, M.H. (1994) The inner world of cell adhesion: integrin cytoplasmic domains. *Trends Cell Biol.* **4**, 109–112

73. O'Toole, T.E., Katagiri, Y., Faull, R.J., Peter, K., Tamura, R., Quaranta, V., Loftus, J.C., Shattil, S.J. and Ginsberg, M.H. (1994) Integrin cytoplasmic domains mediate inside-out signal transduction. *J. Cell Biol.* **124**, 1047–1059

74. O'Toole, T.E., Mandelman, D., Forsyth, J., Shattil, S.J., Plow, E.F. and Ginsberg, M.H. (1991) Modulation of the affinity of integrin $\alpha_{IIb}\beta_3$ (GPIIb-IIIa) by the cytoplasmic domain of α_{IIb}. *Science* **254**, 845–847

75. Gailit, J. and Ruoslahti, E. (1988) Regulation of the fibronectin receptor affinity by divalent cations. *J. Biol. Chem.* **263**, 12927–12932

76. Neugebauer, K.M. and Reichardt, L.F. (1991) Cell-surface regulation of β 1-integrin activity on developing retinal neurons. *Nature (London)* **350**, 68–71

77. Kovach, N.L., Carlos, T.M., Yee, E. and Harlan, J.M. (1992) A monoclonal antibody to β 1 integrin (CD29) stimulates VLA-dependent adherence of leukocytes to human umbilical vein endothelial cells and matrix components. *J. Cell Biol.* **116**, 499–509

78. van de Wiel-van Kemenade, E., van Kooyk, Y., de Boer, A.J., Huijbens, R.J., Weder, P., van de Kasteele, W., Melief, C.J. and Figdor, C.G. (1992) Adhesion of T and B lymphocytes to extracellular matrix and endothelial cells can be regulated through the β subunit of VLA. *J. Cell Biol.* **117**, 461–470

79. Faull, R.J., Kovach, N.L., Harlan, J.M. and Ginsberg, M.H. (1993) Affinity modulation of integrin $\alpha_5\beta_1$: regulation of the functional response by soluble fibronectin. *J. Cell Biol.* **121**, 155–162

80. Arroyo, A.G., Garcia-Pardo, A. and Sanchez-Madrid, F. (1993) A high affinity conformational state on VLA integrin heterodimers induced by an anti-β 1 chain monoclonal antibody. *J. Biol. Chem.* **268**, 9863–9868

81. Danilov, Y.N. and Juliano, R.L. (1989) Phorbol ester modulation of integrin-mediated cell adhesion: a postreceptor event. *J. Cell Biol.* **108**, 1925–1933

82. Tapley, P., Horwitz, A., Buck, C., Duggan, K. and Rohrschneider, L. (1989) Integrins isolated from Rous sarcoma virus-transformed chicken embryo fibroblasts. *Oncogene* **4**, 325–333

83. Wang, N., Butler, J.P. and Ingber, D.E. (1993) Mechanotransduction across the cell surface and through the cytoskeleton. *Science* **260**, 1124–1127

84. Ignotz, R.A., Heino, J. and Massague, J. (1989) Regulation of cell adhesion receptors by transforming growth factor-β. Regulation of vitronectin receptor and LFA-1. *J. Biol. Chem.* **264**, 389–392

85. Heino, J., Ignotz, R.A., Hemler, M.E., Crouse, C. and Massague, J. (1989) Regulation of cell adhesion receptors by transforming growth factor-β. *J. Biol. Chem.* **264**, 380–388

86. Santala, P. and Heino, J. (1991) Regulation of integrin-type cell adhesion receptors by cytokines. *J. Biol. Chem.* **266**, 23505–23509

87a. Åhlén, K. and Rubin, K. (1995) *Exp. Cell. Res.*, **215**, 347–353

87. Enenstein, J., Waleh, N.S. and Kramer, R.H. (1992) Basic FGF and TGF-β differentially modulate integrin expression of human microvascular endothelial cells. *Exp. Cell. Res.* **203**, 499–503

88. Klein, S., Giancotti, F.G., Presta, M., Albelda, S.M., Buck, C.A. and Rifkin, D.B. (1993) Basic fibroblast growth factor modulates integrin expression in microvascular endothelial cells. *Mol. Biol. Cell* **4**, 973–982

89. Janat, M.F., Argraves, W.S. and Liau, G. (1992) Regulation of vascular smooth muscle cell integrin expression by transforming growth factor β_1 and by platelet-derived growth factor-BB. *J. Cell. Physiol.* **151**, 588–595

90. Chen, J.D., Kim, J.P., Zhang, K., Sarret, Y., Wynn, K.C., Kramer, R.H. and Woodley, D.T. (1993) Epidermal growth factor (EGF) promotes human keratinocyte locomotion on collagen by increasing the α2 integrin subunit. *Exp. Cell. Res.* **209**, 216–223

91. Elsdale, T.R. and Bard, J.B.L. (1972) Collagen substrata for studies on cell behavior. *J. Cell Biol.* **54**, 626–637

92. Bell, E., Ivarsson, B. and Merrill, C. (1979) Production of a tissue-like structure by contraction of collagen lattices by human fibroblasts of different proliferative potential *in vitro*. *Proc. Natl. Acad. Sci. U.S.A.* **76**, 1274–1278

93. Stopak, D. and Harris, A.K. (1982) Connective tissue morphogenesis by fibroblast traction. *Dev. Biol.* **90**, 383–398

94. Buttle, D.J. and Ehrlich, H.P. (1983) Comparative studies of collagen lattice contraction utilizing a normal and a transformed cell line. *J. Cell. Physiol.* **116**, 159–166

95. Grinnell, F. and Lamke, C.R. (1984) Reorganization of hydrated collagen lattices by human skin fibroblasts. *J. Cell Sci.* **66**, 51–63

96. Nusgens, B., Merrill, C., Lapiere, C. and Bell, E. (1984) Collagen biosynthesis by cells in a tissue equivalent matrix in vitro. *Collagen Relat. Res.* **4**, 351–363

97. Mauch, C., Hatamochi, A., Scharffetter, K. and Krieg, T. (1988) Regulation of collagen synthesis in fibroblasts within a three-dimensional collagen gel. *Exp. Cell. Res.* **178**, 493–503

98. Nakagawa, S., Pawelek, P. and Grinnell, F. (1989) Extracellular matrix organization modulates fibroblast growth and growth factor responsiveness. *Exp. Cell. Res.* **182**, 572–582

99. Tingstrom, A., Heldin, C.H. and Rubin, K. (1992) Regulation of fibroblast-mediated collagen gel contraction by platelet-derived growth factor, interleukin-1 α and transforming growth factor-β1. *J. Cell Sci.* **102**, 315–322

100. Lin, Y.C. and Grinnell, F. (1993) Decreased level of PDGF-stimulated receptor autophosphorylation by fibroblasts in mechanically relaxed collagen matrices. *J. Cell Biol.* **122**, 663–672

101. Tomasek, J.J. and Hay, E.D. (1984) Analysis of the role of microfilaments and microtubules in acquisition of bipolarity and elongation of fibroblasts in hydrated collagen gels. *J. Cell Biol.* **99**, 536–549

102. Gullberg, D., Tingstrom, A., Thuresson, A.C., Olsson, L., Terracio, L., Borg, T.K. and Rubin, K. (1990) β_1 integrin-mediated collagen gel contraction is stimulated by PDGF. *Exp. Cell. Res.* **186**, 264–272

103. Klein, C.E., Dressel, D., Steinmayer, T., Mauch, C., Eckes, B., Krieg, T., Bankert, R.B. and

Weber, L. (1991) Integrin $\alpha_2\beta_1$ is upregulated in fibroblasts and highly aggressive melanoma cells in three-dimensional collagen lattices and mediates the reorganization of collagen I fibrils. *J. Cell Biol.* **115**, 1427–1436

104. Hunt, R.C., Pakalnis, V.A., Choudhury, P. and Black, E.P. (1994) Cytokines and serum cause $\alpha_x\beta_1$ integrin-mediated contraction of collagen gels by cultured retinal pigment epithelial cells. *Invest. Ophthalmol. Vis. Sci.* **35**, 955–963

105. Ehrlich, H.P. and Wyler, D.J. (1983) Fibroblast contraction of collagen lattices in vitro: inhibition by chronic inflammatory cell mediators. *J. Cell. Physiol.* **116**, 345–351

106. Van Bockxmeer, F.M., Martin, C.E. and Constable, I.J. (1984) Effect of cyclic AMP on cellular contractility and DNA synthesis in chorioretinal fibroblasts maintained in collagen matrices. *Exp. Cell. Res.* **155**, 413–421

107. Ehrlich, H.P., Rockwell, W.B., Cornwell, T.L. and Rajaratnam, J.B. (1991) Demonstration of a direct role for myosin light chain kinase in fibroblast-populated collagen lattice contraction. *J. Cell. Physiol.* **146**, 1–7

108. Guidry, C. (1993) Fibroblast contraction of collagen gels requires activation of protein kinase C. *J. Cell. Physiol.* **155**, 358–367

109. Montesano, R. and Orci, L. (1988) Transforming growth factor β stimulates collagen-matrix contraction by fibroblasts: implications for wound healing. *Proc. Natl. Acad. Sci. U.S.A.* **85**, 4894–4897

110. Clark, R.A., Folkvord, J.M., Hart, C.E., Murray, M.J. and McPherson, J.M. (1989) Platelet isoforms of platelet-derived growth factor stimulate fibroblasts to contract collagen matrices. *J. Clin. Invest.* **84**, 1036–1040

111. Guidry, C. and Hook, M. (1991) Endothelins produced by endothelial cells promote collagen gel contraction by fibroblasts. *J. Cell Biol.* **115**, 873-880

112. Gillery, P., Coustry, F., Pujol, J.P. and Borel, J.P. (1989) Inhibition of collagen synthesis by interleukin-1 in three-dimensional collagen lattice cultures of fibroblasts. *Experientia* **45**, 98–101

113. Grinnell, F. (1994) Fibroblasts, myofibroblasts, and wound contraction. *J. Cell Biol.* **124**, 401–404

114. Rodt, S.Å., Reed, R.K., Ljungström, M., Gustafsson, T.O. and Rubin, K. (1994) *Circ. Res.* **75**, 942–948

4

Lymphatic safety factor

Aubrey E. Taylor*‡, Timothy M. Moore*, Anthony Rizzo† and Pavel L. Khimenko*

Departments of *Physiology and †Surgery, University of South Alabama, College of Medicine, Mobile, AL 36688-0002, U.S.A.

Introduction

For many years physiologists have known that elevating microvascular pressure results in increased lymph flow due to an increased filtration occurring across the microvascular (or capillary) walls. However, the mechanisms responsible for signalling the lymphatic system to increase its ability to accommodate the increased fluid entering the tissues are poorly understood.

Several mechanisms have been proposed to explain the lymph flow responses that occur with changes in microvascular fluid filtration: (1) Fluid entering the tissues increases interstitial fluid pressure, which elevates the pressure gradient acting between the interstitium and the small lymphatic capillaries, resulting in greater lymphatic filling [1]. (2) The lymphatics are known to have an intrinsic ability to contract and many factors can affect both their rate of contraction and the magnitude of the force generated, e.g. the increased intralymphatic pressure caused by the greater lymphatic filling could elucidate a myogenic response by the smooth muscle in larger lymphatics, causing them to contract more forcefully thus propelling lymph in a forward direction, opening the lymphatic valves towards the tissues and decreasing the intralymphatic pressure in small tissue lymphatics which increases their filling pressure [2–4]. (3) Tissue motion can also accelerate lymph flow and is an important means of increasing lymph flow in organs such as muscle and lungs [5–8]. (4) When fluid enters the interstitium, the tissue spaces expand and fluid can more easily move through the tissues to enter the lymphatics. However, tissues usually do not swell appreciably with moderate elevations in microvascular filtration, yet lymph flow increases [9]. (5) Lymph flow increases when the microvascular walls are damaged by some unknown mechanisms. This last phenomenon, which causes lymph flow to increase as a result of damaged microvascular membranes, is the focus of this chapter, and necessitates a brief review of transmicrovascular filtration as presented in the following sections [10,11].

Transvascular fluid filtration

Physiologists at the time of E. Starling knew that microvascular pressures could be elevated substantially yet no apparent oedema resulted [12,13]. In fact, this observation led Starling to assess the roles

‡To whom correspondence should be addressed.

of plasma and tissue proteins, tissue pressure and lymph flow in preventing oedema formation in tissues. Starling defined the hydrostatic transmicrovascular filtration pressure as the difference between the gradient of microvascular hydrostatic (P_{mv}) and tissue fluid hydrostatic (P_t) pressures and the protein osmotic pressures of plasma (π_p) and tissue (π_t) fluids. Starling hypothesized that when microvascular pressure was increased π_t decreased. Conversely, when microvascular pressure was decreased π_t increased. Thus, changes in microvascular pressure caused the protein osmotic pressure gradient ($\pi_p - \pi_t$) to change in a direction to oppose capillary pressure changes, i.e. transmicrovascular filtration is a self-limiting process [12] as defined by the following equation which is referred to as Starling's Law of the Capillaries:

$$P_{mv} - P_t = \pi_p - \pi_t \tag{1}$$

Starling postulated from his data that only the transmicrovascular plasma protein osmotic pressure gradient changed in a direction to oppose changes in microvascular pressures. He also thought, correctly, that positive tissue pressure would increase the pressure surrounding the veins and increase the microvascular pressure by a like amount, with the result being no change in the transmicrovascular hydrostatic pressure gradient [12].

However, Starling did define the ability of the lymphatics to remove capillary filtrate in terms of the transmicrovascular pressure drop $[(P_{mv} - P_t) - (\pi_{mv} - \pi_t)]$ associated with a given lymph flow (LF) as the lymph flow divided by the filtration coefficient of the microvascular wall (K_{fc}):

$$\text{Lymph flow pressure drop} = LF/K_{fc} \tag{2}$$

The filtration coefficient is a measure of the volume conductance of the microvascular wall and is a function of the permeability of water in the microvascular barrier and the surface area available for fluid exchange. K_{fc} can be low in some organs and very large in others, e.g. the K_{fc} is 0.015 (ml/min per mmHg per 100 g of tissue) in skeletal muscle and 0.250 in lungs. Since K_{fc} is multiplied by the trans-microvascular pressure drop, then for the same microvascular pressure drop in both organs, more lymph would flow from the lung compared with skeletal muscle. However, their lymphatic safety factors are identical, since the absolute magnitude of lymph flow does not determine the lymphatic safety factor when calculated by eqn. (2); but the lymphatic safety factor is a function of the ratio of lymph flow to filtration coefficient, i.e. the pressure drop across the microvascular wall is responsible for producing the lymph. Assume that $LF = 0.15$ ml/min for skeletal muscle and $LF = 2$ ml/min in the lung. The transvascular pressure drop for each case would be 0.15/0.015 = 10 mmHg and 0.02/0.2 = 10 mmHg for skeletal muscle and lung respectively. Although lymph flow was much lower in skeletal muscle, the lymph flow safety factor is identical to that of the lung.

Since lymph flow was very small in Starling's study, he thought that under normal physiological conditions the imbalance in the filtration forces was much smaller than K_{fc} and would not be an important factor opposing oedema until oedema fluid had begun to accumulate and lymph flow was increased [12].

A small imbalance in transmicrovascular filtration forces has been measured in a variety of tissues, as shown in Table 1. Note that large imbalances in transmicrovascular forces occur in tissues that are either absorbing large amounts of fluid (absorbing intestine and renal peritubular capillaries) or filtering large amounts of fluid (glomerular capillaries). However, most organs in the body have imbalances in forces of about 1 mmHg under normal conditions [14]. The exceptions are the glomerular capillaries, which are always filtering, and the brain microvessels. The brain microvessels are almost impermeable to water, resulting in almost no transmicrocirculatory filtration even with this large negative imbalance in forces, i.e. the brain microvessels should be absorbing. The physiological significance of this large imbalance in transmicrovascular forces in the brain is not presently known, but it may indicate that some microvessels in the brain remove small amounts of tissue fluid.

The ability of the lymphatic system to remove tissue fluids and oppose oedema was not re-examined until Landis' classical paper in 1927 [15] and his review article on capillary fluid transport [16]. Landis observed that oedema did not develop in many different tissues until microvascular pressures were elevated by 15–20 mmHg and defined the term 'margin of safety' to describe this phenomenon. Again, like Starling, Landis thought that the increased plasma protein osmotic pressure gradient $(\pi_{mv} - \pi_t)$ associated with increased transmicrovascular filtration was the major force that regulated fluid movement into the interstitium when microvascular pressures were changed. Landis also

Table 1

Tissue	P_{mv} (mmHg)	P_t (mmHg)	π_p	π_t	LF (ml/min per 100 g)	ΔP (mmHg)
Subcutaneous	13	−5	21	4	0.015	+1
Skeletal muscle	9	−3	20	8	0.005	0
Brain	11	7	14	0	—	−10
Intestine (normal)	16	2	23	10	0.08	+1
Intestine (absorbing)	16	3	23	5	0.10	−5
Liver	7	6	22	20	0.10	−1
Lung	7	−5	23	12	0.10	+1
Cardiac muscle	23	15	21	13	0.12	0
Glomerular	50	15[a]	28	0[a]	2.0	+7
Renal peritubular	25	7	32	7	2.0	−7

Starling forces for selected tissues

Modified from [38] with permission. P_{mv}, P_t, π_p, π_t and LF denote microvascular and tissue hydrostatic pressures, plasma and tissue protein osmotic pressures, and lymph flow respectively. ΔP is the sum of the forces $[(P_c - P_t) - (\pi_p - \pi_t)]$ and represents filtration when negative. A sum of zero indicates no filtration or absorption.

[a]*This represents tubular pressures rather than renal interstitial pressure.*

proved Starling's Law of the Capillaries in individual capillaries by showing that capillary filtration was a linear function of microvessel pressure and became zero when $P_{mv} = \pi_p$. However, Landis also thought that lymph flow could remove a substantial amount of transmicrovascular filtrate in some tissues and also serve as a deterrent to excessive oedema formation [16].

Several other research groups have also studied the functional aspects of the lymphatics relative to oedema formation. In Australia, Yoffey and Courtice's group provided many new studies on the lymphatics and also wrote a wonderful and most useful book on the subject [17]. The Hungarian group of Foldi, Rusznyak, Sazbo and Papp studied the lymphatic drainage patterns of many organs in health and disease and much of our present knowledge of the physiology of the lymphatic system was developed by this group and published in a classical book written in English [18]. Of specific interest to this chapter was their development of a concept that the lymphatic system had a maximal capacity to remove microvascular filtrate. As Rusznyak *et al.* studied lymph flow after elevating microvascular pressures they noted that only small amounts of oedema formed with moderate elevations in venous outflow pressures because lymph flow increased sufficiently to remove most of the transmicrovascular filtration. However, when microvascular pressures were elevated to levels that produced maximal lymph flows then oedema fluid rapidly accumulated in the tissues. These investigators coined the term 'lymphatic over-whelming' to explain the development of oedema (i.e. the lymphatic system in many organs can remove most of the transvascular filtrate before observable oedema occurs, and serves as the major factor opposing oedema formation as microvascular pressures increase, when organs are doing their routine physiological functions; therefore once the lymphatic system is over-whelmed then oedema formation continues almost unabated).

Another condition that produces high lymph flows, that are not maintained even as oedema develops, is seen when microvascular pressure is increased by elevating venous outflow pressures. Figure 1 shows venous (P_v) and tissue (P_t) pressures and lymph flow (LF) after increasing venous outflow pressure by 25 mmHg in an isolated dog hind-paw preparation [9]. Note that lymph flow and tissue pressure increased very rapidly with the maximum lymph flow effect occurring after about 5 min. Tissue pressure also increased rapidly, but then increased at a much lower rate. By approximately 10 min, lymph flow decreased from the maximal value of 40×10^{-2} ml/min to 20×10^{-2} ml/min. Oedema was developing; but lymph flow decreased below its maximal obtainable rate by 50%.

Oedema safety factors

Figure 2 shows the accumulation of oedema fluid in an organ as a function of microvascular pressure. Note the curve represented by the solid line. As transvascular pressure increased, almost no fluid accumulated in the tissues until the pressure exceeded 25–30 mmHg. This figure is similar to that in the classical study of Guyton and Lindsey

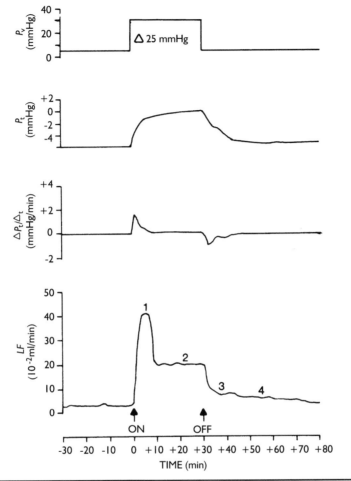

Figure I

Effect of increasing venous pressure by 25 mmHg in an isolated dog paw

P_v, P_t and LF refer to venous pressure, tissue pressure and lymph flow respectively. I, 2, 3 and 4 refer to maximal, steady-state, rapid-off-transient and new baseline lymph flows after increasing venous pressure and then returning it to baseline values. Reproduced from [9] with permission.

obtained during the formation of pulmonary oedema in dog lungs [19]. When the plasma protein osmotic pressure was also lowered in that study, the microvascular pressure at which the tissues became oedematous decreased, as shown by the broken curve in Figure 2. Guyton interpreted these findings as indicating that the protein osmotic gradient ($\pi_{mv} - \pi_t$) increased as transmicrovascular filtration increased and opposed the increased microvascular pressure, i.e. transvascular filtration is self-regulating as predicted by Starling's Law of the Capillaries [eqn. (1)].

In the early 1960s Guyton and co-workers discovered that interstitial pressure was subatmospheric and, importantly, it increased by

Figure 2

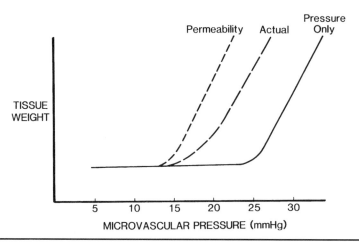

Plot of tissue weight (oedema formation) as a function of
microvascular pressure for normal tissues (Pressure Only),
decreased plasma proteins or increased vascular permeability
(Permeability) and actual lymph flow when tissues are damaged and
lymph flow becomes large due to oedema-dependent lymph factors
(Actual)

5–10 mmHg during oedema formation [20]. Guyton used the new
concept of a dynamic tissue pressure to define an 'oedema safety factor'.
This parameter defined all factors in an organ that could respond to
increased transvascular filtration by changing in a direction to oppose
the formation of oedema. These factors are increases in lymph flow,
tissue fluid pressure and the protein osmotic gradient acting across the
microvascular wall [21].

The reason that oedema did not develop until microvascular
pressures became high, which are depicted for normal tissues as 'pressure
only' in Figure 2, is that the oedema safety factors can change by
20–30 mmHg before oedema develops. We had originally thought that
the safety factors in damaged microvessels would respond in a manner
similar to decreasing plasma proteins, which is shown as 'permeability' in
Figure 2. The logic we used was that decreasing plasma protein levels
caused $(\pi_p - \pi_t)$ to decrease and consequently produced a smaller plasma
protein osmotic safety factor. When the microvascular exchange vessels
are damaged, the $(\pi_p - \pi_t)$ is less because π_t is higher, but in addition it
is not fully expressed because the actual plasma osmotic pressure must
be multiplied by a factor which describes the selectivity of the microvascular exchange vessels to plasma proteins. This factor is the reflection coefficient for the plasma proteins at the microvessel wall. For
normal microvessels, this factor is approximately 1; however, when the
microvessels are damaged, the factor can be reduced to values as low as
0.3–0.4.

We now know, however, that damage to microvascular walls and
plasma protein dilution with isotonic solutions results in very large
lymph flows and these conditions will produce a curve more similar to
that shown in Figure 2 as 'actual'. Thus, in conditions associated with

damage to microvessels, oedema does begin to accumulate at lower pressures, but the high lymph flow removes greater amounts of transmicrovascular filtration and less oedema develops for a given microvascular pressure [21].

Since Guyton's definition of the oedema safety factors, several studies have been conducted in different organs using this concept. Some of these studies are presented in Table 2 which shows the percentage change in each safety factor as microvascular pressure was changed by 20 mmHg in several different tissues [22]. Note that the transvascular protein osmotic pressure is the major factor opposing oedema in organs with low permeability to plasma proteins, such as lung, small intestine and colon; but this factor is unimportant when the tissue protein concentration is low, which occurs in hind paw, or in the tissues that are very permeable to plasma proteins such as heart and liver.

Interestingly, tissues in which the transvascular protein osmotic pressure cannot substantially change rely on lymph flow and tissue pressure increases to oppose oedema formation. The lymph flow factor is highest in liver, and the increased tissue pressure is the major safety factor opposing oedema development in heart, liver and hind paw. It is important to realize that the oedema safety factor explains how an excessive build up of tissue fluid is prevented under conditions that occur from moment to moment in normally functioning tissues, but different forces are responsible for opposing oedema formation in different tissues [22].

Lymphatic safety factor when microvascular walls are damaged

The discussion presented above shows very convincing data indicating that the lymph flow factor is an important safety factor against oedema formation in some organs. However, over the years it has become quite clear that lymph flow could increase to astronomical levels under certain experimental conditions. For example, lymph flows become higher

Tissue	Increased $(\pi_p - \pi_t)$ (%)	Increased lymph flow (%)	Increased P_t (%)	Table 2
Lung	50	17	33	
Hind paw	14	24	62	
Small intestine	45	20	35	
Colon	52	4	44	
Liver	0	42	58	
Heart	7	12	81	

Safety factors in various tissues
Modified from [38] with permission. $\pi_p - \pi_T$ is the absorptive force and P_t is the tissue fluid pressure. The values are shown as percentages of the total safety factor measured when capillary pressure was increased 20 mmHg above control values.

following large vascular expansions with isotonic saline [1], the initial effect on lymph flow of increased microvascular pressure [9], and when microvascular barriers are damaged. This led our group to develop the concept of 'oedema-dependent lymphatic factors' to describe the phenomenon associated with producing these high lymph flows [10].

The importance of this phenomenon can be better appreciated by calculating how these large lymph flows reduce the amount of fluid accumulating in the tissues, since the result produces a more efficient blood–tissue oxygen-exchange barrier because the diffusion distance between blood exchange vessels and tissue cells is decreased. In addition the increased lymph flow will also provide an overflow system that produces a larger plasma volume at a smaller extracellular volume, i.e. the

Figure 3

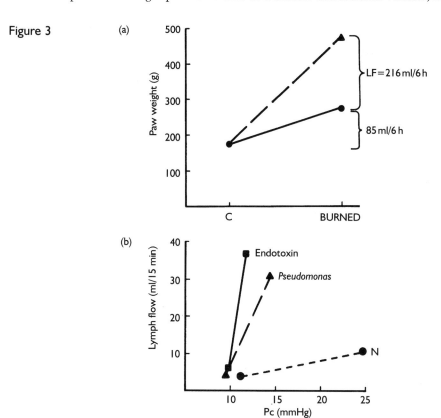

Effects of (a) damaged tissue on lymph flow and paw weight in a dog, and (b) sepsis on lymph flow in sheep (compared with only increasing microvascular pressure)

(a) C refers to inital weight following increasing venous pressure to 50 mmHg. The solid line shows how much oedema actually formed after a burn injury and the broken line shows how much oedema would have formed if lymph flow had not increased to such high levels. This occurred because lymph flow increased by an additional 216 ml/6 h. (b) Effect of sepsis on lymph flow as compared with only increasing microvascular pressure. Reproduced from [10] with permission. Data from Dyess et al. [24] and Brigham et al. [25].

lymphatic system simply returns more microvascular filtrate back into the circulation, decreasing oedema formation and plasma volume loss.

Figure 3(a) shows oedema formation in a dog hind-paw preparation that was subjected to a scald burn. In this study venous outflow pressure was increased to 50 mmHg to obtain the maximal lymph flow that normally occurs in this tissue when microvascular pressures are increased. The maximal lymph flow that occurred with this increased microvascular pressure averaged 90 ml/6 h and the organ weight was 180 g (solid line). Following burn injury to the paw, the lymph flow increased by 216 ml/6 h, but the paw weight only increased by 85 g although the microvascular walls were severely damaged, as shown by the solid line. Without this large increase in lymph flow the amount of oedema formed would have been 216 ml greater, as shown by the upper broken line in the Figure! [24].

Why did this large increase in lymph flow occur? At first, we had thought that microvascular pressure increased; but that should not cause an increased lymph flow above that produced by the high venous pressure. Figure 3(b) shows how damaged microvascular walls alter lymph flow from a sheep lung challenged with sepsis. Shown on this Figure are lymph flows obtained from sheep lungs in the presence of endotoxin and *Pseudomonas* sp., both of which severely damage the microvessel walls of the lung in this experimental preparation [25]. These lymph flows are compared with those in normal lungs when microvascular pressure was increased in steps (lower broken line). Note that lymph flow increased 8–10-fold with sepsis, but only 2-fold when pressure was increased to 25 mmHg in normal lungs. From these results it is clear that lymph flow can increase to very high levels in organs with damaged microvascular walls although microvascular pressures were not significantly affected by sepsis. Also, recall Chen *et al.*'s study (Figure 1) in which lymph flow increased to higher levels when venous pressure was elevated then was maintained at each new steady state. Thus lymph flow is not usually maximized. What causes these large increases in lymph flow? Why does lymph flow not function at these levels in organs at all times to prevent oedema from occurring?

Oedema-dependent lymph factors

There is absolutely no doubt that damage to microvascular endothelial barriers results in large lymph flows in many organs. As increases in microvascular pressures can be ruled out as the causative factor, then this phenomenon must reflect either a change in the pumping capability of the lymphatic system, or an enhancement of lymphatic filling [10]. Figure 4 shows schematically the various factors that could be the mechanism responsible for producing the large lymph flows occurring in damaged tissues.

The lymphatics could fill more easily if the tissue resistance decreases as tissues swell (shown as $R_T\downarrow$). If tissue compliance decreases ($C_T\uparrow$) then tissue pressure would not increase to levels which compress these initial lymphatic vessels and prevent the gradient for lymphatic filling from attaining a constant value because of a waterfall-type effect,

Figure 4

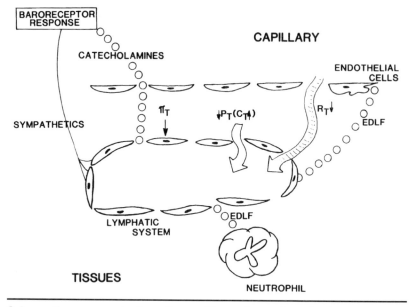

**Schematic representation of a capillary–tissue–lymphatic system
showing various mechanisms that could cause large lymph flows in
damaged tissues**
*Reproduced from [11] with permission. Abbreviation: EDLF, oedema-dependent
lymph factor.*

i.e. intralymphatic pressure increases to the same extent as tissue
pressure and filling pressure is maximized.

In addition the lymphatics are innervated and respond to
hormonal factors and various endothelial factors that are activated or
released when damaged. The most plausible hypothesis to explain these
huge lymph flows is that some substance(s) is released by the damaged
endothelial cell or other tissue cells, such as neutrophils and macrophages, which increases the pumping capability of the entire lymphatic
system (shown as an oedema-dependent lymph factor). In fact, Smith
[11] has data indicating that increased plasma proteins increase
lymphatic pumping capabilities.

Table 3 shows the effects of various vasoactive compounds on
isolated lymphatic vessels. We have not indicated the species or lymphatic vessel type, but the interested reader can refer to the cited papers
for additional information, since species and different lymphatics can
respond differently to these substances. Table 3 is presented here in
order to emphasize the number of compounds that can affect the rate
and force of lymphatic contraction [26–36]. Many compounds increase
both rate and force of contraction and if these are released by either
endothelial or tissue cells they will increase lymph flow. There is no
doubt that many of these substances are released in damaged tissue.

When the lymphatic vessels are preconstricted, many compounds
cause them to relax, which is simular to the behaviour of vascular
smooth muscle in the circulations of many organs. This indicates that
lymphatic vessels have a Ying and Yang system which modulates their

Substance	Rate	Force	Table 3
Isolated lymphatics normal tone	I	I	
Distension [28,35]	I	I	
Bradykinin [30]	I	I	
Noradrenaline [26]	I	I	
Prostaglandin $F_{2\alpha}$	I	I	
Prostaglandins I_2 and E_2 [29]	—	D	
5-Hydroxytryptamine–histamine [29]	I	I	
Histamine (low doses HI) [31]	I	I	
Acetylcholine [27]	D	D	
Removal of endothelium [27,28]	—	—	
Isolated lymphatics precontracted			
Atrial natriuretic peptide [32]	D	D	
Vasoactive intestinal peptide [34]	D	D	
Isoprenaline [33]	D	D	
Histamine (H2) [31]	D	D	
Adenosine [29]	—	D	
Nitroprusside [29]	—	D	
Acetylcholine (atropine, NO inhibitors and removal of endothelium blocks) [29]	—	D	

Effects of various vasoactive substances on rate and force of contractions on isolated lymphatic vessels [29]
I, D, and — refer to increase, decrease and no change respectively.

tone and intrinsic pumping capabilities both in an up- and down-regulation pattern. An interesting case in point is the apparent differences seen between acetylcholine's effects on normal and toned lymphatic vessels. This same effect is seen in the pulmonary circulation of rats relative to the release of nitric oxide by acetylcholine. When acetylcholine is placed into the circulation of normal rat lungs perfused with a plasma–saline solution, blood vessel dilation does not occur. However, if the lung's circulation is toned, say with thromboxane, then acetylcholine will cause an endothelial-dependent blood vessel relaxation that can be blocked by nitric oxide inhibitors [37]. This indicates that low-pressure systems such as the lung and lymphatics do not have a sufficient wall stress to cause nitric oxide release by endothelial cells. This effect may explain why lymphatic vessels dilate with acetylcholine, but removal of endothelial cells does not affect lymphatic contractility or rate in vivo.

Obviously, lymph flow from an organ can be modulated by many compounds, but we do not presently understand which compound(s) prevents the lymphatic system from attaining its maximal flow rate. Our aim in this chapter was to stimulate more research in this area, since the data clearly indicate that lymph flow can obtain astronomical levels in some experimental conditions. An understanding of the mechanisms that regulate lymph flow will provide new insight into the development of new therapies to use in various forms of tissue damage to lessen the degree of tissue oedema and provide a more stable plasma volume and better tissue oxygenation.

References

1. Taylor, A.E., Gibson, H., Granger, H.J., et al. (1973) The interaction between intracapillary forces in the overall regulation of interstitial volume. Lymphology 6, 192–208
2. Hall, J.G., Morris, B. and Woolley, G. (1965) Intrinsic rhythmic propulsion of lymph in the unanesthetized sheep. J. Physiol. (London) 180, 336–349
3. McHale, N.G. and Roddie, I.C. (1976) The effect of transmural pressure on pumping activity in isolated bovine lymphatic vessels. J. Physiol. (London) 261, 255–269
4. Ohhashi, T., Azuma, T. and Sakaguchi, M. (1980) Active and passive mechanical characteristics of bovine mesenteric lymphatics. Am. J. Physiol. 239, H88–H95
5. White, J.C., Field, M.E. and Drinker, C.K. (1933) On the protein content and normal flow of lymph from the foot of the dog. Am. J. Physiol. 103, 34–44
6. McMaster, P.D. (1937) Changes in the cutaneous lymphatics of human beings and in the lymph flow under normal and pathological conditions. J. Exp. Med. 65, 347–372
7. Courtice, F.C. and Morris, B. (1953) The effect of diaphragmatic movement on the absorption of protein and of red cells from the pleural cavity. Aust. J. Exp. Biol. Med. Sci. 31, 227–238
8. Morris, B. (1953) The effect of diaphragmatic movement on the absorption of protein and of red cells from the peritoneal cavity. Aust. J. Exp. Biol. Med. Sci. 31, 239–246
9. Chen, H.I., Granger, H.J. and Taylor, A.E. (1991) Lymph flow transients following elevation of venous pressure in the dog hindpaw. Lymphology 24, 155–160
10. Taylor, A.E. (1991) The lymphatic edema safety factor: the role of edema dependent lymphatic factors (EDLF). Lymphology 23, 111–123
11. Smith, C.-S. and Taylor, A.E. (1991) Increased initial lymphatic uptake in high-flow high-protein oedema: an additional safety factor against tissue oedema. Lymphology 24, 2–6
12. Starling, E.H. (1886) On the absorption of the fluids from the connective tissue spaces. J. Physiol. (London) 19, 312–316
13. Heidenhain, R. (1894) Neue Versuche Uber die Anfsaugung im Dunndarm. Arch. Ges. Physiol. 56, 579–631
14. Taylor, A.E. (1981) Starling forces. Circ. Res. 49, 557–575
15. Landis, E.M. (1927) Microinjection studies of capillary permeability. II. The relationship between capillary pressure and the rate at which fluid passes through the walls of single capillaries. Am. J. Physiol. 82, 217–238
16. Landis, E.M. (1934) Capillary pressure and capillary permeability. Physiol. Rev. 14, 404–481
17. Yoffey, J.M. and Courtice, F.C. (1970) Lymphatics, Lymph and the Lymphomyeloid Complex, 3rd edn., Academic Press, London
18. Rusznyak, I., Foldi, M. and Szabo, G. (1967) Lymphatics and Lymph Circulation, 2nd edn., Pergamon Press, Oxford
19. Guyton, A.C. and Lindsey, A.W. (1959) Effect of elevated left atrial pressure and decreased plasma protein pressure concentration on the development of pulmonary edema. Circ. Res. 649–657
20. Guyton, A.C., Taylor, A.E. and Granger, H.J. (1975) Circulatory Physiology II. Dynamics and Control of Body Fluids, W.B. Saunders, Philadelphia, PA
21. Guyton, A.C. and Coleman, T.G. (1968) Regulation of interstitial fluid volume and pressure. Ann. N. Y. Acad. Sci. 150, 537–547
22. Aukland, K. and Nicolaysen, G. (1981) Interstitial fluid volume: local regulating mechanisms. Physiol. Rev. 61, 556–583
23. Nicoll, P.A. and Taylor, A.E. (1977) Lymph formation and flow. Annu. Rev. Physiol. 39, 73–92
24. Dyess, D.L., Ardell, J.L., Townsley, M.I., Taylor, A.E. and Ferrara, J.J. (1992) Effects of hypertonic saline and dextran-70 resuscitation on microvascular permeability after burn. Am. J. Physiol. 262, H1832–H1837
25. Brigham, K., Woolverton, W., Blake, L., et al. (1974) Increased lung vascular permeability caused by pseudomonas bacteremia. J. Clin. Invest. 54, 792–804
26. Ohhashi, T. and Azume, T. (1984) Varied effects of prostaglandins on spontaneous activity in bovine mesenteric lymphatics. Microvasc. Res. 27, 71–80
27. Yokoyama, S. and Ohhashi, T. (1993) Effects of acetylcholine on spontaneous contractions in isolated bovine mesenteric lymphatics. Am. J. Physiol. 264, H1460–H1464
28. Hanley, C.A., Ellas, R.M. and Johnston, M.G. (1992) Is endothelium necessary for transmural pressure-induced contractions of bovine truncal lymphatics? Microvasc. Res. 43, 134–146
29. Ohhashi, T. (1993) Mechanisms for regulating tone in lymphatic vessels. Biochem. Pharmacol. 45, 1941–1945
30. Azuma, T., Ohhashi, T. and Roddie, I.C. (1983) Bradykinin-induced contractions of bovine mesenteric lymphatics. J. Physiol. (London) 342, 217–227
31. Watanabe, N., Kawai, Y. and Ohhashi, T. (1988) Dual effects of histamine on spontaneous activity in isolated bovine mesenteric lymphatics. Microvasc. Res. 36, 239–249
32. Ohhashi, T., Watanabe, N. and Kawai, Y. (1990) Effects of atrial natriuretic peptide on isolated

bovine lymph vessels. *Am. J. Physiol.* **259**, H42–H47

33. Ohhashi, T., Kawai, Y. and Azume, T. (1978) The response of lymphatic smooth muscles to vasoactive substances. *Pfluegers Arch.* **375**, 183–188

34. Ohhashi, T., Olschowka, J.A. and Jacobowitz, D.M. (1983) Vasoactive intestinal peptide inhibitory innervation in bovine mesenteric lymphatics. *Circ. Res.* **53**, 535–538

35. Ohhashi, T. and Roddie, I.C. (1981) Relaxation of bovine mesenteric lymphatics in response to transmural stimulation. *Am. J. Physiol.* **240**, H498–H504

36. Ohhashi, T. (1987) Regulation of motility of small collecting lymphatics. In *Advances in Microcirculation* (Staub, N.C., Hogg, J.C. and Hargens, A.R., eds.), pp. 171–183, Karger, Basel, Switzerland

37. Wilson, P.S., Barnard, J.W., Ward, R.A., Thompson, W.J. and Taylor, A.E. (1992) Nitric oxide release attenuates thromboxane-mediated increased vascular and airway resistance in rat lungs. *Circulation* **86**, I604

38. Taylor, A.E. (1991) *Encyclopedia of Human Biology*, p. 35, Academic Press, New York

5

A study of compressive properties of cartilage using unconfined compression: example of an experimental and theoretical approach

Alice Maroudas*, Joseph Mizrahi and Eric Benaim
Julius Silver Institute of Biomedical Engineering Sciences, Department of Biomedical Engineering, Technion, Israel Institute of Technology, Haifa 32000, Israel

Introduction

Cartilaginous tissues such as articular cartilage and the intervertebral disc are called upon to function under very high compressive loads. They can do this owing to the special properties of the matrix and in particular to the interplay between its three major components, i.e. proteoglycans (PGs), collagen and water.

Articular cartilage is an avascular tissue, with a very low cell density. The cell population in human articular cartilage occupies less than 1% of the total tissue volume. Water containing dissolved solutes accounts for 65–85% of the tissue volume, depending on age and location. Collagen constitutes about 70% of the dry weight, PG about 20% and other proteins and electrolytes the remaining 10%. The collagen fibrils form a network capable of resisting tension but not compression. These fibrils are embedded in an aqueous concentrated PG solution. The PGs are flexible polyelectrolytes of high fixed charge density (FCD) which endow the tissue with a high osmotic pressure and a low hydraulic permeability, enabling the tissue to remain hydrated in the face of high applied pressures. The collagen mesh with its high tensile strength resists swelling, thus making it possible for the PG–water mixture to exist as a concentrated solution.

When an external compressive stress is applied to cartilage the tissue deforms and two effects result: (1) the rearrangement of the polymer network, which leads to a change in the shape of the specimen at constant volume; and (2) creep associated with the loss of fluid from the matrix, which causes a decrease in the total volume of the tissue and hence a closer packing of the solid constituents. Effect 1 is thought to be associated with the very rapid bulk movement of the PG–water gel, which is resisted by the collagen fibre network [1]. Effect 2 is much slower than effect 1 since it involves the movement of fluid relative to the very fine pores formed by the PG molecules. In this chapter we will concern ourselves with both of these effects. In particular, we shall show how it is possible to relate cartilage creep to fluid flow, which in turn

*To whom correspondence should be addressed.

can be quantitatively described in terms of the hydraulic permeability and the osmotic pressure of the matrix. Our approach is based on a two-compartment model of the cartilage matrix with which we shall deal first.

Two-compartment model of cartilage

A schematic view of the matrix of a cartilaginous tissue is shown in Figure 1: because of their size the PGs cannot penetrate into the intrafibrillar (IF) space. The matrix thus consists of two compartments: the space within the collagen fibrils, from which the PGs are excluded, and the extrafibrillar (EF) space, the properties of which are determined chiefly by the presence of the PGs. At physiological pH the IF compartment has no effective charge while the EF compartment has a high concentration of negatively charged groups.

The IF compartment contains a small quantity of 'bound' water, the rest consisting of 'free' water (the quantity of which is controlled

Figure I

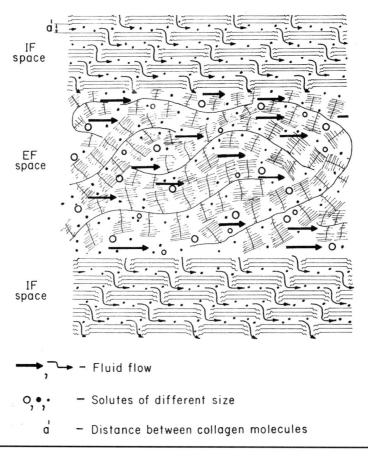

IF space

EF space

IF space

$\longrightarrow$ $\rightsquigarrow$ – Fluid flow

$O, \bullet, \cdot$ – Solutes of different size

d' – Distance between collagen molecules

Schematic representation of the two-compartment model of the cartilage matrix

partly by the intermolecular repulsion forces, the precise nature of which is at present not clear, and partly by the osmotic pressure gradients between the outside and the inside of the fibril) [2,3].

It is an oversimplification to consider the matrix as consisting of only two compartments, as clearly other heterogeneities exist. However, at present not enough information is available to take into account differences within the EF compartment with regard to the PG concentration.

In order to characterize the EF compartment, particularly in relation to its polyelectrolyte behaviour, the concentration of the PGs and their FCD must be expressed on the basis of the EF water alone (this will be referred to as the 'effective value') rather than on the total tissue water (often referred to as the 'overall value'). It should be noted that if the concentration of the PG is based on total water in the tissue it will be underestimated, while if its effective value is used the properties of the matrix such as osmotic pressure can be deduced directly from the properties of solutions of isolated PG at the same concentration.

If one wishes to calculate the fraction of EF water corresponding to a given set of conditions, the fraction of IF water must be known. It has been shown recently that the latter is not a constant, but itself varies.

Maroudas *et al.* [3] have shown, using X-ray diffraction data, that the intercollagen spacing in cartilage is regulated by the magnitude of the pressure gradient existing between the outside and the inside of the fibril; thus the ratio of IF water to dry collagen decreases with an increase in the osmotic pressure existing in the EF compartment and can be expressed as a unique function of the latter, that is:

$$\frac{\phi_{IF}}{\phi_{coll}} = f(\pi) \tag{1}$$

where ϕ_{IF} = volume fraction of the specimen representing IF water; ϕ_{coll} = volume fraction of collagen in the specimen, either initially or during compression; $f(\pi)$ has been determined empirically [3] for both human and bovine cartilage.

With regard to fluid flow, it is necessary to know not only the relative sizes of the EF and IF compartments, but also the dimensions of the component networks. Thus, the EF compartment can be pictured as a random assembly of very fine rods [glycosaminoglycans (GAG) and protein core] — diameter of the order of 0.5 nm — in which are embedded the very much thicker rods, namely the collagen fibrils (50–100 nm). Except when the PG concentration is very low, the main resistance to flow is offered by the 'thin' rods, the collagen fibrils acting more or less as a 'dead' volume. The actual flow of fluid and diffusion of solutes takes place through passages between the 'thin' rods. These passages or 'pores' are approximately 2–3 nm in radius (as determined by several methods — see Maroudas [4] and Byers *et al.* [5]).

It should be borne in mind that fluid exchange also takes place between the EF and IF compartments and that there is fluid flow through the IF compartment in parallel with that through the EF space, although at a very much lower rate [6–8].

Cartilage swelling pressure

It has been shown that the main factor responsible for resisting external compression, be it mechanical or osmotic, is the osmotic pressure of the PG within the cartilage [4,7–9]. When cartilage is not subjected to an externally applied pressure, the swelling tendency of the PG is exactly balanced by the elastic tension in the collagen network. The latter decreases very rapidly as soon as the tissue begins to shrink in volume. When the decrease in volume is equal to, or more than, approximately 5%, the collagen tension becomes negligible in relation to the osmotic pressure of the PG. Under such conditions, the swelling pressure of cartilage is equal to the osmotic pressure, π, of the PG constituent [10]. It should be noted that during weight-bearing, cartilage loses fluid and, as a result, the concentration of PG in the EF compartment increases, leading to a gradual increase in the swelling pressure.

Provided we know the pressure–concentration relationship for PG and the effective PG concentration in cartilage, based on the space which they actually occupy (i.e. on the EF compartment), we can predict the swelling pressure of the tissue for any degree of hydration. The osmotic pressure of the PGs extracted from cartilage has been studied both experimentally and theoretically ([11,12]; A. Maroudas, S. Erlich, K.H. Parker, C.P. Winlove and R. Schneiderman, unpublished work). The experimental determination of π has been based on equilibrium dialysis against polyethylene glycol solutions of known osmotic pressure [13–15]. Theoretical studies to predict the electrostatic component of the osmotic pressure were initially based on the Donnan model [11] which, however, consistently overestimated the osmotic pressure. More recently, Parker and colleagues (K.H. Parker, C.P. Winlove, A. Maroudas, R. Schneiderman and S. Erlich, unpublished work; see also [12]) have developed a theoretical treatment based on a rod-in-cell model, using the Poisson–Boltzmann equation. While this work was in progress a similar analysis was published by Buschmann and co-workers [16]. The analysis of Parker *et al.* applies to a wider range of conditions: the PGs are modelled as a mixture of two kinds of rods with different linear FCDs corresponding to keratan and chondroitin sulphates (KS and CS) and uncharged rods representing the protein. Addition of bivalent ions is also incorporated.

For PGs containing different proportions of KS to CS, both theory and experiment show, for a given FCD, an increase in π with an increasing KS to CS ratio. Addition of Ca^{2+} at physiological concentration depresses π by some 10% for both CS and PG solutions. In spite of the assumptions underlying the theory and the uncertainty in the choice of some of the basic parameters, the comparison between theory and experiment is very encouraging and can help in data interpretation. It should be noted that the theoretical model underestimates the osmotic pressure by an amount which is nearly independent of ionic strength. We suggest that this difference represents the non-ionic contributions to π. They account for 20–40% of the total π at physiological ionic strength, thus constituting a factor which cannot be altogether neglected.

We have shown experimentally, that the total osmotic pressure of PG solutions including both the electrostatic and the excluded-volume contributions can be expressed by an equation of the form [11,15]:

$$\pi_{PG} = B\,(FCD)^2 \tag{2}$$

For cartilage PGs, B=26.6 at 4°C and 29.0 at 37°C [15]. If we assume that PG within the tissue obeys the same equation we have:

$$(\pi)_{cart} = B\,(FCD_{EF})^2 \tag{3}$$

where FCD_{EF} refers to the fixed charge density in the extrafibrillar compartment. Using this relationship, together with information on overall FCD, total hydration and the proportions of IF and EF water, we can estimate the osmotic pressure within the cartilage matrix at any stage of compression.

Hydraulic permeability

A second property of cartilage matrix which determines the rate of volume decrease during compression is the hydraulic permeability. As in the case of the swelling pressure, we have made an attempt to estimate theoretically the hydraulic permeability; the model we used is based on short lengths of polymer chains being oriented obliquely to flow [6,17].

It should be noted that in our case, the simplified geometrical model has to take into account the two matrix compartments; flow is assumed to take place in parallel through these compartments, each consisting of rod-like molecules (GAG and collagen, respectively) and each presenting its own resistance to flow depending on rod diameter and the fractional volume of solids [6].

We took the composition of cartilage by weight to be as follows [18]: collagen content = 16%; PG = 10% (GAG = 6%; protein = 4%) H_2O = 72%. The FCD corresponding to this composition is approximately 0.23 meq./g of tissue water. The corresponding fraction of IF water was taken as $1.1 \times$ collagen weight [19]. From these data we obtained the following values: fractional volume occupied by collagen and IF water is 0.33; fractional volume occupied by PG and EF water is 0.67. In the EF compartment the fractional volume of solids (PG) is 0.1. We took the mean radius of GAG chains to be 0.45 nm. The radius for the core protein was assumed to be the same for lack of better data.

For the IF compartment, the fractional volume of solids (collagen) is 0.4 and the rod radius (radius of collagen molecule) was taken as 0.62 nm.

The hydraulic permeability estimated from the above data was around 5×10^{-13} cm$^3 \cdot$s$\cdot$g^{-1} or 5×10^{-16} m$^4 \cdot$N$^{-1} \cdot$s^{-1} for fully hydrated tissue, reducing to about one-third of this value for a 30% reduction in tissue volume.

Compressive properties of cartilage: unconfined compression

Mechanical testing of articular cartilage in compression can be carried out by one of the following methods: indentation, confined compression or unconfined compression. Each of these methods has its own advantages and drawbacks. Testing the cartilage on the joint surface by indentation may be the closest to the physiological loading conditions. However, the results obtained are difficult to analyse and interpret. On the other hand, experiments involving compression of excised plugs of cartilage, while further removed from the physiological situation, can yield unambiguous data on the material properties of cartilage.

We have investigated cartilage plugs in unconfined compression [7,8,20,21] (J. Mizrahi, E. Benaim and A. Maroudas, unpublished work), as this method of testing can yield information on both volume change due to fluid loss and lateral shape change due to matrix deformation. On the basis of such measurements it is possible to analyse the deformation process and to attempt to clarify the respective roles of the collagen network and the PG–water solution in resisting the compressive stresses to which cartilage is subjected. We shall briefly describe our experimental and theoretical approaches.

Theoretical model

A basic assumption in our model is that collagen fibrils cannot transmit compressive stresses. The meaning of this assumption is that in the loading (vertical) direction, the contribution of the collagen network to load bearing decreases with increasing deformation: it becomes zero at a given deformation and remains zero at higher deformations. It should be noted that although from this stage on there is no tension in the vertical fibrils, the horizontal fibrils are under tensile forces. As the specimen creeps, it decreases in volume and changes it shape. The latter change is accompanied by a change in orientation of the fibrils in the collagen network.

The constitutive model of the collagen network introduces two parameters: the fibril stiffness (in tension) and a shape parameter. This latter parameter describes the ability of the collagen network to change the angle between the families of the collagen fibrils while under load. The two parameters can be obtained experimentally from the changes in the surface area of the specimen during compression.

The decrease in volume is due to fluid flow out of the loaded specimen: the rate of fluid loss obeys a modified Darcy equation in which the rate of flow is proportional to the permeability coefficient and the overall pressure gradient, the latter being the difference between the hydrostatic and the osmotic pressures. As the fluid loss proceeds, both the permeability coefficient and the pressure gradient decrease, the latter because of the increase in the osmotic pressure. A final stage will be reached at which the osmotic pressure becomes equal to the hydrostatic (i.e. the applied) pressure and flow will cease.

It should be noted that during flow the hydrostatic pressure profile depends on the deformation of the matrix in the radial direction and is not necessarily parabolic.

Experimental system and method

The experimental system we developed consisted of the following components: (i) loading apparatus, for applying a step-loading compression to the specimen; (ii) specimen cell — the top surface of the specimen was compressed against a transparent rigid plunger so that it could be observed throughout the creep phase; (iii) a microscope used to view the deforming top surface; to the microscope, a stills camera and a video camera were attached; (iv) a linear displacement transducer (LVDT) for measuring the thickness of the specimen; and (v) a computer, used to control the sequence of on-line data collection, to sample and to process the data obtained. A diagram of the apparatus is shown in Figure 2.

Cylindrical specimens of cartilage, about 5 mm in diameter, from human hip and knee joints obtained at autopsy were used. Each specimen was loaded for 24 h, during which period its dimensions were measured continuously. The dimensions measured included the diameters in directions parallel and perpendicular to the prick-line pattern of the top surface, the specimen thickness and the specimen profile.

In addition to the mechanical data, wet weight, dry weight and overall FCD, as well as the collagen content of each test specimen, were measured. Some of these measurements were made before and some after the mechanical tests.

Illustrative results
Diameter deformations

Diameter deformation as a function of time is shown in Figure 3. Two distinct phases characterized the deformation obtained: (i) the instantaneous phase, in which there is a marked change in shape, with no change in volume; and (ii) the creep phase, in which fluid is squeezed out of the specimen. In this phase, the volume decrease is characterized by a significant decrease in thickness, with a minor increase in the surface area of the specimen. The diameter deformation of the specimen is always bigger in a direction perpendicular to the prick-lines as

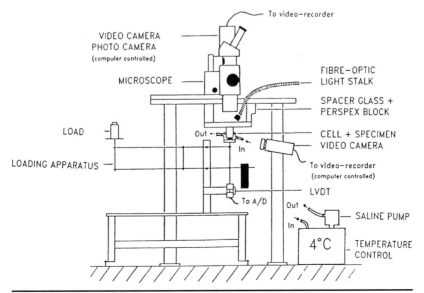

Figure 2

Diagram of the experimental set-up for the determination of mechanical parameters characterizing unconfined compression

Figure 3

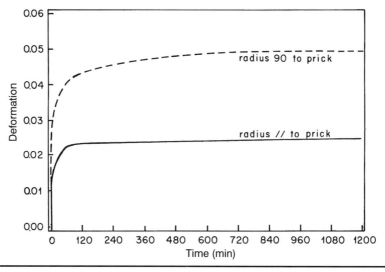

Radius deformation of the cartilage surface as a function of time

compared with the diameter deformation in a direction parallel to the prick-lines.

Creep — initial stages

Figure 4 shows the initial portion of a typical curve of creep versus time for an unconfined specimen of femoral head cartilage; the contribution of the constant volume bulk deformation (given by surface strain) has been subtracted, so that a net volume decrease due to fluid outflow can be calculated ([8]; J. Mizrahi, E. Benaim and A Maroudas, unpublished work). It can be seen that the rate of creep rapidly decreases with decrease in volume. This is due to both an increase in the osmotic pressure of the PG and a decrease in the hydraulic permeability, as predicted from the theoretical model.

Derivation of hydraulic permeability from creep measurements

Using Darcy's law, we were able to calculate the hydraulic permeability during the course of creep, from fluid flux and from a knowledge of the hydrostatic and the osmotic pressure gradients. Fluid flux is obtainable from volume measurements alone; osmotic pressure is determined from volume measurements, as well as from the overall FCD and the calculated effective FCD; the calculation of the hydrostatic pressure profile depends on the assumptions made. We have assumed (a) a parabolic pressure profile, and (b) a profile based on our model, incorporating the mechanical characteristics of the collagen network. The values of permeability thus obtained could be compared with those predicted, for different water contents, from the geometrical model (already described in this chapter). Figure 5 shows the curves of permeability calculated using our creep results and those estimated from the geometrical model. It can be seen that after a short initial period where considerable differences are observed, all three estimates yield similar values [21].

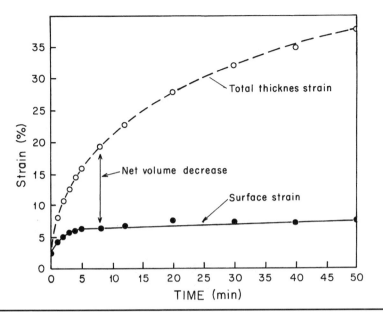

Figure 4

Typical graph of cartilage creep versus time for an applied pressure of 6 atm

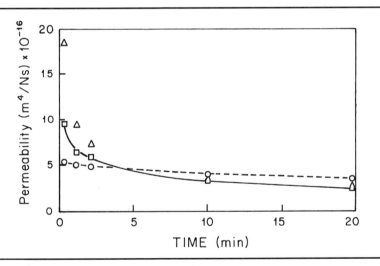

Figure 5

Variation of hydraulic permeability with time during the initial creep period
The hydraulic permeability was calculated from: ○, a geometrical model; △, creep measurements and Darcy's law using a parabolic pressure profile; and □, a pressure profile based on our theoretical model.

Comparison between applied pressure and osmotic pressure of the PGs at final equilibrium: physiological implications

In all experiments in which the mechanical loading pressure was higher than the initial osmotic pressure, the final values of the osmotic pressure,

Figure 6

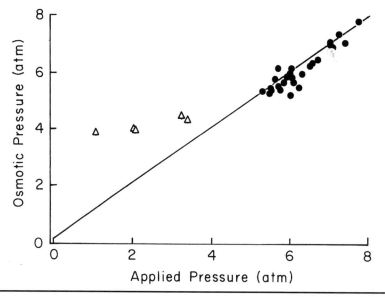

Comparison between applied and PG osmotic pressure at final equilibrium

$\triangle$, $P_{applied} > \pi$; $\bullet$, $P_{applied} < \pi$.

π, tended to coincide with the applied pressure, as shown in Figure 6. This indicates that in the final equilibrium state the applied pressure is resisted only by the osmotic pressure of the PG and that the collagen fibrils do not therefore take part in bearing the compressive load. Thus, one of the basic assumptions underlying our theoretical model is experimentally justified.

Knowing that in the final equilibrium state the compressive stress in the direction of load application is resisted only by the osmotic pressure in the EF compartment, we can estimate the amount of water which will remain in the latter compartment for any given applied stress. We also know how the hydration of the IF compartment varies with compression and we can, therefore, predict its water content for a given pressure [3]. Hence we can predict the total amount of water at final equilibrium for a given applied stress. For instance, for a pressure of 50 atm (5 MPa), corresponding to the physiological pressure range as assessed by modern measurements, we estimate that at equilibrium the amount of water retained within human femoral head cartilage will be equal to approximately 90% of its dry weight and the total volume of the tissue will be reduced by some 50% of its initial value.

It should be borne in mind, however, that *in vivo*, except if a person is standing still for a long time, equilibrium is rarely achieved. Hence, it is essential to be able to provide a description of what happens during the non-steady-state process, such as the creep phase of the deformation described above.

References

1. Weightman, B. and Kempson, G.E. (1979) Load carriage. In *Adult Articular Cartilage* (Freeman, M.A.R., ed.), 2nd edn., pp. 291–333, Pitman Medical, London
2. Katz, E.P., Wachtel, E.J. and Maroudas, A. (1986) Extrafibrillar proteoglycans osmotically regulate the molecular packing of collagen in cartilage. *Biochim. Biophys. Acta* **882**, 136–139
3. Maroudas, A., Wachtel, E., Grushko, G., Katz, E.P. and Weinberg, P.D. (1991) Osmotic and mechanical pressures in water partitioning in articular cartilage. *Biochim. Biophys. Acta* **1073**, 285–294
4. Maroudas, A. (1979) Physico-chemical properties of articular cartilage. In *Adult Articular Cartilage* (Freeman, M.A.R., ed.), pp. 215–290, Pitman Medical, London
5. Byers, P.D., Bayliss, M.T., Maroudas, A., Urban, J. and Weightman, B. (1983) Hypothesising about joints. In *Studies in Joint Disease* (Maroudas, A. and Holborow, J., eds.), vol. 2, pp. 241–276, Pitman Medical, London
6. Maroudas, A., Mizrahi, J., Ben Haim, E. and Ziv, I. (1987) Swelling pressure in cartilage. *Adv. Microcirc.* **13**, 203–212
7. Benaim, E. (1989) Biomechanical model for cartilage creep in compression. D.Sc. Thesis, Technion, Haifa, Israel
8. Benaim, E., Mizrahi, J. and Maroudas, A. (1990) Shape and volume changes in cartilage during creep in unconfined compression. *Trans. Orthop. Res. Soc.* **15**, 153
9. Grushko, G., Schneiderman, R. and Maroudas, A. (1989) Some biochemical and biophysical parameters for the study of the pathogenesis of osteoarthritis: a comparison between the processes of ageing and degeneration in human hip cartilage. *Connect. Tissue Res.* **19**, 149–176
10. Maroudas, A. and Bannon, C. (1981) Measurement of swelling pressure in cartilage and comparison with the osmotic pressure of constituent proteoglycans. *Biorheology* **18**, 619–632
11. Urban, J., Maroudas, A., Bayliss, M.T. and Dillon J. (1979) Swelling pressures of proteoglycans at the concentrations found in cartilaginous tissues. *Biorheology* **16**, 447–464
12. Maroudas, A., Erlich, S., Parker, K.H., Winlove, C.P., Johnston, P. and Schneiderman, R. (1995) *Trans. Orthopaedic Soc.* **20**, in the press
13. Erlih, S. (1995) MSc. Thesis, Technion, Haifa, Israael
14. Parsegian, V.A., Rand, R.P., Ruller, N.L. and Rau, D.C. (1986) Osmotic stress for the direct measurement of intermolecular forces. *Methods Enzymol.* **127**, 400–416
15. Maroudas, A. and Grushko, G. (1990) Measurement of swelling pressure of cartilage. In *Methods in Cartilage Research* (Maroudas, A. and Kuettner, K., eds.), pp. 298–301, Academic Press, London
16. Buschmann, M.D., Gluzband, Y.A., Grodzinsky, A.J., Kimura, J.H. and Hunziker, E.K. (1993) Proteoglycan-associated electrostatic forces and the development of functional mechanical properties in chondrocytes/agarose gel cultures. *Trans. Orthop. Res.* **18**, 74
17. Jackson, G.W. and James, D.F. (1982) The hydrodynamic resistance of hyaluronic acid and its contribution to tissue permeability. *Biorheology* **19**, 317–330
18. Maroudas, A., Bayliss, M.T. and Venn, M.F. (1980) Further studies on the composition of human femoral head cartilage. *Ann. Rheum. Dis.* **39**, 514–523
19. Wachtel, E., Maroudas, A. and Schneiderman, R. (1995) Age related changes in collagen packing in human articular cartilage. *Biochim. Biophys. Acta*, in the press
20. Mizrahi, J., Maroudas, A., Lanir, Y., Ziv, I. and Webber, T.J. (1986) The instantaneous deformation of cartilage: effects of collagen fiber orientation and osmotic stress. *J. Biorheol.* **23**, 311–330
21. Mizrahi, J., Maroudas, A. and Benaim, E. (1990) Unconfined compression for studying cartilage creep. In *Methods in Cartilage Research* (Maroudas, A. and Kuettner, K., eds.), pp. 293–298, Academic Press, London

compressive load altered the pattern of proteoglycans produced by the fibrocartilaginous region of bovine flexor tendon [47]; with no compressive load, cultured tendon explants produced mainly small proteoglycans, but after only 4 days of compressive loading, synthesis of large proteoglycans was induced.

The cells of cartilages also respond to *in vitro* loading, with the response depending on loading pattern. Static loading of articular cartilage explants (reviewed in [48,71]) and of chondrocytes cultured in agarose gels [72] invariably produces a decrease in matrix synthesis rates, the decrease being proportional to the applied load or compression. The response to cyclic loading, however, depends on frequency. While low-amplitude compressive strains do not affect synthesis in 3-mm-diam. explants subjected to unconfined compression at low frequencies (<0.001 Hz), synthesis is stimulated [49] at higher frequencies (>0.01 Hz) (Figure 3). Similar results were seen upon cyclic compression of chondrocytes in agarose gel culture [72]. Load affects the synthesis of other matrix macromolecules such as fibronectin [50], and can also affect matrix turnover and stability. Prolonged (12 h) static compression can retard the rate at which proteoglycans are able to form stable aggregates with hyaluranon [51]. Higher amplitude compressions can increase the rate at which matrix breakdown products are formed and released into the external medium [52]. After release from static loading, synthesis of small proteoglycans and link protein recovers within hours, but synthesis of the large aggregating proteoglycan aggrecan did not return to control values for 2–3 days [53].

Little work has been carried out on intervertebral disc explants, principally because of the difficulty of handling the tissue *in vitro*, since it swells and loses proteoglycans on exposure to aqueous solutions [54]. However, static loading of bovine coccygeal discs affected protein and proteoglycan synthesis rates. At low loads the discs were swollen and synthesis rates were low. Synthesis rates increased with increase in load and were at a maximum under loads which held the tissue near its *in vivo* level of hydration; furthermore, loading which expressed fluid

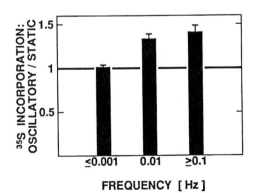

Figure 3

Effect of frequency on proteoglycan synthesis rates in articular cartilage explants
Data taken from [71].

decreased synthesis rates in a manner similar to that seen in articular cartilage [55].

Possible extracellular signals

From the results showing that the effect of load on matrix synthesis depends critically on load duration and magnitude, it has been apparent that cartilage cells respond not to mechanical stress as such, but to the compression-induced changes in deformation, hydrostatic pressure, fluid and ion content, and fluid flow (with associated streaming potentials) which occur in their immediate environment (Figure 4).

Under static loading, fluid is lost from the tissue and proteoglycan concentration increases, leading to an increase in extracellular cation concentrations and osmolality and a decrease in extracellular pH. These effects have been studied independently of changes in hydration by altering the ionic strength and pH of the medium in which disc or cartilage slices or isolated chondrocytes are suspended.

Figure 4

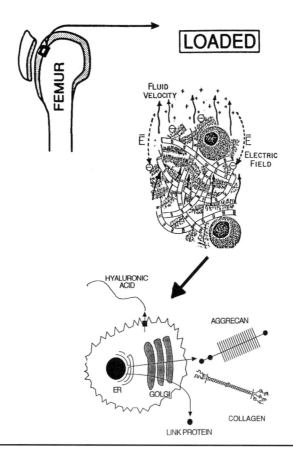

Schematic of fluid flow and streaming potential fields caused by dynamic compression of cartilage, which is known to regulate cell synthesis of matrix molecules including aggrecan, link protein, hyaluronan and collagen

Matrix synthesis rates in cartilage explants are very sensitive to pH, and decreased with decreasing pH below pH 6.9–7.0 [49,56]. Similar results were seen in the disc [57], although here the maximum synthesis rate was found at pH 7.0–7.1 rather than at pH 7.4. An increase in extracellular osmolality also induced a dose-dependent decrease in synthesis rates in cartilage explant, in isolated chondrocytes and in disc [54,59] (Figure 5). The fall in synthesis rates induced by increasing extracellular osmolality and reducing pH in this way is very similar to that resulting from fluid loss as the result of cartilage compression. It thus appears that the cells respond to changes in extracellular ion concentrations and osmolality rather than to changes in hydration as such.

Hydrostatic pressures of the orders seen in cartilage and disc can affect many cellular processes; for example, pressures of 5–15 MPa can cause a reduction in exocytosis, reduce RNA and protein synthesis, or affect the activity of the Na,K-ATPase [60]. It is thus not surprising that the changes in hydrostatic pressure seen on loading can also affect metabolism in cartilaginous tissues. In cartilage and disc, 20 s applications of hydrostatic pressures lead to an increase in the rate of sulphate and amino acid incorporation over the following 2 h [61,62]; the effective levels which stimulated synthesis were much higher in cartilage than in disc (7.5–15.0 MPa for cartilage explants [62,63] compared with 1.0–2.5 MPa for disc [61]). Isolated chondrocytes reacted to even lower levels of hydrostatic pressure [63]. Longer applications of the same levels of pressure reduced the stimulation seen, and synthesis could even be depressed after several hours of applied pressure [62,63]. These results suggest that hydrostatic pressure has at least two different effects on the synthetic pathway, one stimulatory and the other inhibitory, the net effect depending on the relative contribution of each pathway.

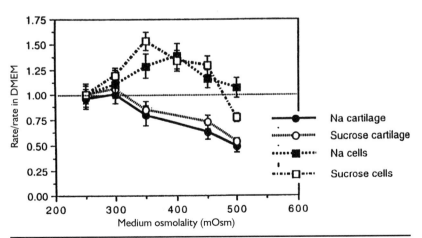

Figure 5

Effect of changing medium osmolality on sulphate incorporation rates

Rates are given relative to incorporation in standard tissue culture medium. (○,●) Cartilage explants; (□, ■) chondrocytes. DMEM, Dulbecco's modified Eagle's medium.

Fluid flow itself (Figure 4) has also been found to affect synthesis rates. When cartilage plugs were exposed to dynamic loads and the profile of synthetic activity was mapped across the plug cross-section, synthetic rates were found to be highest in regions experiencing the highest fluid flows [64]. Many other cells have been found to respond to fluid flow [65,66]. Fluid flow also induces streaming potentials (see below), and it is thus of interest to note that several investigators have found that protein and proteoglycan synthesis in cartilage and chondrocytes respond to imposed oscillating electrical fields [67,68].

Although some extracellular signals which influence mechano-transduction in cartilage cells are now understood, little work has been carried out on intracellular pathways. Some early work showed that exposure to hydrostatic pressure altered intracellular cyclic AMP and also caused influx of Ca^{2+} [69], but this work has so far not been extended. It will be of interest to see if the pathways induced by load in cartilage are similar to those mapped out for endothelial cells for instance [70].

Cartilage electromechanics: forces and flows in the ECM

During the past two decades, investigators have found that mechanical-to-electrical transduction interactions within the ECM play a significant role in the physiology and structure–function relationships of connective tissues. As described above, they may also play a role as mediators of cell metabolism. We therefore summarize some recent results in cartilaginous tissues with emphasis on forces and flows at the molecular level in the immediate environment of the cells.

When cartilage is compressed in a cyclic fashion, electric fields and their associated electrical potential differences are produced [73–75]. The mechanism for this response is now known to be a 'streaming' or electrokinetic effect: mechanical deformation of the cartilage matrix causes a flow of interstitial fluid and entrained counterions relative to the fixed charge groups of the matrix (Figure 4). Fluid convection of counterions tends to separate these ions from the oppositely charged macromolecules of the ECM, giving rise to a voltage gradient or 'streaming potential' [75,76]. This phenomenon was observed in a series of experiments [76,77] using cylindrical discs of adult bovine femoro-patellar groove cartilage that were compressed between two silver chloride electrodes in a uniaxial confined compression geometry. A small amplitude sinusoidal compression superimposed on a static offset compression produced a sinusoidal potential whose amplitude and phase varied with frequency in a manner that was consistent with an electro-kinetic mechanism [77]. (Mechanically generated streaming potentials have also been studied as an important phenomenon in bone [78–80].) Investigators have studied the possibility that streaming potentials are important signals that regulate cell metabolism in connective tissues [67,71,73,78–81]; however, it has been difficult experiment-ally to isolate the effect of streaming potentials from that of the associated fluid flow, since both physical phenomena are inextricably coupled.

The molecular constituents responsible for electrokinetic phenomena in cartilage have been studied by examining the dependence of compression-induced streaming potentials on bath pH and ionic strength [76]. At physiological pH, the proteoglycan molecules were found to be the predominant source of the potentials. Hence, the transduction response is seated in the ECM. Streaming potentials have been demonstrated in living cartilage [75,81].

More recently, a converse electrokinetic phenomenon has been observed in cartilage: current-generated stress [76]. Application of a sinusoidal electrical current to cartilage discs (e.g. in the one-dimensional geometry of Figure 6a) exerts an electrophoretic force on the negatively charged solid matrix and an opposite force on the positively charged interstitial fluid causing electro-osmotic fluid flow. [These mechanisms are analogous to gel electrophoresis, with the collagen network playing the role of acrylamide. Negatively charged proteoglycans tend to migrate downward in Figure 6(a). If constrained by collagen, a downward mechanical stress is generated; however, if proteoglycans are absent or disaggregated and mobile, the mechanical stress is lower or absent.] This combination of forces produces a deformation within the matrix and a mechanical stress that can be measured by a sensor at the tissue surface (Figure 6a). The stress amplitude and phase have been modelled successfully [77] by combining linear electrokinetic coupling laws with laws [82,83] that relate stress, strain and fluid flow in cartilage.

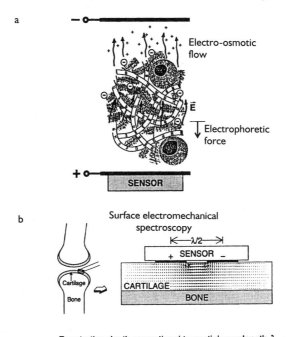

Figure 6

(a) Schematic of current-generated stress produced in cartilage by an applied current density and (b) the configuration of the surface probe for non-destructive measurement of cartilage electrokinetic properties (adapted from [88])

Cartilage degradation affects electrokinetic transduction

Since electrokinetic effects such as streaming potential and current-generated stress are directly proportional to proteoglycan charge density, the early loss of proteoglycans in diseases such as osteoarthritis could be detectable by such measurements. This hypothesis was tested by Hoch et al. [84], who compared early biochemical, mechanical and electromechanical changes in the knee joint cartilage of ambulating rabbits as a function of time after surgical removal of the left medial meniscus, a well-established surgical model for osteoarthritis-like cartilage degradation [85]. Hoch et al. [84] consistently found early, focal loss of proteoglycan in the medial tibial plateau cartilage, and an associated decrease in the streaming potential measured from cartilage plugs removed from the same joint surface. In an *in vitro* model for cartilage degradation, Frank et al. [86] found that enzymic extraction of proteoglycan from discs of adult bovine cartilage resulted in a decrease in dynamic stiffness and a significantly greater relative reduction in streaming potential. Thus, electrokinetic measurements were found to provide a more sensitive indicator of molecular-level cartilage degeneration than purely mechanical tests.

Surface detection of cartilage degeneration via electromechanical spectroscopy

Previous measurements of current-generated stress and streaming potential utilized a uniaxial configuration, in which it was necessary to access two opposite surfaces of an excised cartilage disc (e.g. Figure 6a). Theoretical analysis [87], however, suggested that a spatially periodic standing wave of current applied to the articular surface of cartilage could also produce a bulk mechanical stress, measurable at the surface. Figure 6(b) illustrates a configuration in which current-generated stress induced and measured at the tissue surface may be used as a diagnostic for early cartilage degeneration, potentially useful in arthroscopic applications [88]. A small current is applied to the cartilage surface using silver chloride electrodes; the spacing between electrodes (about 2.5 mm for the device of Figure 6b) defines the half-spatial wavelength of the applied current density. Since this current can be applied at different frequencies, both wavelength and frequency can be independently specified. The use of this variable-frequency wavelength or 'modal' approach [89] has been motivated in part by recent advances in interdigitated electrode sensor technology and materials characterization. In classical dielectric spectroscopy, for example, dielectric measurements made over a wide frequency range are used to infer properties about a homogeneous medium placed between two electrodes. It has now been found that surface excitations, applied by an interdigitated electrode structure with an imposed spatial wavelength (determined by the electrode geometry) and temporal frequency, can also yield information about bulk material properties of dielectric materials [90]. The use of this approach for measuring electrokinetic properties of connective tissues has been called electromechanical spectroscopy [88].

The three-dimensional current-generated stress distribution within the bulk of the tissue in Figure 6(b) is complex, but is related to that of the current density. The normal stress at the cartilage surface has the same spatial periodicity as the current excitation but is out of phase in time [87]. A description of the spatial distribution of matrix displacement, fluid velocity, hydrostatic pressure, and electric and stress fields produced by an idealized spatially sinusoidal current applied to the surface of an idealized charged, isotropic, homogeneous layer of cartilage is given in [87].

The surface spectroscopic approach, with variable imposed spatial wavelength and temporal frequency, offers several distinct advantages in characterizing the properties of normal and degraded tissue in intact joints. First, surface electrodes may be used to make measurements on cartilage non-destructively. Secondly, the technique introduces micro-structural spatial sensitivity into such measurements. When electrode spacing is very small, the resulting current density has a very short wavelength (λ), and the amplitude of the applied current will decay within a short distance ($\leq \lambda/3$) from the electrodes into the bulk tissue. Therefore, the current-generated stress response will reveal the quality (e.g. proteoglycan content) of the superficial cartilage layer. Longer wavelength excitations will generate fields that penetrate further into the medium, and can therefore probe the quality of cartilage in the deeper zones. Hence, this approach is capable of resolving differences between surface properties and those deeper within the tissue, and of probing spatial non-uniformities in the bulk.

Connective-tissue electromechanics: porous media theory

The application of porous media theories to describe streaming potentials in hydrated media appears to have begun in the area of soil mechanics. Frenkel [91] studied 'seismoelectric potentials' associated with the propagation of longitudinal waves in moist soil. He used electrokinetic theory associated with quasistatic Poiseuille flow in charged, cylindrical capillaries to model the induced potentials. Biot [92] found that electrokinetic coupling to acoustic waves contributed to the dissipation of acoustic energy in soils. Chandler [93] measured and modelled streaming potentials in fluid-saturated porous rock in response to acoustic stimuli. Frank and Grodzinsky [77] derived a poroelastic model for electrokinetic transduction in cartilage that combines linear electrokinetic coupling laws with poroelastic [82,83] material laws (A similar approach was also used [94] to model stress-generated potentials in cortical bone.) This poroelastic–electrokinetic model was recently extended [87] for the case of variable-frequency-wavelength excitation via surface electrodes as in Figure 6(b). Lai et al. [95] incorporated electrochemical tissue behaviour into their mixture theory for cartilage biomechanics. All the above models have been limited to the case of isotropic, homogeneous media.

Electromechanical spectroscopy of chemically modified cartilage

A hallmark of degenerated cartilage (e.g. in osteoarthritis) is the loss of the highly charged proteoglycans which are the source of the high fixed-charge density and associated electromechanical and physico-chemical properties of the tissue under physiological conditions. To evaluate the sensitivity of the spectroscopic approach of Figure 6(b) in detecting changes in charge density within cartilage tissue, we measured the current-generated stress response of cartilage discs before, during and after the cartilage was subjected to controlled chemical modifications. Previously, the effects of altered bath pH on the electrokinetic transduction response of cartilage was characterized in uniaxial confined compression [86]. Lowering bath pH neutralizes the negative fixed-charge groups (sulphate and carboxyl groups) of cartilage, and thereby decreases the amplitude of streaming potential and current-generated stress response.

Figure 7 shows the dependence of current-generated stress on bath pH measured by the spectroscopic surface probe of Figure 6(b) [88]. At each frequency, the amplitude of the measured current-generated stress has been normalized to that at approx. pH 7. For clarity, data from a single cartilage disc is shown; the normalized responses for all five discs tested were qualitatively similar. As the bath pH was lowered from its initial value of pH 7, the stress amplitude decreased markedly, reaching a minimum at a value that varied monotonically with frequency but was always in the pH range 2.4–2.8 (Figure 7a). As the pH was lowered beyond this point, the stress amplitude increased, while the phase angle underwent an abrupt 180° transition (Figure 7b), indicating that the direction of the current-generated stress had reversed. These results suggest that the isoelectric

Figure 7

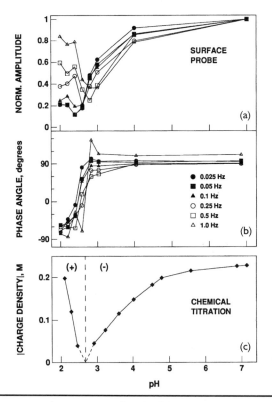

Current-generated stress amplitude (a) and phase (b) measured in adult bovine cartilage versus bath pH (from [88]), and (c) magnitude of the fixed-charge density of adult bovine cartilage measured by chemical titration (from [96])

pH, the pH value at which the tissue is electrically neutral, was in the pH range 2.4–2.8 for each disc. Independent determination of the fixed-charge density of specimens of adult bovine femoropatellar cartilage by means of chemical titration as a function of bath pH [96], shown in Figure 7(c), confirmed that the isoelectric pH lies within this pH range. (Direct chemical measurement showed that changing bath pH in these experiments did not result in loss of proteoglycan constituents [88], but only a change in their net charge.) It is seen from Figure 7 that the amplitude of the current generated measured by the surface probe changed with pH in a manner markedly similar to that produced by direct pH alteration of cartilage charge density, showing the sensitivity of electrokinetic transduction to the molecular-level charge associated with matrix proteoglycans.

Conclusions

Articular cartilage and the intervertebral disc both carry high compressive loads and are essential in the functioning of joints in the musculoskeletal system. However, they have different roles, in that articular cartilage acts as a stiff, low-friction surface to the bones, while the intervertebral discs link the vertebral bodies and provide flexibility to the spinal column. Though their composition is similar, their structural organization is very different and relates to their different functional roles. The cells of both tissues respond to mechanical stimuli, but how mechanical signals result in the production and maintenance of an appropriate extracellular matrix is still unknown.

Support for this research was provided by grants from the Arthritis and Rheumatism Council U0501 (J.P.G.U.), NIH Grant AR33236, NSF Grant BCS-9111401, and VA Grant V525P-1743 (A.J.G.).

References

1. Heinegard, D. and Oldberg, A. (1989) Structure and biology of cartilage and bone matrix non-collagenous macromolecules. *FASEB J.* **3**, 2042–2051
2. Broom, N. and Marra, D. (1985) New structural concepts of articular cartilage demonstrated with a physical model. *Connect. Tissue Res.* **14**, 1–8
3. Maroudas, A. (1979) Physico-chemical properties of articular cartilage. In: *Adult Articular Cartilage* (Freeman, M., ed.), pp. 215–290, Pitman Medical, London
4. Grodzinsky, A.J. (1983) Electromechanical and physicochemical properties of connective tissue. *CRC Crit. Rev. Bioeng.* **9**, 133–199
5. Eyre, D.R., Apone, S., Wu, J.-J., Ericsson, L.H. and Walsh, K.A. (1987) Collagen type IX, evidence for covalent linkages to type II collagen in cartilage. *FEBS Lett.* **220**, 337–341
6. Vogel, K.G. and Trotter, J.A. (1987) The effect of proteoglycans on the morphology of collagen fibrils formed in vitro. *Collagen. Rel. Res.* **7**, 105–114
7. Buckwalter, J.A. (1982) The fine structure of the intervertebral disc. in: *Idiopathic Low Back Pain*, (White, A.A. and Gordon, S.L., eds.), pp. 108–143, C.V. Mosby, St. Louis
8. Coventry, M.B., Ghormley, R.K. and Kernohan, J.W. (1945) The intervertebral disc: Its microscopic anatomy and pathology; anatomy, development and physiology. Part 1. *J. Bone Joint Surg.* **27**, 105–112
9. Beadle, O.A. (1931) *The intervertebral discs. Observations on their normal and morbid anatomy in relation to certain spinal deformities*, HMSO, London
10. Viidik, A. (1973) Functional properties of collagenous tissues. *Int. Rev. Connect. Tissue Res.* **6**, 127–215
11. Takeda, T. (1975) Three-dimensional observations of collagen framework of human lumbar discs. *J. Jpn. Orthop. Assoc.* **49**, 45–57
12. Stockwell, R.A. (1979) *Biology of Cartilage Cells*, Cambridge University Press, Cambridge

13. Broom, N.D. and Marra, D.L. (1986) Ultrastructural evidence for fibril-to-fibril associations in articular cartilage and their functional implication. *J. Anat.* **146**, 185–200
14. Maroudas, A. and Bannon, C. (1981) Measurement of swelling pressure in cartilage and comparison with the osmotic pressure of constituent proteoglycans. *Biorheology* **18**, 619–632
15. Maroudas, A. (1976) Balance between swelling pressure and collagen tension in normal and degenerate cartilage. *Nature (London)* **260**, 808–809
16. Weightman, B. and Kempson, G. (1979) Load carriage. In: *Adult Articular Cartilage* (Freeman, M.A.R., ed.), pp. 291–332, Pitman Medical, London
17. Nachemson, A. and Elfstrom, G. (1970) Intravital dynamic pressure measurements in lumbar discs. A study of common movements, manouvers and exercises. *Scand. J. Rehabil. Med.* **2** (Suppl. 1), 1–40
18. Nachemson, A. and Morris, J.M. (1964) In vivo measurements of interdiscal pressure. *J. Bone Joint Surg.* **46A**, 1077–1092
19. Afoke, A., Hutton, W.C. and Byers, P.D. (1990) Pressure measurement in the human hip joint using Fujifilm. In: *Methods in Cartilage Research,* (Maroudas, A. and Kuettner, K., eds.), pp. 281–287, Academic Press, London
20. Hodge, W.A., Fuan, R.S., Carlson, K.L., Burgess, R.G., Harris, W.H. and Mann, R.W. (1986) Contact pressures in the human hip joint measured in vivo. *Proc. Natl. Acad. Sci. U.S.A.* **83**, 2879–2883
21. Athanasiou, K.A., Rosenwasser, M.P., Buckwalter, J.A., Malinin, T.I. and Mow, V.C. (1993) Interspecies comparison of in situ intrinsic mechanical properties of distal femoral cartilage. *J. Orthop. Res.* **9**, 330–340
22. Boos, N., Wallin, A., Gbedegbegnon, T., Aebi, M. and Boesch, C. (1993) Quantitative MR imaging of lumbar intervertebral disks and vertebral bodies: influence of diurnal water content variations. *Radiology* **188**, 351–354
23. Lipson, S. and Muir, H. (1981) Proteoglycans in experimental disc degeneration. *Spine* **6**, 194–201
24. Muir, H. and Carney, S.L. (1987) Pathological and biochemical changes in cartilage and other tissues of the canine knee resulting from induced joint instability. In: *Joint Loading: Biology and Health of Articular Structures,* (Helminen, H.J., Kiviranta, I., Tammi, M., Saamanen, A.-M., Paukkonen, K. and Jurvelin, J., eds.), pp. 47–63, Wright, Bristol
25. Tyler, J.A., Bolis, S., Dingle, J.T. and Middleton, J.F.S. (1992) Mediators of Matrix Catabolism. in: *Articular Cartilage and Osteoarthritis,* (Kuettner, K.E., Schleyerbach, R., Peyron, J. and Hascall, V., eds.), pp. 251–264, Raven Press, New York
26. Morales, T.I. (1992) Polypeptide regulators of matrix homeostasis in articular cartilage. In: *Articular Cartilage and Osteoarthritis* (Kuettner, K., Schleyerbach, R., Peyron, J. and Hascall, V., eds.), pp. 265–280, Raven Press, New York
27. Demer, L.L. (1992) Mechanical factors in artery wall function and atherogenesis. *Monogr. Hum. Genet.* **14**, 82–97
28. Mukherjee, D. and Sen, S. (1990) Collagen phenotypes during development and regression of myocardial hypertrophy in spontaneously hypertensive rats. *Circ. Res.* **67**, 1474–1480
29. Gillard, G.C., Reilly, H.C., Bell-Booth, P.G. and Flint, M.H. (1979) The influence of mechanical forces on the glycosaminoglycan content of the rabbit flexor digitorum profundus tendon. *Connect. Tissue Res.* **7**, 37–46
30. Slowman, S.D. and Brandt, K.D. (1986) Composition and glycosaminoglycan metabolism of articular cartilage from habitually loaded and habitually unloaded sites. *Arthritis Rheum.* **29**, 88–94
31. Roberts, S., Weightman, B., Urban, J.P.G. and Chapell, D. (1986) Mechanical and biochemical properties of human articular cartilage in osteoarthritic femoral heads and in autopsy specimens. *J. Bone Joint Surg.* **68B**, 278–288
32. Jurvelin, J., Helminen, H., Lauritsalo, S., et al. (1985) Influences of joint immobilization and running exercise on articular cartilage surfaces of young rabbits. *Acta Anat.* **122**, 62–68
33. Tammi, M., Paukkonen, K., Kiviranta, I., Jurvelin, J., Saamanen, A.-M. and Helminen, H.J. (1987) Joint loading induced alterations in articular cartilage. In: *Joint Loading. Biology and Health of Articular Cartilage,* (Helminen, H.J., Kiviranta, I., Saamanen, A.-M., Tammi, M., Paukkonen, K. and Jurvelin, J., eds.), pp. 64–88, Wright, Bristol
34. Palmoski, M., Perricone, E. and Brandt, K.D. (1979) Development and reversal of a proteoglycan aggregation defect in normal canine knee cartilage after immobilization. *Arthritis Rheum.* **22**, 508–517
35. Palmoski, M., Colyer, R.A. and Brandt, K.D. (1980) Joint motion in the absence of normal loading does not maintain normal articular cartilage. *Arthritis Rheum.* **23**, 325–334
36. Arokoski, J., Kiviranta, I., Jurvelin, J., Tammi, M. and Helminen, H.J. (1993) Long-distance running causes site-dependent decrease of cartilage glycosaminoglycan content in the knee joints of beagle dogs. *Arthritis Rheum.* **36**, 1451–1459
37. Puustjarvi, K., Lammi, M., Kiviranta, I., Helminen, H.J. and Tammi, M. (1993) Proteoglycan synthesis in canine intervertebral discs after long distance running training. *J. Orthop. Res.* **11**, 738–746
38. Paukkonen, K., Selkainaho, K., Jurvelin, J. and Helminen, H.J. (1985) Cells and nuclei of articular cartilage chondrocytes in young rabbits enlarged after non-strenuous physical exercise. *J. Anat.* **142**, 13–20
39. Kiviranta, I., Tammi, M., Jurvelin, J., Arokoski, J., Saamanen, A.-M. and Helminen, H. (1988) Moderate running exercise augments glycosaminoglycans and thickness of articular cartilage in the knee joint of young beagle dogs. *J. Orthop. Res.* **6**, 188–195

40. Burton-Wurster, N., Todhunter, R.J. and Lust, G. (1993) Animal models of Osteoarthritis. In: *Joint Cartilage Degradation: Basic and Clinical Aspects*, (Woessner, J.F. and Howell, D.S., eds.), pp. 347–384, Marcel Dekker, New York

41. Holm, S. and Nachemson, A. (1983) Variation in the nutrition of the canine intervertebral disc induced by motion. *Spine* **8**, 866–874

42. Higuchi, M., Abe, K. and Kaneda, K. (1983) Changes in the nucleus pulposus of the intervertebral disc in bipedal mice: A light and electron microscopic study. *Clin. Orthop.* **175**, 251–257

43. Cassidy, J., Yong-Hing, M., Kirkaldy-Willis, W. and Wilkinson, A. (1988) A study of the effects of bipedalism and upright posture on the lumbosacral spine and paravertebral muscles of the wistar rat. *Spine* **13**, 301–308

44. Holm, S. and Nachemson, A. (1982) Nutritional changes in the canine intervertebral disc after spinal fusion. *Clin. Orthop.* **169**, 243–258

45. Sumpio, B.E., Banes, A.J., Link, W.G. and Johnson, G. (1988) Enhanced collagen production by smooth muscle cells during repetitive mechanical stretching. *Arch. Surg.* **123**, 1233–1236

46. Jones, D.B., Nolte, H., Scholubbers, J.-G., Turner, E. and Veltel, D. (1991) Biochemical signal transduction of mechanical strain in osteoblast-like cells. *Biomaterials* **12**, 101–110

47. Koob, T.J., Clark, P.E., Hernandez, D.J., Thurmond, F.A. and Vogel, K.G. (1992) Compression loading in vitro regulates proteoglycan synthesis by tendon fibrocartilage. *Arch. Biochem. Biophys.* **298**, 303–312

48. Gray, M.L., Pizzanelli, A.M., Lee, R.C., Grodzinsky, A.J. and Swann, D.A. (1989) Kinetics of the chondrocyte biosynthetic response to compressive loading and release. *Biochim. Biophys. Acta* **991**, 415–425

49. Sah, R.L., Kim, Y.L., Doong, J.-Y.H., Grodzinsky, A.J., Plaas, A.H.K. and Sandy, J.D. (1989) Biosynthetic response of cartilage explants to dynamic compression. *J. Orthop. Res.* **7**, 619–639

50. Burton-Wurster, N., Vernier-Singer, M., Farquhar, T. and Lust, G. (1993) Effect of compressive loading and unloading on the synthesis of total protein, proteoglycan and fibronectin by canine cartilage explants. *J. Orthop. Res.* **11**, 717–729

51. Sah, R.L., Grodzinsky, A.J., Plaas, A.H.K. and Sandy, J.D. (1990) Effects of tissue compression on the hyaluronate binding properties of newly synthesized proteoglycans in cartilage explants. *Biochem. J.* **267**, 803–808

52. Sah, R.L., Doong, J.-Y.H., Grodzinsky, A.J., Plaas, A.H.K. and Sandy, J.D. (1991) Effects of compression on the loss of newly synthesized proteoglycans and proteins from cartilage explants. *Arch. Biochem. Biophys.* **286**, 20–29

53. Kim, Y.J., Grodzinsky, A.J., Plaas, A.H.K. and Sandy, J.D. (1992) The differential effects of static compression on the synthesis of specific cartilage matrix components. *Trans. Am. Orthop. Res. Soc.* **17**, 108

54. Bayliss, M.T., Urban, J.P.G., Johnstone, B. and Holm, S. (1986) In vitro method for measuring synthesis rates in the intervertebral disc. *J. Orthop. Res.* **4**, 10–17

55. Ohshima, H., Urban, J.P.G. and Bergel, D.H. (1995) Effect of static load on matrix synthesis rates in the intervertebral disc measured *in vitro* by a new perfusion technique. *J. Orthop. Res.*, **13**, 22–29

56. Gray, M.L., Pizzanelli, A.M., Grodzinsky, A.J. and Lee, R.C. (1988) Mechanical and physiochemical determinants of the chondrocyte biosynthetic response. *J. Orthop. Res.* **6**, 777–792

57. Ohshima, H. and Urban, J.P.G. (1992) Effect of lactate concentrations and pH on matrix synthesis rates in the intervertebral disc. *Spine* **17**, 1079–1082

58. Urban, J.P.G., Hall, A.C. and Gehl, K.A. (1993) Regulation of matrix synthase rates by the ionic and osmotic environment of articular chondrocytes. *J. Cell. Physiol.* **154**, 262–270

59. Urban, J.P.G. and Bayliss, M.T. (1989) Regulation of proteoglycan synthesis rate in cartilage in vitro: influence of extracellular ionic composition. *Biochim. Biophys. Acta* **992**, 59–65

60. Jannasch, H.W., Marquis, R.E. and Zimmerman, A.M. (1987) *Current Perspectives in High Pressure Biology*, Academic Press, London

61. Ishihara, H., Urban, J.P.G. and Hall, A.S. (1993) The effect of physiological hydrostatic pressures on synthesis in different regions of the intervertebral disc. *J. Physiol. (London)* **467**, 214

62. Hall, A.C., Urban, J.P.G. and Gehl, K.A. (1991) The effects of hydrostatic pressure on matrix synthesis in articular cartilage. *J. Orthop. Res.* **9**, 1–10

63. Parkkinen, J.J., Ikonen, J., Lammi, M.J., Laakonen, J. and Helminen, H.J. (1993) Effects of cyclic hydrostatic pressure on proteoglycan synthesis in cultured chondrocytes and articular cartilage explants. *Arch. Biochem. Biophys.* **300**, 458–465

64. Kim, Y.J., Sah, R.L., Grodzinsky, A.J., Plaas, A.H.K. and Sandy, J.D. (1994) Mechanical regulation of cartilage biosynthetic behavior: physical stimuli. *Arch. Biochem. Biophys.* **311**, 1–12

65. Davies, P.F. (1989) How do vascular endothelial cells responds to flow? *News Pharmaceut. Sci.* **4**, 22–25

66. Reich, K.M. and Frangos, J.F. (1991) Effect of flow on prostaglandin E2 and inositol triphosphate levels in osteoblasts. *Am. J. Physiol.* **261**, C428–C432

67. MacGinitie, L.A., Gluzband, Y.A. and Grodzinsky, A.J. (1994) Electric field stimulation can increase protein synthesis in articular cartilage explants. *J. Orthop. Res.* **12**, 151–160

68. Lee, R.C., Rich, J.B., Kelley, K.M., Weiman, D.S. and Mathews, M.B. (1982) A comparison of in vitro cellular responses to mechanical and electrical stimulation. *Am. Surgeon* **48**, 567–574

69. Bourret, L.A. and Rodan, G.A. (1988) The role of calcium in the inhibition of cAMP accumulation in epiphyseal cartilage cells exposed to cartilage pressure. *J. Cell. Physiol.* **88**, 353–362

70. Davies, P.F. and Tripathi, S.C. (1993) Mechanical stress mechanisms and the cell. *Circ. Res.* **72**,

239–245

71. Sah, R.L.-Y., Grodzinsky, A.J., Plaas, A.H.K. and Sandy, J.D. (1992) Effects of static and dynamic compression on matrix metabolism in cartilage explants. In: *Articular Cartilage Biochemistry and Osteoarthritis* (Kuettner, K.E., Hascall, V.C. and Schleyerbach, R., eds.), pp. 373–392, Raven Press, New York

72. Buschmann, M.D., Gluzband, Y.A., Grodzinsky, A.J. and Hunziker, E.B. (1995) Mechanical compression modulates matrix biosynthesis in chondrocyte/agarose culture. *J. Cell Sci.*, in the press

73. Bassett, C.A.L. and Pawluk, R.J. (1972) Electrical behavior of cartilage during loading. *Science* **178**, 982–983

74. Lotke, P.A., Black, J. and Richardson, S.J. (1974) Electromechanical properties in human articular cartilage. *J. Bone Joint Surg.* **56A**, 1040–1046

75. Grodzinsky, A.J., Lipshitz, H. and Glimcher, M.J. (1978) Electromechanical properties of articular cartilage during compression and stress relaxation. *Nature (London)* **175**, 448–450

76. Frank, E.H. and Grodzinsky, A.J. (1987) Cartilage electromechanics I : electrokinetic transduction and the effects of pH and ionic strength. *J. Biomechanics* **20**, 615–627

77. Frank, E.H. and Grodzinsky, A.J. (1987) Cartilage electromechanics II: a continuum model of cartilage electrokinetics and correlation with experiments. *J. Biomechanics* **20**, 629–639

78. Gross, D. and Williams, W.S. (1982) Streaming potential and the electromechanical response of physiologically moist bone. *J. Biomechanics* **15**, 287–295

79. Pienkowski, D. and Pollack, S.R. (1983) The origin of stress-generated potentials in fluid-saturated bone. *J. Orthop. Res.* **1**, 30–41

80. Otter, M.W., Palmieri, V.R., MacGinitie, L.A., and Cochran, G.V.B. (1990) A canine tibia model for comparison of streaming potentials in vivo and in vitro. *Trans. Bioelec. Repair Growth Soc.* **10**, 8

81. Kim, Y.J., Bonassar, L.J. and Grodzinsky, A.J. (1995) The role of cartilage streaming potential, fluid flow and pressure in the stimulation of chondrocyte biosynthesis during dynamic compression. *J. Biomechanics*, in the press

82. Biot, M.A. (1955) Theory of elasticity and consolidation for a porous anisotropic solid. *J. Appl. Phys.* **26**, 182–185

83. Mow, V.C., Kuei, S.C., Lai, W.M. and Armstrong, C.G. (1980) Biphasic creep and stress relaxation of articular cartilage in compression: theory and experiments. *J. Biomech. Eng.* **102**, 73–84

84. Hoch, D.H., Grodzinsky, A.J., Koob, T.J., Albert, M.L. and Eyre, D.R. (1983) Early changes in material properties of rabbit articular cartilage after meniscectomy. *J. Orthop. Res.* **1**, 4–12

85. Moskowitz, R.W., Howell, D.S., Goldberg, V.M., Muiz, O. and Pita, J.C. (1979) Cartilage proteoglycan alterations in an experimentally induced model of rabbit osteoarthritis. *Arthritis Rheum.* **22**, 155–163

86. Frank, E.H., Grodzinsky, A.J., Koob, T.J. and Eyre, D.R. (1987) Streaming potentials: a sensitive index of enzymatic degradation in articular cartilage. *J. Orthop. Res.* **5**, 497–508

87. Sachs, J.R. and Grodzinsky, A.J. (1989) A mathematical model of an electromechanically coupled poroelastic medium driven by an electric current. *PhysicoChem. Hydrodynamics*, **11**, 585–614

88. Berkenblit, S.I., Frank, E.H., Salant, E.P. and Grodzinsky, A.J. (1994) Nondestructive detection of cartilage degeneration using electromechanical surface spectroscopy. *J. Biomech. Eng.* **116**, 384–392

89. Melcher, J.R. (1981) *Continuum Electromechanics*. MIT Press, Cambridge, U.S.A.

90. Zaretsky, M.C., Li, P. and Melcher, J.R. (1989) Estimation of thickness, complex bulk permittivity and surface conductivity using interdigital dielectrometry. *IEEE Trans. Insul.* **24**, 1159–1166

91. Frenkel, J. (1944) On the theory of seismic and seismoelectric phenomena in a moist soil. *J. Phys. U.S.S.R.* **8**, 230–241

92. Biot, M.A. (1962) Generalized theory of acoustic propagation in porous dissipative media. *J. Accoust. Soc. Am.* **34**, 1254–1264

93. Chandler, R. (1981) Transient streaming potential measurements on fluid-saturated porous structures: an experimental verification of Biot's slow wave in the quasi-static limit. *J. Accoust. Soc. Am.* **70**, 116–121

94. Salzstein, R.A., Pollack, S.R., Mak, A.F.T. and Petrov, N. (1987) Electromechanical potentials in cortical bone: I. a continuum approach. *J. Biomechanics* **20**, 261–270

95. Lai, W.M., Hou, J.S. and Mow, V.C. (1991) A triphasic theory for the swelling and deformation behaviors of articular cartilage. *J. Biomech. Eng.* **113**, 245–258

96. Frank, E.H., Grodzinsky, A.J., Phillips, S.L. and Grimshaw, P.E. (1990) Physicochemical and bioelectrical determinants of cartilage material properties. In: *Biomechanics of Diarthrodial Joints* (Mow, V.C., Ratcliffe, A. and Woo, S.L.-Y., eds.), pp. 261–282, Springer-Verlag, New York

7

Interstitial fluid pressure

Rolf K. Reed

Department of Physiology, University of Bergen, Årstadveien 19, N-5009 Bergen, Norway

Introduction

The interstitium is the loose connective-tissue compartment found in all organs of the body. The interstitium as dealt with and discussed in this chapter is focused on, and refers to, data and experiments on skin unless otherwise specified.

The structural components of the interstitium and the physico-chemical properties are dealt with in detail in other sections of this book, and only a brief survey will be given here on some aspects of this issue. The major structural component in loose connective tissues is collagen, which in skin accounts for about 15% of the wet weight [1]. The glycosaminoglycans constitute the other main structural component of which hyaluronan in skin makes up about 50%, resulting in a concentration of somewhat less than 1 mg/ml, i.e. a concentration where the individual molecules show entanglement and become physically intertwined and will also exhibit exclusion towards other macro-molecules [1,2].

The interstitial fluid volume

The interstitium contains the interstitial fluid volume which is otherwise defined as the extracellular and extravascular fluid compartment and which is formed by ultrafiltration of plasma through the capillary wall. The interstitial fluid normally has a protein concentration and a colloid osmotic pressure which is about half that of plasma, and the protein concentration and composition is determined by the properties of the capillary wall and the transcapillary fluid filtration rate [3]. The electrolyte composition of the interstitial fluid is similar to that of plasma, but modified relative to plasma according to a Donnan equi-librium due to the lower plasma protein concentration in the interstitial fluid.

The interstitial fluid volumes in skin and skeletal muscle constitute 40% and 10% of the wet weight respectively, and are controlled by the balance between the capillary fluid filtration and the lymph flow (Figure 1). At steady state interstitial fluid volume is constant and these two fluid fluxes are equal. The capillary fluid filtration is generated by the net capillary filtration pressure which in peripheral tissues like skin and skeletal muscle is approx. 0.5 to 1 mmHg (Figure 1). The transcapillary pressure gradient is generated by the imbalance in colloid osmotic pressure in plasma (approx. 20 mmHg in experimental animals) and interstitial fluid (approx. half that of plasma colloid osmotic pressure), and capillary and interstitial hydrostatic

Figure 1

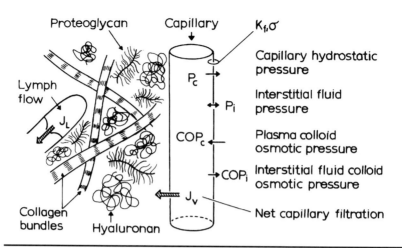

Schematic drawing of the interstitium with the major structural components, a lymphatic and the colloid osmotic pressure (COP) and hydrostatic pressure (P) acting across the capillary wall
Subscripts c and i denote capillary and interstitial respectively. K_f and σ are the capillary filtration coefficient and capillary reflection coefficient for proteins respectively. Reproduced from [14] with permission.

pressures. The fluid filtration rate is the product of this pressure gradient and the capillary filtration coefficient, which is the 'water permeability' of the capillary wall. The resulting fluid filtration will determine the interstitial fluid volume together with the lymph flow, and thereby also the hydrostatic pressure in the interstitial fluid as discussed below.

Interstitial fluid pressure

The interstitial fluid pressure (P_{if}) is the pressure which can be measured through a fluid-filled catheter inserted into the interstitium and connected to a pressure transducer or water manometer [4]. This pressure is crucial in the control of the interstitial fluid volume since it is the filling pressure for the initial lymphatics and participates in capillary fluid exchange. The concept of a negative P_{if} originates from the experiments of Guyton [5] in the early 1960s reporting that P_{if} in chronically implanted perforated capsules was -6 to -8 mmHg after about 6 weeks of implantation [4,5]. Prior to this time several attempts had been made to measure P_{if} using needles, and in several cases using an infusion of fluid through the needle (for references see [1,6]). The pressures recorded with these techniques were above ambient pressure, in retrospect explained by the infusion used to keep the needles open [6]. It has been argued that the more negative P_{if} reported with chronically implanted capsules could be caused by the connective tissue lining the capsule and acting as a semipermeable membrane since measurements of the reflection coefficient of the capsule yielded values of 0.3–0.6 [7]. However, in a steady-state situation, this should not restrict protein diffusion to an extent which creates gradients in protein concentration; therefore protein concentration and P_{if} should be the same in the capsule and surrounding tissue.

Following the reports of the chronically implanted capsules, several techniques were developed to allow measurement of P_{if} shortly (minutes) after introduction of the probe into the tissue since this is not possible with the chronically implanted capsules. The first of these methods was the wick technique developed by Scholander, Hargens and Miller [8] who used a cotton wick which was introduced into the interstitium through a needle. Aukland and his collaborators developed the wick-in-needle technique [9] and were also able to employ the micropuncture technique for measurement of P_{if} using sharpened glass capillaries (tip diameter around 5 μm) connected to a servocontrolled counterpressure system [10].

The concept of a negative P_{if} gradually became accepted. However, there remained a controversy on the magnitude of negativity of P_{if} since the chronically implanted capsules in general gave pressures several mmHg more negative than the needle and wick techniques. This controversy was solved by a series of experiments performed by Wiig [11,12] who measured P_{if} simultaneously with several techniques in controls, as well as after acute changes in the fluid balance in the tissues induced by intravenous saline infusion, locally increased venous pressure and peritoneal dialysis. These experiments showed that the chronically implanted capsules described by Guyton [5], a chronically implanted porous capsule made from polyethylene [13], the wick-in-needle technique and the micropuncture technique all yielded the same pressure in controls (Figure 2). With acute changes in tissue hydration, the chronically implanted capsules overestimated the changes in P_{if} compared with the micropuncture and wick-in-needle techniques. However, if allowed enough time (about 2–3 h), the different techniques again gave the same pressure in overhydration. A similar time response was seen in dehydration with the exception that the chronically implanted perforated capsule did not reattain the pressure of the other three devices. Two conclusions were drawn from these experiments. First, the different techniques used for measurement of P_{if} yielded the same pressure in controls under identical experimental conditions. Secondly, with acute changes in interstitial hydration the chronically implanted capsules responded more slowly and transiently overestimated the response in P_{if}, probably due to the dense connective tissue formed during the weeks of implantation acting as a semipermeable membrane with a rather low reflection coefficient [14].

Solid and total interstitial pressures

The earlier discrepancy between P_{if} measured with needles and the 5–10 mmHg more negative pressure measured with chronically implanted capsules led to the introduction of the term 'solid tissue pressure'. The solid tissue pressure is a stress exerted between the formed elements in a tissue. Since it is a stress, it has a direction which

Figure 2

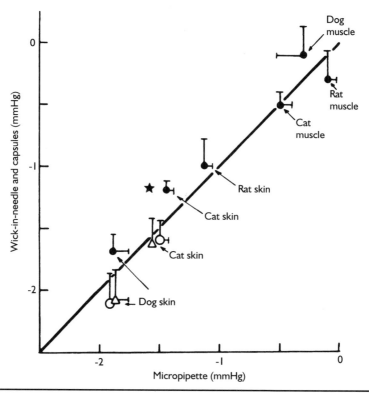

**Interstitial fluid pressure in skin/subcutis and skeletal muscle
measured with fluid equilibration techniques in normally hydrated
cats, rats and dogs using the micropipette technique [10], wick-in-
needle (●) [9], perforated hollow capsule (○) [5], and perforated
porous capsules (△) [13]**
*Results are given as mean ±S.E.M. Significant difference for cats (P<0.05)
denoted by filled star. Line of identity is shown. Reproduced from [14] with
permission.*

distinguishes it from a hydrostatic pressure, but at the same time it can
be converted into a hydrostatic pressure when the solids through which
it is exerted encroach upon the fluid volume.

As discussed in detail elsewhere [1], there seems little reason to
continue to use the term solid tissue pressure since the P_{if} measured by
different fluid equilibration techniques simultaneously yields the same
values under identical experimental conditions (Figure 2). Thus, the solid
tissue pressure will be zero if it is taken as the difference between the P_{if}
measured with needles and that measured with chronically implanted
capsules. However, there may still be stresses within individual fibres or
fibre networks in the tissue. According to Meyer's concept [15–17] the
swelling tendency of the tissue is due to its content of hyaluronan.
Furthermore, there is a microfibril network which restrains an expanding
network of collagen fibres. According to this concept, overhydration of
the tissue will allow the collagen network to expand and thereby lower
its stress while at the same time the stress in the restraining microfibril

network will increase. The increasing interstitial volume will also increase P_{if}, so that in a new steady state the stresses in the network will again balance P_{if}. Once the degree of hydration of the tissue is determined by transcapillary fluid‾flux and lymph flow, P_{if} is determined and will balance the stresses in the fibres and fibre networks. Thus, if the tissue volume increases or decreases as a result of altered tissue hydration the stresses will readjust, but the relationship between the stresses, the P_{if} and interstitial fluid volume will all be contained in the interstitial volume–pressure relationship (see below). However, it should be mentioned that a solid tissue pressure might exist in the kidney and the basis for this and its consequences are discussed in detail elsewhere [18].

The total tissue pressure is the sum of the P_{if} and the solid tissue pressure. However, as discussed above, as long as there is little reason to maintain the concept of a solid tissue pressure, the total tissue pressure will equal P_{if}.

Interstitial compliance

Normally, P_{if} will participate in maintaining a constant interstitial fluid volume. The relative importance of P_{if} in control of interstitial fluid volume is contained in the term compliance which is defined as the ratio between a change in interstitial fluid volume divided by the corresponding change in P_{if}, i.e. the derivative of the interstitial volume–pressure relationship with respect to pressure. A low compliance implies that a small change in interstitial fluid volume will generate a large change in P_{if}. In the case of enhanced capillary filtration, the increased filtration and interstitial volume will raise P_{if}, which in turn will act across the capillary wall to limit capillary filtration and thereby further changes in interstitial fluid volume. The interstitial volume–pressure relationship which is shown in Figure 3 is similar in rats [19,20], cats [21] and dogs [22]. The following features should be noted about this relationship. First, the curve is linear in dehydration and the initial part of overhydration, and interstitial compliance in skin and skeletal muscle is about 10–15% per mmHg, i.e. with a 10–15% change in interstitial fluid volume, P_{if} will change by 1 mmHg [14,19–22]. Secondly, in overhydration, compliance soon increases and above 50–100% overhydration compliance approaches infinity since there is very little change in P_{if} despite large changes in interstitial fluid volume. Finally, the increase in interstitial volume from control interstitial volume to the virtually horizontal part of the curve is of the order of 2–3 mmHg in skin and skeletal muscle.

Normal control of interstitial fluid volume

Normal control of interstitial fluid volume is achieved by automatic readjustment of interstitial colloid osmotic and hydrostatic pressures in response to the altered capillary filtration. With increased capillary filtration the protein concentration in the capillary filtrate will fall [3,23]. With an increase in interstitial fluid volume of 10–15%, P_{if} will increase

Figure 3

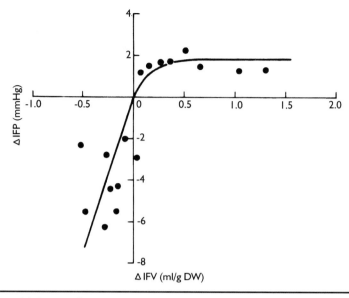

Interstitial compliance
The change in interstitial fluid volume (ΔIFV) versus the change in interstitial fluid pressure (ΔIFP) is shown for dog skin. The data points represent individual experiments. Normal IFV and IFP in dog skin was 1.45 ml/g DW (dry weight) and − 1.9 mmHg respectively. Reproduced from [22] with permission.

by 1 mmHg (see above) and at the same time lower the interstitial protein concentration and thereby the interstitial colloid osmotic pressure from 10–12 mmHg by about 1 mmHg. The effect of these changes across the capillary wall is principally similar as both will lower the net capillary filtration pressure. The increased net capillary filtration pressure will therefore be compensated by a rise in P_{if} and a fall in interstitial colloid osmotic pressure, and thereby tend to keep the net capillary filtration pressure and fluid filtration constant. Thus, around control interstitial volume an increased capillary filtration will be counteracted by a lowering of interstitial colloid osmotic pressure and increased P_{if}. Furthermore, these changes will be quantitatively of the same importance in maintaining a constant interstitial volume as compliance is around 10–15% per mmHg. The changes in dehydration will be opposite to those described above, but again the interstitial hydrostatic and colloid osmotic pressures are of quantitatively the same importance in maintaining a constant interstitial fluid volume.

Although P_{if} and interstitial fluid colloid osmotic pressure are of equal importance in normal control of interstitial fluid volume, their individual capacity to limit excessive increases in capillary filtration and thereby oedema formation is very different. The capacity of P_{if} to counteract increased filtration is limited to the rise from normal control to the virtually horizontal level of the interstitial volume–pressure curve, i.e. 2–3 mmHg. However, the capacity of interstitial colloid osmotic pressure to limit excessive filtration is around 10 mmHg since interstitial fluid colloid osmotic pressure can fall from its normal value of

10–12 mmHg to a colloid osmotic pressure which is virtually zero. The lowest colloid osmotic pressure which can be obtained corresponds to the plasma protein concentration times $(1-\sigma)$ where σ is the capillary reflection coefficient for protein [3]. The relative importance of P_{if} may differ between tissues, and in encapsulated tissues the importance of an increased P_{if} will greatly exceed that of a lowering of colloid osmotic pressure in normal control of interstitial fluid volume [24]. Finally, it needs to be mentioned that with longstanding increased capillary filtration an enhanced lymph flow is required to lower the interstitial protein content (for references see [1]).

To summarize, the role of P_{if} in the control of normal interstitial volume is to maintain a constant volume and this is achieved by changes in P_{if} acting to oppose the changes in transcapillary filtration pressure.

Lymph flow

P_{if} will also participate in control of interstitial fluid volume through its influence on lymph flow, since P_{if} is normally considered to serve as the filling pressure of the initial lymphatics. Fluid flux from the capillaries through the interstitium to the initial lymphatics will have to occur down a hydrostatic pressure gradient to provide filling of the initial lymphatics from the interstitial fluid volume, as there is no evidence for an active fluid and solute transport across the lymphatic endothelium [25]. The previous controversy of an uphill pressure gradient on this stretch seems to originate from measurements in different species in different laboratories: the very negative values for P_{if} have been replaced with values around ambient pressure. The few studies with simultaneous measurement of P_{if} and pressure in the initial lymphatics have been performed by Hogan and colleagues [26,27], who demonstrated a down-hill pressure gradient from the interstitium to the initial lymphatics during part of the contraction cycle of the lymphatic, thus providing the necessary pressure gradient for filling the lymphatics. For a more detailed discussion on the filling of the initial lymphatics reference should be made to recent reviews [1,25].

Burn injury

The normal role of P_{if} in maintaining a constant interstitial volume as described above was challenged by observations showing that following a burn injury to the skin P_{if} fell to values as low as -150 mmHg (Figure 4) [28,29]. The increased negativity of P_{if} will, in this situation, 'actively' enhance capillary filtration and no longer prevent an increase in interstitial fluid volume. The magnitude of the lowering of P_{if} was dependent upon the hydration of the tissue (Figure 4): when supplying intravenous fluid substitution, the lowered P_{if} returned to control and eventually to positive values. When fluid movement into the injured area and oedema formation was prevented by inducing circulatory arrest and introducing a diffusion barrier towards the underlying skeletal muscle, P_{if} values as low as -150 mmHg were observed. Studies of the

Figure 4

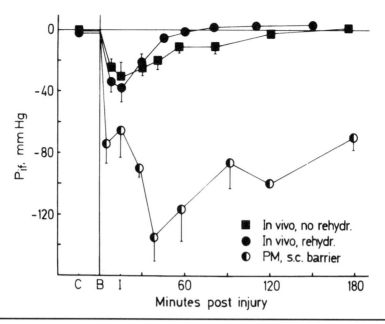

Effect of a full thickness burn injury covering 40% of the body surface on interstitial fluid pressure (P$_{if}$) in skin

C, B and I denote control measurement, burn injury and start of infusion respectively. 'In vivo, no rehydr.' implies that no intravenous fluid resuscitation was given (■). Intravenous fluid resuscitation (5 ml/h) was given to the group denoted 'In vivo, rehydr.' (●). In the last group, 'PM, s.c. barrier' (◐), the burn injury (20% of body surface) was inflicted after circulatory arrest and placement of a diffusion barrier between the skin and the underlying skeletal muscle. Values are means ±S.E.M. Reproduced from [28] with permission.

molecular events involved in creating the increased negativity of P$_{if}$ in burn injury suggested that collagen denaturation was an important event in this process [29].

The low P$_{if}$ measured by Lund *et al.* [28,29] offers an explanation to an experimental observation by Artursson and Mellander [30], who estimated from the rate of fluid accumulation and the capillary filtration coefficient that a net capillary filtration pressure of 2–300 mmHg was required to explain the rapidity of oedema formation in a second-degree burn injury. The net filtration pressure was ascribed to an increase in osmolarity, but the experimental data of Artursson and Mellander [30] fit well with the observed lowering of P$_{if}$. Furthermore, Artursson and Mellander [30] measured a 2–3-fold increase in the capillary filtration coefficient, which has been confirmed in studies on burn injuries [31,32] as well as other inflammatory processes [33]. The observation that increased capillary net filtration pressure is the major pathophysiological change required to explain the rapid oedema formation is in contrast to the commonly accepted notion that large changes in capillary permeability explain the rapidly forming oedema in acute inflammation [34]. The lowering of P$_{if}$ in burn injury therefore points out two principally important issues. First, a considerable increase in net capillary filtration pressure is required to rapidly generate inflammatory oedemas. Secondly, it shows that the loose connective tissues can be 'active' participants in generation of the rapidly forming oedema in burn injury.

Inflammation

After the initial observation of increased negativity of P_{if} in burn injury, several inflammatory reactions characterized by rapid oedema formation have been studied with respect to principally similar changes in P_{if}. Since visible oedema requires doubling of interstitial fluid volume, and the interstitial fluid in skin normally turns over in 12–24 h, formation of visible oedema in 5–10 min implies that capillary filtration is increased at least 100-fold above control levels. Again, the capillary filtration coefficient is increased by 2–3 times above control [33] and a dramatic increase in capillary net filtration pressure is therefore required to explain the rapidity of the oedema formation. Increased negativity of P_{if} has been observed in several inflammatory reactions, although the negativity of P_{if} is less pronounced than that seen in burn injury. Thus, a lowering of P_{if} from -1 to between -5 and -10 mmHg has been observed after xylene application to the skin [35], in carrageenan-induced inflammation [36] and in complement-induced oedema formation [37]. Furthermore, several of the acute inflammatory reactions which have been studied with respect to increased negativity of P_{if} involve mast cell degranulation: dextran anaphylaxis in rats will induce oedema formation in the paws and the airways and is accompanied by an increased negativity of P_{if} in skin [38] (see Figure 5) and trachea [39]. In trachea the mast-cell-degranulating substances C48/80 and polymyxin B

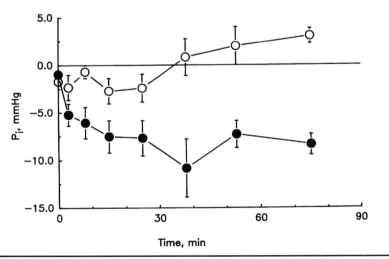

Figure 5

Effect of dextran anaphylaxis on interstitial fluid pressure (P_i) in rat paw skin

Open circles denote intact circulation, closed circles denote circulatory arrest. Values are given as mean $\pm$ S.E.M. Reproduced from [38] with permission.

will lower P_{if} from -1 to approx. -5 to -10 mmHg [40]. Finally, neurogenic inflammation in trachea, i.e. the inflammation seen after stimulation of C-fibres and release of neuropeptides [41,42], is also associated with a rapid lowering of P_{if} from -1 to -10 mmHg, starting within 1 min of nerve stimulation and completed within a few minutes (Figure 6) [43]. The involvement of neuropeptides in this situation is verified by the lack of response after denervation of C-fibres with depletion of neuropeptides by capsaicin, which abolished the lowering of P_{if} upon electrical stimulation of the vagal nerve (Figure 6).

Cellular participation in control of P_{if}

Although degranulation of the mast cells is involved in creating increased negativity of P_{if}, this does not convey information about the physical and/or structural events which take place in this process.

Figure 6

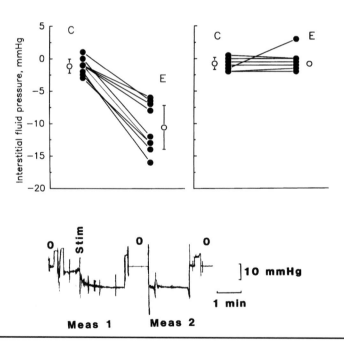

Interstitial fluid pressure in rat trachea in neurogenic inflammation
Upper panel, left-hand side: interstitial fluid pressure in control (C) and after electrical stimulation of the vagal nerve (E) in control rats. Upper panel, right-hand side: interstitial fluid pressure in control (C) and after vagal nerve stimulation (E) in rats subjected to capsaicin denervation of the sensory C-fibres. Values are given as mean ± S.D. Lower panel. Meas 1: interstitial fluid pressure measured in control and during electrical stimulation of the vagal nerve (Stim). Meas 2: repeated measurement after control of zero-level (0) of the servocontrolled counterpressure technique. Reproduced from [43] with permission.

Information on this comes from separate experiments. First, the balance between capillary filtration and lymph flow is what normally keeps the tissues in a slightly dehydrated state. When a piece of loose connective tissue is removed and soaked in saline, it will imbibe fluid and eventually reach a fluid content and volume which is about twice that of the intact tissue [15–17]. This property is associated with hyaluronan as the swelling is abolished if the tissue is treated with hyaluronidase or soaked in a solution of hyaluronan with a concentration corresponding to that in the interstitial fluid of the tissue sample. Based on studies of the swelling properties of umbilical cord and selective enzymic digestion of specific connective-tissue components, Meyer and colleagues [15–17] concluded that the tendency of loose connective tissues to swell when allowed free access to saline is caused by hyaluronan and that around the control interstitial volume a microfibril network is restraining an expanding network of collagen fibres.

Secondly, *in vivo* experiments suggest that the connective-tissue cells participate in control of P_{if} mediated via the receptors for their attachment to the structural components of the loose connective tissue, the integrins [44–47]. A detailed survey on integrin function is given in Chapter 3 in this book [48], and only a few comments on their structure and function will be given here. The integrins are heterodimeric receptors consisting of an α- and a β-subunit in which the specificity towards the connective-tissue component is determined by the specific α- and β-subunit constituting the receptor. Presently eight α- and 15 β-subunits have been identified, constituting a total of 20 integrins with known functions [48]. Integrins with a β_1-subunit in general attach to structural connective-tissue components, and evidence for the involvement of integrins in the phenomenon of increased negativity of P_{if} in inflammatory reactions has been obtained by using a polyclonal antibody towards the β_1-integrin subunit: subdermal injection of anti-β_1-integrin IgG resulted in rapid oedema formation concomitant with increased negativity of P_{if} with a time course and magnitude similar to that seen in several of the inflammatory reactions described above [49] (Figure 7). The magnitude of lowering of P_{if} was dependent on the dose of anti-β_1-integrin IgG and also specific for this IgG, since preimmune IgG and anti-fibronectin IgG did not change P_{if} (Figure 7).

The use of the collagen gel contraction assay [50–52], in parallel with measurements of P_{if}, has started to provide information also on other aspects of cellular participation in control of P_{if}. Thus, subdermal injection of cyclic AMP lowers P_{if} as well [53] and in the gel contraction assays cyclic AMP will prevent the collagen gel contraction from taking place. This attests further to connective tissues and their cells being able to actively participate in the control of P_{if}.

Based on the above experiments with anti-β_1-integrin IgG it is tempting to suggest that the final step in the chain of events leading to increased negativity of P_{if} in formation of inflammatory oedema involves perturbation of the β_1-integrin function with release of the contact between connective-tissue cells and the connective-tissue fibres, allowing the collagen (or microfibril) network described by Meyer and co-workers [15–17], and thereby also hyaluronan, to expand. This expansion *in situ* will lower P_{if} until the stress in the fibre networks is balanced towards a more negative P_{if} [48].

Mast cells

Mast cells are directly, and possibly also indirectly, involved in creating the increased negativity of P_{if}. Mast-cell degranulation in dextran anaphylaxis [38,39] or by C48/80 or polymyxin B [40] provides a way of inducing increased negativity of P_{if}. It presently seems likely that the constituents of the mast cells act by interference with other connective-tissue cells to perturb the β_1-integrin function. The neurogenic inflammation will act via neuropeptides which in turn exert their

Figure 7

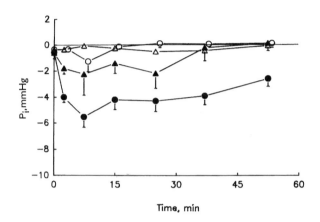

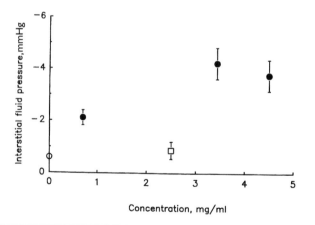

Effect of anti-β_1-integrin antibody on interstitial fluid pressure
Upper panel: Effect on interstitial fluid pressure (P_i) after subdermal injection of anti-β_1 integrin IgG (3.4–4.5 mg/ml; ●) and preimmune IgG (2.5 mg/ml; ○) from the same rabbit. Also shown is the effect of a peptide with an RGD sequence (6 mg/ml; ▲), and anti-fibronectin IgG (2.5 mg/ml; △).
Mean ± S.E.M. Lower panel: Interstitial fluid pressure as a function of concentration of anti-β_1 integrin IgG (●). Also shown is saline control (○) and preimmune IgG (□). Values are given as mean ± S.E.M. Reproduced from [43] with permission.

action either directly on the connective-tissue cells carrying the β_1-integrin receptors or via the mast cells. There are several studies which alone, and together, suggest a functional relationship between the nervous system and mast cells. First, mast cells swell [54] or degranulate [55] in response to vagal nerve stimulation and this reaction is abolished after denervation with capsaicin, which will deplete the sensory nerves of neuropeptides [55]. Secondly, substance P [56,57] and acetylcholine [58] will induce mast-cell degranulation *in vitro*, suggesting that these substances may act as transmitters to induce mast-cell degranulation. Thirdly, there is a close association between mast cells and sensory nerve fibres *in vivo* [59,60], and about two-thirds of the mast cells have a sensory nerve fibre located within a few micrometres [43,61]. Taken together, these studies would seem to suggest a functional pathway between the sensory C-fibres and the loose connective tissue via the mast cell. This pathway would constitute one of several possible ways to act on connective-tissue cells and participate in control of and induction of increased negativity of P_{if}.

Hyaluronan

The inherent tendency of a loose connective tissue to swell in saline as described above is related to the tissue's content of hyaluronan [15–17]. Previously, hyaluronan was considered to turn over slowly and to be catabolized completely within the tissue. However, recent experiments show that the turnover of hyaluronan is rapid and that the catabolism also takes place outside the tissue, as discussed in detail in the chapter by Laurent elsewhere in this book [2,62]. In short, hyaluronan is removed from the tissue by the lymphatics [63–69] to become catabolized in lymph nodes [64,70] and liver endothelial cells [71].

Hyaluronan flux out of the tissue increases with increasing fluid flux through the interstitium (measured as lymph flow) [65–69,72–74] and the increased lymphatic removal of hyaluronan will imply an increased turnover rate of hyaluronan in the tissues. The importance of the lymphatic removal in catabolism of hyaluronan seems to differ between tissues. In skin about 5% of the total amount was drained by the lymphatics per day [66,69] and in the small intestine of rats as much as 50% was removed by the same pathway [73]; with the lung the level is in between these values [65,68,72]. The effect on the hyaluronan content of the tissue has only been studied in a few long-term experiments. In the lung Pou *et al.* [72] were able to drain 30% of the total hyaluronan each day over a period of one week. In short-term experiments in the intestine it has been possible to lower hyaluronan content to 40% of control in 4–6 h by applying increased venous pressure to raise interstitial fluid flux (measured as lymph flow) [67]. In the rat small intestine, approx. 50% of the hyaluronan is removed by the lymphatics in 24 h [73]. However, increasing the lymph flow and thereby the lymphatic flux of hyaluronan to twice normal levels over a period of several days in hypoproteinaemic rats did not alter the content of hyaluronan in the intestine [74]. Thus, in situations with increased interstitial fluid flux and hyaluronan removal, priority is seemingly given to raising synthesis and maintaining a constant amount of hyaluronan in the loose connective tissues, which would imply that the swelling properties, hydraulic conductivity and other interstitial transport properties of the tissues are kept constant.

Summary

This review has summarized our present knowledge of the role of P_{if} in fluid balance in loose connective tissues. P_{if} will normally act as a 'passive controller' to counteract changes in the interstitial fluid volume. In several acute inflammatory reactions P_{if} becomes more negative and will thereby enhance capillary fluid filtration and oedema formation. Thus, the loose connective tissues become 'active' participants in the transcapillary fluid exchange rather than 'passive' controllers of their interstitial fluid volume. The chain of events leading to increased negativity of P_{if} seems to involve the receptors towards structural connective-tissue components, the integrins, as well as connective-tissue cells.

References

1. Aukland, K. and Reed, R.K. (1993) Interstitial-lymphatic mechanisms in the control of extracellular fluid volume. *Physiol. Rev.* **73**, 1–78
2. Reed, R.K. and Laurent, U.B.G. (1992) Turnover of hyaluronan in the microcirculation. *Am. Rev. Respir. Dis.* **146**, S37–S39
3. Taylor, A.E. and Granger, D.N. (1984) Exchange of macromolecules across the capillary wall. In: *Handbook of Physiology. The Cardiovascular System. Microcirculation*. Section 2, vol. IV, pp. 467–520, Am. Physiol. Soc., Bethesda, MD
4. Guyton, A.C., Granger, H.J. and Taylor, A.E. (1971) Interstitial fluid pressure. *Physiol. Rev.* **51**, 527–563
5. Guyton, A.C. (1963) A concept of negative interstitial fluid pressures based on pressures measured in implanted perforated capsules. *Circ. Res.* **12**, 399–414
6. Aukland, K. and Nicolaysen, G. (1981) Interstitial fluid volume: Local regulatory mechanisms. *Physiol. Rev.* **61**, 556–643
7. Granger, H.J. and Taylor, A.E. (1975) Permeability of connective tissue linings isolated from implanted capsules. *Circ. Res.* **36**, 222–228
8. Scholander, P.R., Hargens, A.R. and Miller, S.L. (1968) Negative pressure in the interstitial fluid in animals. *Science* **161**, 321–328
9. Fadnes, H.O., Reed, R.K. and Aukland, K. (1977) Interstitial fluid pressure in rats measured with a modified wick technique. *Microvasc. Res.* **14**, 27–36
10. Wiig, H., Reed, R.K. and Aukland, K. (1981) Micropuncture measurement of interstitial fluid pressure in rat subcutis and skeletal muscle: Comparison to wick-in-needle technique. *Microvasc. Res.* **21**, 308–319
11. Wiig, H. (1985) Comparison of methods for measurement of interstitial fluid pressure in cat skin/subcutis and muscle. *Am. J. Physiol.* **249**, H929–H944
12. Wiig, H., Reed, R.K. and Aukland, K. (1985) Measurement of interstitial fluid pressure in dogs: Evaluation of methods. *Am. J. Physiol.* **253**, H283–H290
13. Ott, C.E., Navar, L.G. and Guyton, A.C. (1971) Pressures in static and dynamic states from capsules implanted in the kidney. *Am. J. Physiol.* **221**, 394–400
14. Wiig, H. (1990) Evaluation of methodologies for measurement of interstitial fluid pressure (P_i): physiological implications of recent P_i data. *Crit. Rev. Biomed. Eng.* **18**, 27–54
15. Meyer, F.A., Laver-Rudich, Z. and Tanenbaum, R. (1983) Evidence for a mechanical coupling of glycoprotein microfibrils with collagen fibrils in Wharton's jelly. *Biochim. Biophys. Acta* **755**, 376–387
16. Meyer, F.A. (1983) Macromolecular basis of globular protein exclusion and swelling pressure in loose connective tissue (umbilical cord). *Biochim. Biophys. Acta* **755**, 388–399
17. Meyer, F.A. (1986) Distribution and transport of fluid as related to tissue structure. In *Tissue Nutrition and Viability* (Hargens, A.R., ed.), pp. 25–46, Springer Verlag, New York
18. Ofstad, J. and Aukland, K. (1985) Renal circulation. In *The Kidney: Physiology and Pathophysiology* (Seldin, G.W. and Giebisch, G., eds.), pp. 471–496, Raven Press, New York
19. Reed, R.K. and Wiig, H. (1981) Compliance of the interstitial space in rats. I. Studies on skeletal

muscle. *Acta Physiol. Scand.* **113**, 297–305

20. Wiig, H. and Reed, R.K. (1981) Compliance of the interstitial space in rats. II. Studies on skin. *Acta Physiol. Scand.* **113**, 307–315
21. Wiig, H. and Reed, R.K. (1985) Interstitial compliance and transcapillary Starling pressures in cat skin and skeletal muscle. *Am. J. Physiol.* **248**, H666–H673
22. Wiig, H. and Reed, R.K. (1985) Volume-pressure relationship (compliance) of interstitium in dog skin and muscle. *Am. J. Physiol.* **253**, H291–H298
23. Michel, C.C. (1984) Fluid movement through capillary walls. In: *Handbook of Physiology. The Cardiovascular System. Microcirculation.* Section 2, vol. IV, pp. 375–409, Am. Physiol. Soc., Bethesda, MD
24. Aukland, K. (1987) Interstitial fluid balance in experimental animals and man. *Adv. Microcirc.* **13**, 110–123
25. Schmid-Schoenbein, G. (1990) Microlymphatics and lymph flow. *Physiol. Rev.* **70**, 987–1028
26. Hogan, R.D. (1981) The initial lymphatics and interstitial fluid pressure. In *Tissue Fluid and Composition* (Hargens, A.R., ed.), pp. 155–163, Academic Press, Baltimore
27. Hogan, R.D. and Unthank, J.L. (1986) The initial lymphatics as sensors of interstitial fluid volume. *Microvasc. Res.* **31**, 317–324
28. Lund, T., Wiig, H. and Reed, R.K. (1988) Acute postburn edema: role of strongly negative interstitial fluid pressure. *Am. J. Physiol.* **255**, H1069–H1074
29. Lund, T., Onarheim, H., Wiig, H. and Reed, R.K. (1989) Mechanisms behind increased dermal imbibition pressure in acute burn edema. *Am. J. Physiol.* **256**, H940–H948
30. Artursson, G. and Mellander, S. (1964) Acute changes in capillary filtration and diffusion in experimental burn injury. *Acta Physiol. Scand.* **62**, 457–463
31. Pitt, R.M., Parker, J.C., Jurkovich, G., Taylor, A.E. and Curreri, P.W. (1987) Analysis of altered capillary pressure and permeability after thermal injury. *J. Surg. Res.* **42**, 693–702
32. Dyess, D.L., Ardell, J.L., Townsley, M.I., Taylor, A.E. and Ferrara, J.J. (1992) Effects of hypertonic saline and Dextran 70 rescucitation on microvascular permeability after burn. *Am. J. Physiol.* **262**, H1832–H1837
33. Korthuis, R.J., Wang, C.Y. and Scott, J.B. (1982) Transient effects of histamine on microvascular fluid movement. *Microvasc. Res.* **23**, 316–328
34. Movat, H.Z. (1985) *The Inflammatory Reaction*, p. 365, Elsevier Publishing, Amsterdam
35. Rodt, S.Å., Wiig, H. and Reed, R.K. (1990) Increased negativity of interstitial fluid pressure contributes to development of oedema in rat skin following application of xylene. *Acta Physiol. Scand.* **140**, 581–586
36. Rodt, S.Å. and Reed, R.K. (1993) Interstitial fluid pressure in rat skin becomes more negative in the initial phase of carrageenan-induced edema. *Int. J. Microcirc. Clin. Exp.* **12**, 299–312
37. Østgaard, G. and Reed, R.K. (1993) Increased negativity of interstitial fluid pressure in rat skin contributes to edema formation induced by Zymosan. *Microvasc. Res.* **46**, 283–292
38. Reed, R.K. and Rodt, S.Å. (1991) Increased negativity of interstitial fluid pressure during the onset stage of inflammatory edema in rat skin. *Am. J. Physiol.* **260**, H1985–H1991
39. Koller, M.-E. and Reed, R.K. (1992) Increased negativity of interstitial fluid pressure in rat trachea in dextran anaphylaxis. *J. Appl. Physiol.* **72**, 53–57
40. Koller, M.-E., Woie, K. and Reed, R.K. (1993) Increased negativity of interstitial fluid pressure (P$_i$) in trachea after mast cell degranulation. *J. Appl. Physiol.* **74**, 2135–2139
41. Lundberg, J.M., Brodin, E., Hua, X. and Saria, A. (1984) Vascular permeability changes and smooth muscle contraction in relation to capsaicin-sensitive substance P afferents in the guinea pig. *Acta Physiol. Scand.* **120**, 217–227
42. Lundberg, J.M. and Saria, A. (1982) Capsaicin-sensitive vagal neurons involved in control of vascular permeability in rat trachea. *Acta Physiol. Scand.* **115**, 521–523
43. Woie, K., Koller, M.-E., Heyeraas, K. and Reed, R.K. (1993) Neurogenic inflammation in rat trachea is accompanied by increased negativity of interstitial fluid pressure. *Circ. Res.* **73**, 839–845
44. Hemler, M.E. (1990) VLA proteins in the integrin family: structures, functions, and their role on leukocytes. *Annu. Rev. Immunol.* **8**, 365–400
45. Springer, T.A. (1991) Adhesion receptors of the immune system. *Nature (London)* **346**, 425–434
46. Hynes, R.O. (1992) Integrins: Versatility, modulation and signalling in cell adhesion. *Cell* **69**, 11–25
47. Rouslahti, E. (1991) Integrins. *J. Clin. Invest.* **87**, 1–5
48. Rubin, K., Åhlen, K., Sundberg, C. and Reed, R.K. (1994) Integrins: transmembrane links between the extracellular matrix and cell interior. In *Interstitium, Connective Tissue and Lymphatics* (Reed, R., McHale, N., Bert, J., Winlove, P. and Laine, G., eds.), pp. 29–40, Portland Press, London
49. Reed, R.K., Rubin, K., Wiig, H. and Rodt, S.Å. (1992) Blockade of β$_1$-Integrins in skin causes edema through lowering of interstitial fluid pressure. *Circ. Res.* **71**, 978–983
50. Gullberg, D., Tingström, A., Thuresson, A.-C., Olsson, L., Terracio, L., Borg, T.K. and Rubin, K. (1990) β$_1$ Integrin-mediated collagen gel contraction is stimulated by PDGF. *Exp. Cell. Res.* **186**, 264–272
51. Bell, E., Ivarsson, B. and Merrill, C. (1979) Production of a tissue-like structure by contraction of collagen lattices by human fibroblasts of different proliferative potential in vitro. *Proc. Natl. Acad. Sci. U.S.A.* **76**, 1274–1278
52. Guidry, C. and Grinnell, F. (1985) Studies on the mechanism of hydrated collagen gel reorganization by human skin fibroblasts. *J. Cell Sci.* **79**, 67–81
53. Rodt, S.Å., Reed, R.K., Ljungström, M., Gustafsson, T. and Rubin, K. (1994) The

anti-inflammatory agent α-trinositol exerts its edema preventing effect through modulation of β_1 integrin function. *Circ. Res.* **75**, 942–948

54. Rotschild, A.M., Gomes, E.L.T. and Rossi, M.A. (1991) Reversible rat mesenteric mast cell swelling caused by vagal stimulation or sham-feeding. *Agents Actions* **34**, 295–301

55. Kierman, J.A. (1990) Degranulation of mast cells in the trachea and bronchi of the rat following stimulation of the vagus nerve. *Int. Arch. Allergy Appl. Immunol.* **91**, 398–402

56. Stead, R.H. and Bienenstock, J. (1990) Cellular interactions between the immune system and mast cells. In *Cell to Cell Interaction* (Burger, M.M., Sordat, B. and Zinkernagel, R.M., eds.), pp. 170–187, Karger, Basel

57. Schultheiss, H. and Hörig, J. (1985) Histamine release from rat peritoneal cells by substance P antagonists and fragments - A study of structure activity relationship. In *Tachykinin Antagonists* (Hükanson, R. and Sundler, F., eds.), pp. 413–420, Elsevier, Amsterdam

58. Fantozzi, R., Masini, E., Blandina, P., Mannaioni, P.F. and Bani-Sacchi, T. (1978) Release of histamine from rat mast cells by acetylcholine. *Nature (London)* **273**, 473–474

59. Bienenstock, J., MacQueen, G., Sestibi, P., Marshall, J.S., Stead, R.H. and Perdue, M.H. (1991) Mast cell/nerve interactions *in vitro* and *in vivo*. *Am. Rev. Respir. Dis.* **143**, S55–S58

60. Ferrante, F., Ricci, A., Cavalotti, C. and Amenta, A. (1990) Suggestive evidence for a functional association between mast cells and sympathetic nerves in meningeal membranes. *Acta Histochem. Cytochem.* **23**, 637–646

61. Nilsson, G., Alving, K., Ahlstedt, S., Hökfelt, T. and Lundberg, J.M. (1990) Peptidergic innervation of rat lymphoid tissue and lung: Relation to mast cells and sensitivity to capsaicin and immunization. *Cell Tissue Res.* **262**, 125–133

62. Laurent, T.C. (1994) Structure of the extracellular matrix. In *Interstitium, Connective Tissue and Lymphatics* (Reed, R., McHale, N., Bert, J., Winlove, P. and Laine, G., eds.), pp. 1–12, Portland Press, London

63. Laurent, U.B.G. and Laurent, T.C. (1981) On the origin of hyaluronate in blood. *Biochem. Int.* **2**, 195–199

64. Fraser, J.R.E., Kimpton, W.G., Laurent, T.C., Cahill, R.N.P. and Vakakis, N. (1988) Uptake and degradation of hyaluronan in lymphatic tissue. *Biochem. J.* **256**, 153–158

65. Lebel, L., Smith, L., Risberg, B., Gerdin, B. and Laurent, T.C. (1988) Effect of increased hydrostatic pressure on lymphatic elimination of hyaluronan from sheep lung. *J. Appl. Physiol.* **64**, 1327–1332

66. Reed, R.K., Laurent, T.C. and Taylor, A.E. (1990) Hyaluronan in prenodal lymph from skin: changes with lymph flow. *Am. J. Physiol.* **259**, H1097–H1100

67. Reed, R.K., Townsley, M.I., Laurent, T.C. and Taylor, A.E. (1992) Hyaluronan flux from cat intestine: changes with lymph flow. *Am. J. Physiol.* **262**, H457–H462

68. Townsley, M.I., Reed, R.K., Ishibashi, M., Parker, J.C., Laurent, T.C. and Taylor A.E. (1995) Hyaluronan efflux from canine lung with increased hydrostatic pressure and saline loading. *Am. J. Respir. Crit. Care Med.*, **150**, 1605–1611

69. Reed, R.K., Townsley, M.I., Zhao, Z., Ishibashi, M., Laurent, T.C. and Taylor, A.E. (1994) Lymphatic hyaluronan from skin increases during increased lymph flow induced by intravenous saline loading. *Int. J. Microcirc.* **14**, 56–61

70. Laurent, U.B.G., Dahl, L.B. and Reed, R.K. (1991) Catabolism of hyaluronan in rabbit skin takes place locally, in lymph nodes and liver. *Exp. Physiol.* **76**, 695–703

71. Smedsrød, B., Pertoft, H., Eriksson, S., Fraser, J.R.E. and Laurent, T.C. (1984) Studies *in vitro* on the uptake and degradation of sodium hyaluronate in rat liver endothelial cells. *Biochem. J.* **223**, 617–626

72. Pou, N.A., King, G., Atchley, P.C., Conary, J.T., Parker, R.E. and Roselli, R.J. (1992) Lymphatic clearance of hyaluronan (HA) increases during and after pulmonary air embolism in sheep. *FASEB J.* **6**, A1533

73. Østgaard, G. and Reed, R.K. (1993) Hyaluronan turnover in the rat small intestine. *Acta Physiol. Scand.* **149**, 237–244

74. Østgaard, G. and Reed, R.K. (1994) Increased lymphatic hyaluronan output and preserved hyaluronan content of the rat small intestine in prolonged hypoproteinemia. *Acta Physiol. Scand.* **H152**, 51–56

8

Interstitial fluid transport

Joel L. Bert* and Mark Martinez
Department of Chemical Engineering, University of British Columbia,
2216 Main Mall, Vancouver, BC, V6T 1Z4, Canada

Introduction

The interstitium (i.e. the extravascular and extracellular connective tissue space) is a porous medium comprised of cellular, fibrous and gel-like materials organized into a complex heterogeneous architecture. Historically, the interstitium has been considered to behave as a homogeneous medium. Although this simplified description does not consider the heterogeneous nature of tissue architecture, a significant number of useful applications have resulted.

This chapter will review and discuss descriptions of interstitial transport. After a review of phenomenological relationships such as Darcy's law and the Debye–Brinkman equation, more fundamental fluid mechanics and novel network models are presented. Speculations about the nature and usefulness of these approaches to describe connective tissue interstitial transport are offered throughout this chapter.

Phenomenological relationships

Darcy's law

Darcy related the volumetric flow rate, Q, of a fluid flowing through a porous medium of cross-sectional area A, directly to the energy loss in the form of a pressure drop, ΔP, inversely to the length, L, of the medium and proportional to a factor called the hydraulic conductivity, K [1].

Darcy's law (as reviewed in Greenkorn [1]) when expressed as:

$$Q = KA \frac{\Delta P}{L} \tag{1}$$

is empirical in that it is not derived from first principles but rather resulted from experimental observation. Although Darcy's law is

*To whom correspondence should be addressed.
Nomenclature: A, cross-sectional area of porous medium (m^2); c, constant of proportionality (dimensionless); D_p, diameter of a particle in the porous medium (m); F, body force (N); H, hydration of the tissue (mass of fluid/mass of tissue); k, intrinsic permeability (m^2); K, hydraulic conductivity (m$^3 \cdot$s$\cdot$kg^{-1}); L, length of porous medium (m); P, pressure (Pa); p, probability of a conduit or junction being open (dimensionless); p_c, critical probability for which there is no flow through the porous media (dimensionless); Q, volumetric flow rate through the porous medium (m^3/s); r, radius of the cylindrical conduit (m); r_h, equivalent hydraulic radius (m); Re_p, Reynolds number (dimensionless); S_o, specific surface area of the solid in contact with the fluid (m^{-1}); u, fluid velocity (m/s); ε, porosity (dimensionless); Θ, Kozeny constant (dimensionless); μ, viscosity of the fluid (Pa$\cdot$s); ρ_f, density of the fluid (kg/m^3).

empirical, DeWiest [2] has demonstrated that it is a limiting form of the rigorous equations of motion of a fluid (i.e. the Navier–Stokes equations) which will be discussed later. Darcy's law is usually considered valid for creeping flow where the Reynolds number (Re_p, a dimensionless parameter which describes the ratio of inertial to viscous forces):

$$Re_p = \frac{\rho_f D_p u}{\mu} \tag{2}$$

is less than about unity [1]. Eqn. (2) is based on a characteristic diameter of a fibre in the medium, D_p, while ρ_f and μ are the density and viscosity of the fluid. The superficial velocity, u, defined by Q/A, is not the actual fluid velocity that exists within the medium but rather an average across the entire cross-sectional area. For flow in the interstitium, one may anticipate that Re_p will be significantly less than unity for all but the most extreme conditions.

The hydraulic conductivity, K, defined by Darcy's law is dependent on the properties of the fluid, as well as on the architecture (pore structure) of the medium. The hydraulic conductivity can be written in terms of the intrinsic permeability (k) which is based only on architecture, and the properties of the fluid as follows:

$$K = \frac{k}{\mu} \tag{3}$$

Darcy's law can also be written in differential form (i.e. at a point in space), so that in one dimension:

$$\frac{Q}{A} = u = -\frac{k}{\mu}\frac{dP}{dx} \tag{4}$$

The minus sign results from the definition of ΔP in eqn. (1), which is in the opposite sense of dP [1]. Porous media, which are characterized by eqn. (4), contain both a solid phase and a fluid phase. Continuous fluid pathways exist through these materials and the relative distribution of fluid and solid volume is referred to as porosity (ε=fluid volume/total volume). For a simplistic use of Darcy's law, k/μ is assumed to be constant throughout the medium and a property of both the medium and the fluid.

Determination of k/μ

Hydraulic conductivity is usually determined experimentally by passing a known volume of fluid through a porous medium of known length and cross-sectional area. For a given pressure drop, the hydraulic conductivity (an overall value for the system) can be calculated from eqn. (1). By use of this equation it is assumed that the fluid does not influence the arrangement of solid materials in the porous medium (i.e. the interstitium is non-deformable).

In a review by Levick [3], a comprehensive summary of flow conductivities is presented for a number of connective tissues. Little new information has been reported since the review by Levick [3]. Lai Fook and his group [4] have measured the flow conductivity of pulmonary interstitia and our group is currently investigating specific aspects of the flow resistance of dermis.

Clearly, hydraulic conductivity, k/μ, depends on interstitial composition and architecture. Levick [3] has reviewed the contribution to hydraulic conductivity of the non-interacting interstitial components (i.e. collagen, glycosaminoglycans, proteoglycans, etc.) which were assumed to have a superimposing effect. That is, if one component is removed, the remaining materials maintain their relative configuration. At the very least, and as discussed by Levick [3], the materials which comprise the interstitium will exclude each other and create local regions of increased concentration (i.e. compared with their apparent concentration).

Hierarchical organization among tissue components and large-scale tissue heterogeneities must also be considered. Materials such as collagenous and elastin fibres, hyaluronan and glycosaminoglycans can be arranged in a number of different architectures which would affect the hydraulic conductivity of the tissue. As an example, collagen can exist in interstitia in a number of geometrical configurations ranging from molecular structures of the order of nanometres, to fibrillar structures as large as hundreds of micrometres. With regard to tissue heterogeneities, the possibility that 'dead end' fluid volumes or 'free fluid channels' may exist within interstitia cannot be discounted.

Additionally, mobile plasma proteins may also contribute to flow resistance [5] based on the differential velocities with which fluid and mobile proteins move through the interstitium. With limited information about tissue organization, the prediction of k/μ based on apparent tissue content must be considered speculative. However, as demonstrated in other contributions to this volume, our knowledge of the organization and structure of interstitia is improving.

From a practical view, it has nonetheless proven useful to assume that k/μ can be expressed in terms of the apparent concentration of tissue components [3]. Alternatively, one can relate k/μ to the fluid content in a tissue as follows:

$$\frac{k}{\mu} = aH^b \tag{5}$$

where a and b are constants, and H is the hydration of the tissue (mass of fluid/mass of dry tissue). This 'power law' relationship between conductivity and porosity (i.e. hydration is a measure of porosity) is well rooted in the empirical scientific literature. Analogous quantitative relationships, sometimes referred to as Archie's law [6], exist for both heat and electrical conduction. However, this formulation does not yield any insight by itself into the architecture and organization of the interstitium.

Along with experimental considerations and empiricism, there have been theoretical approaches to determining relationships between properties of a porous medium, such as porosity, and hydraulic conductivity. In general the theoretical models can be categorized by two fundamentally different approaches. In the first approach, flow is assumed to occur through the medium in a series of continuous channels. The most popular example of this approach is the fibre matrix theory which yields the familiar Kozeny–Carman equation. In other descriptions of hydraulic conductivity, flow is assumed to occur around solid objects which comprise the porous medium. The particles, fibres, or other structures which form the solid phase of the porous medium dissipate energy as a result of viscous drag forces; this approach is referred to as the drag theory. These approaches are dealt with separately below.

Fibre matrix theory

The application of what is now referred to as the fibre matrix theory to describe the resistance of interstitia to fluid flow began with the work of Curry and Michel [7]. This approach has a strong historical background in relation to flow through other porous media; for example, various forms of filtration and groundwater flows.

In the fibre matrix theory the interstitium is treated as a porous medium idealized as a series of pores which are connected in order to form hypothetical conduits. The cross-section of the conduit may have an extremely complicated shape and a tortuous pathlength but, on average, a constant area. The channels are assumed to be distributed randomly throughout the medium and are considered to be reasonably uniform in size. Through a dimensional analysis it is reasoned that since intrinsic permeability (k) has the dimensions of length squared, it can be related to a characteristic property of the medium with the same dimension, such as the 'equivalent hydraulic radius' of a hypothetical channel (r_h) [8]. A possible measure of r_h would be the ratio of volume of the channel to its surface area. This leads to an expression for hydraulic conductivity of the general form [8]:

$$\frac{k}{\mu} = c \, \frac{r_h^2}{\mu f(\varepsilon)} \tag{6}$$

where $f(\varepsilon)$ is a porosity function; and c is a dimensionless constant. The problem at hand is to give c and $f(\varepsilon)$ physical significance and quantifiable characteristics, if possible. One cannot infer any information about the actual pore structure of the interstitium based upon the concept of equivalent hydraulic radius.

The Kozeny theory represents the most widely accepted explanation of c and $f(\varepsilon)$ [8]. A Hagen–Poiseuille-type equation is used for all channels passing through a cross-section normal to the flow in the porous medium and gives the average pore velocity in the pathways. Additionally, the tortuosity of the pathways is considered statistically and is related to physical properties of the medium such as porosity (ε) and specific surface area of the solid in contact with the fluid (S_o). Finally, hydraulic conductivity (K) is expressed as:

$$K = \frac{k}{\mu} = \frac{\varepsilon^3}{\Theta S_o^2 (1-\varepsilon)^2 \mu} \tag{7}$$

The constant Θ is the Kozeny constant which depends on ε and is usually assigned the value of 5 when $\varepsilon < 0.9$; most physiological tissues fall within this range.

It is difficult to estimate adequately the value of S_o in interstitia. For a simple structure such as a periodic array of collagen fibres of radius r with porosity ε, S_o is clearly defined, i.e.:

$$S_o = \frac{\text{surface area of a fibre}}{\text{volume of a fibre}} = \frac{2}{r} \tag{8}$$

However, if the collagenous material is organized in a random hierarchial structure, then the value of S_o depends very strongly on the geometric relationship and size of the fibres. If several small fibres organize to form a larger fibre (which may contain some fibrillar fluid), then the value of S_o will decrease because the larger 'unit', which contains the same amount of fibrous material, is the apparent structure which resists flow. The situation becomes more complex when one considers the potential for interaction and organization of other materials which comprise the interstitial space.

Drag theory

Another approach to the physical explanation of permeability, different from that by Kozeny, is called the 'drag theory'. In it, the solids are treated as obstacles to the otherwise straight flow through the porous medium. The particles, fibres, or other structures which form the solid phase of the porous medium dissipate energy as a result of viscous drag acting on their surface. The drag of the fluid on a solid surface is estimated from the Navier–Stokes equation (the general equation for flow which will be described later), and the sum of all the drag in the medium is equal to flow resistance (i.e. μ/k). As a specific example, for the case of a random distribution of circular cylindrical fibres of uniform diameter, D_p, the hydraulic conductivity is given by eqn. (9) [8]:

$$K = \frac{k}{\mu} = \frac{3}{16} \left[\frac{2 - \ln(Re)}{4 - \ln(Re)} \right] \frac{\varepsilon D_p^{\,2}}{\mu(1 - \varepsilon)} \tag{9}$$

This approach is different from the Kozeny–Carman formulation, yet the final expression for hydraulic conductivity is of the general form similar to that given in eqn. (6); that is, k/μ is related to a length dimension squared $(D_p^{\,2})$, a porosity function $[f(\varepsilon) = (1 - \varepsilon)/\varepsilon]$, and a constant $\{c = 3[2 - \ln(Re)]/16[4 - \ln(Re)]\}$. For the drag theory model of eqn. (9), the constant c is a weak function of Re for creeping flow. This is in contrast with the Kozeny–Carman formulation in which the constant of proportionality is independent of velocity.

Length scale in a porous medium

Unfortunately, the main problem inherent in using the empirical and theoretical approaches given above in eqns. (7) and (9) is that the required parameters are bulk (i.e. overall) properties and apply to a length scale within the medium that contains enough solid elements to yield an average hydraulic flow conductivity. As an example of the effect of scale, consider the porous medium as shown in Figure 1, which has been divided into four representative elemental volumes. Each elemental volume (referred to hereafter as a slice) in the two-dimensional representation is comprised of the same quantity of rod and randomly coiled material which may represent schematically collagen fibres and hyaluronan respectively. For this scale, therefore, all slices have the same porosity. If we choose to investigate any slice of this material at a smaller length scale, then slices 1 and 3 would be reasonably uniform, but the other slices would be heterogeneous (note the space which contains no solids in the central part of slice 4). At a still much reduced size scale, portions within all of the slices would display different porosities. Consider the hydraulic conductivity for each slice. If hydraulic conductivity is measured for the horizontal plane, then slices 1, 2 and 3 would have similar values. In comparison, slice 4 would have a much higher hydraulic conductivity as a result of the free fluid channel through the middle of the tissue slice. Intuitively, it is apparent that collagenous fibres which are well organized into larger structures, as in slices 2 and 4, offer less resistance to flow then a similar amount of the unorganized smaller fibres. This would be reflected in the Kozeny–Carman formulation in the specific surface area term S_o. For organized structures, S_o would be much less than for an equivalent amount of randomly distributed material [see eqn. (8)]. Since k/μ is inversely proportional to S_o^2 [see eqn. (7)], the organized fibre arrangement would have a much higher value of conductivity than the random array.

The issue of scale and of heterogeneity may be important both on the gross and on the fine level of interstitial organization. These considerations influence the description of flow, and limit the usefulness of characterizing flow resistance of interstitia to an appropriate length scale.

Figure 1

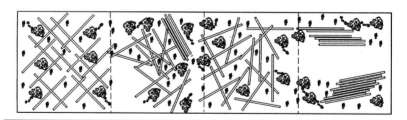

Scale, heterogeneity and k/μ in interstitia

A schematic of the interstitium is shown subdivided into four slices. The rods may represent collagenous fibres while the two sizes of random coils may represent hyaluronan or proteoglycans. The amount of both the rods and coils is the same in each slice. Therefore, the porosity of each slice is equivalent. On a smaller-length scale (i.e. compared with the length scale of each slice) local porosities within each slice may be very different. The organization of individual collagenous fibres into bundles has a strong impact on both local porosity and resistance to flow across the slices in the horizontal direction. The flow conductivities in slices 1–3 may be similar but that of slice 4 will be much greater due to heterogeneity.

Both the fibre matrix and the drag theories of tissue resistivity highlight the very strong dependence of hydraulic conductivity on porosity. An important implication of this occurs during mechanical or flow-induced compression or 'compaction' of tissues.

Effect of compaction on k/μ

Consider the simple experimental arrangement shown schematically in Figure 2. Under the conditions shown, a disc of tissue is supported by

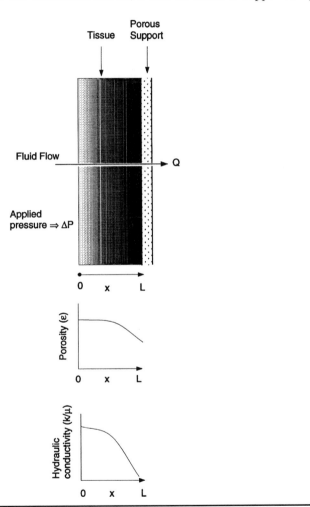

Figure 2

Flow-induced interstitial compaction

The upper part of this schematic depicts the steady-state flow, Q, through a tissue of thickness L, which is held by a porous support. The pressure in the upstream fluid is greater than the downstream condition by ΔP. The tissue is compacted in the direction of flow due to the applied pressure. Consequently, the porosity of the tissue decreases in the direction of flow. The hydraulic conductivity, which may be a strong function of porosity, also decreases in the direction of flow and a considerable fraction of the overall resistance may reside in a narrow band of tissue adjacent to the porous support.

a rigid support and fluid is forced through the tissue under an external pressure head. For a compliant tissue, the fluid content at each point in the tissue in the direction of flow is determined by the upstream cumulative pressure drop through the tissue. The interstitial fluid pressure, defined in the absence of mechanical or flow-induced constraints, is an inverse measure of the ability of the tissue to imbibe fluid relative to the fully swollen standard condition. For the flow conditions described in Figure 2, the flow-induced force supported by the tissue increases in the direction of flow. The tissue at the interface of the porous structure, which holds the tissue in place, supports the full pressure drop across the tissue. At this position the tissue fluid content corresponds to tissue pressure–volume characteristics of the total pressure drop; therefore, the tissue is in a relatively dehydrated state compared with equilibrium with the bathing fluid. If the upstream pressure driving force is removed, the tissue at the porous support will tend to imbibe fluid and return to its equilibrium condition. Tissue rehydration will also occur throughout the tissue proportional to the distance from the tissue–fluid interface. Therefore, under conditions of flow there will be a gradient in tissue fluid content which decreases from the fluid–tissue interface to the tissue–support interface. This condition is the phenomenon known as compaction, which results from the fact that tissues are deformable materials. Concomitant, and determined by the fluid content gradient (i.e. a porosity gradient), is a gradient in k/μ. Under conditions shown in Figure 2, division of the steady-state flow rate across the tissue by the overall driving force yields a space-averaged value of k/μ. At steady state for one dimension, the flow rate through the tissue is constant and Darcy's law applies. Since the fluid content varies through the tissue, so does k/μ. Therefore, an integrated form of Darcy's law, using a relationship such as eqn. (5), in conjunction with knowledge of how interstitial fluid pressure varies with porosity, could be used to describe the average k/μ. Substantial errors in the determination of k/μ as a function of fluid content can result if compaction is not considered but only space-averaged values of k/μ are measured. A significant amount of work describing the flow-dependent or mechanically induced deformation has been reported for materials such as cartilage [9,10] and corneal stroma (see the review of Fatt and Weissman [11]). For the case of cartilage, deformation in response to mechanical loading and the fluid exchange that accompanies it play an important role in the physiology of this tissue. Unfortunately, very few data of this type are available for other deformable connective tissues.

Debye–Brinkman equation

Darcy's law is restricted to uniform velocities throughout the fluid phase. In order to account for the fact that solid surfaces impede fluid motion through viscous effects, the Debye–Brinkman equation was developed. A typical boundary condition employed when describing flow over a solid surface is called the 'no-slip' condition (i.e. the fluid velocity is zero at the solid's surface). In the direction away from the solid surface the fluid velocity increases until, if no other impediments to motion are present, a uniform free stream velocity is attained. For a porous medium, this description of flow where solids may interact and influence the velocity profiles of the fluid is clearly much more complex than that considered by Darcy's law. In the Debye–Brinkman equation, viscosity effects due to flow over solid objects are considered.

The first stage in the description of fluid flow for this analysis is an accounting of the mass of fluid to be investigated. For an incompressible fluid (i.e. interstitial fluid under physiological conditions can be considered to be incompressible), conservation of mass is expressed in vector notation as follows:

$$\nabla \cdot \hat{u} = 0 \tag{10}$$

where $\hat{u}$ represents the actual fluid velocity. The above equation is referred to as the 'continuity equation' and states that all volumetric flow into a control volume of space also leaves that volume.

The second stage of the model formulation of the Debye–Brinkman equation involves a description of energy dissipation in the fluid. This equation is empirical and states that energy dissipation resulting from a pressure drop through a porous medium is converted into a bulk stress which goes into velocity, and viscous dissipation as follows:

$$\nabla P = -\frac{\mu}{k} u + \mu \nabla^2 u \tag{11}$$

The third term in the equation represents the viscous drag. Clearly, by neglecting viscous drag this equation reduces to Darcy's law.

A significant complication in the application of the Debye–Brinkman equation as compared with Darcy's law is that the architecture of the porous medium must be defined clearly. As stated previously, the specific architecture of connective tissue interstitia is generally not well defined, so that application of the Debye–Brinkman equation to interstitia is likewise limited. When the Debye–Brinkman equation is solved for the specific architecture and boundary conditions, the results are in the form of a pressure field and velocity field within the continuous (fluid) phase. Velocities across any plane can be integrated to yield a flow rate through the tissue. This flow rate could be used in Darcy's law with the pressure difference and tissue area to derive an equivalent hydraulic conductivity for the interstitium.

As an example of the use of the Debye–Brinkman equation, Ethier [12] considered an interstitium-type material comprised of two dramatically differently sized materials as shown in Figure 3 (which is a representation of the system that he studied). The randomly distributed smaller solids in this figure may correspond to hyaluronan and proteoglycans while the periodically arranged larger rods could be representative of collagenous fibres. The radii of these materials are different by orders of magnitude. Therefore, the composite system could be considered as one with larger fibres embedded in a matrix which has properties of the smaller solids distributed uniformly in the continuous fluid phase. This is an example of length-scale considerations. That is, the scale of the two sizes of fibres as discussed by Ethier [12] allows for the assumption that the coarse fibres appear to be embedded in a uniform material whose conductivity can be described based upon the

Figure 3

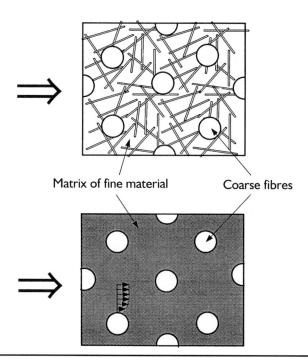

Matrix of fine material   Coarse fibres

Flow through a composite medium
The upper portion of this schematic depicts an interstitium comprised of small-diameter rods randomly oriented and large-diameter rods which are ordered in a dimension perpendicular to the page. Fluid flows through this fibrous arrangement in the direction of the arrow. This representation is an adaptation of the system considered by Ethier [12]. Based on scale considerations, flow through this system can be considered to occur around an ordered array of coarse fibres embedded in a continuum of material whose properties can be related to the concentration of the smaller fibrous rods. This is depicted in the lower figure. A typical fluid velocity profile is shown for the region near one of the large fibres in the lower portion of the figure. Ethier [12] analysed the flow resistance of this system by application of the Debye–Brinkman equation.

concentration of the finer fibres. Ethier [12] concludes that the viscous effects as accounted for in the Debye–Brinkman equation are significant for the range of parameters investigated, which include typical interstitia. This conclusion questions the utility of Darcy's law for describing flow in interstitia.

From the work of Ethier [12] it is apparent that a number of parameters are required to characterize the system that he studied. These include: the size, spacing and organization of the larger fibres; and the size and concentration of smaller fibres. Simplifying assumptions concerning these parameters are invoked in order to describe interstitia in the absence of morphological information. Even with the aid of the simplifying assumption, the solution of the Debye–Brinkman equation is much more complex than for Darcy's law. If a sensitivity analysis is performed in order to assess the relative impact of changing the various parameters, then the computational intensity increases as well.

Navier–Stokes equation

The Navier–Stokes equation, which is applied along with the continuity equation, is a general formulation which describes the motion of a fluid; it is based upon a 'force balance'. For a fluid with constant viscosity and density, the Navier–Stokes equation in a porous medium is:

$$\nabla \cdot \hat{u}\hat{u} = -\frac{1}{\rho}\nabla P + \frac{\mu}{\rho}\nabla^2 \hat{u} + F \qquad (12)$$

The first term in the equation represents the contribution of inertial forces on transport; the second term, the effect of pressure dissipation; the third term, the effect of shear stress (i.e. viscous forces); and the fourth term, the effect of body forces, such as gravity. For creeping flow in interstitia it is generally accepted that inertial forces are insignificant in comparison with the pressure and viscosity forces. Likewise, changes in gravitational effects are assumed to be insignificant in the systems of interest in this work. Therefore, the Navier–Stokes equation can be reduced to a simpler form referred to as the 'Stokes' equation:

$$\nabla P = \mu\nabla^2 \hat{u} \qquad (13)$$

Clearly, the Debye–Brinkman equation, eqn. (11), reduces to the Stokes equation for example when k is very large. Tsay and Weinbaum [13] have solved eqn. (13) in conjunction with the continuity equation, eqn. (10), for periodic arrays of fibres between parallel planes. In their work they investigated the impact of clefts between endothelial cells which contain a glycocalyx and the effect of this material on transcapillary movement of fluid and macromolecules. While the work of Weinbaum and colleagues has focused on the endothelial junction, their work can be generalized to interstitia. The solution of the above equations with appropriate boundary conditions yields a velocity distribution throughout the bounded network under consideration from which the flow as a function of driving forces can be investigated. The complexity involved in setting up and solving the basic fluid mechanics equations, with reasonable simplifying assumptions, can be estimated to be orders of magnitude greater than for the phenomenologically based models.

As a simplification, Tsay and Weinbaum [13] have also used the Debye–Brinkman equation (with the conductivity of the medium determined by the fibres in the cleft, bounded by the close parallel walls of the cells) to simulate results for the same system. For the cross-bridging fibres in the clefts, the results for both types of fluid flow formulations (i.e. Stokes versus the Debye–Brinkman functions) compare favourably with regard to prediction of hydraulic conductivity. There are a considerable number of adjustable parameters in their models and a paucity of specific information about the properties of these clefts. Also, there are a significant number of assumptions which have been invoked in order to develop mathematical descriptions which are both reasonable and tractable mathematically. One such assumption is that the fibres which confer resistance in the cleft are arranged periodically (i.e. ordered packing exists). A similar assumption of periodicity was used by Ethier [12] in his work, which was more directly analogous to interstitia. In a recent theoretical analysis comparing pressure drops and volumetric flow in packed fibrous beds which are slightly perturbed from ordered arrays, it was concluded that significant differences resulted due to channelling of fluid flow through the slightly higher porosity regions [14]. This result, even though the analysis was carried out for a scale of porous medium (i.e. hollow fibres surrounded by fluid) much greater than that typical of an interstitium, questions the validity of the results for fluid flow through assumed ordered arrays of fibres. Nonetheless, the approaches taken by Weinbaum and his colleagues [13] and by Ethier [12] are powerful tools, which may serve as a model for further studies on interstitial exchange.

Network models

Conduit networks

A completely different way to investigate flow in porous media is through network modelling. In this approach, the flow of fluid in the porous medium occurs in an interconnected lattice of pores and capillaries. Network models have made significant impact in many fields, most notably soil science and reservoir theory. The network junctions can have an irregular lattice and the capillary segments which connect these can be distributed over the network in any particular fashion. In Figure 4 several different qualitative networks are shown. The conducting pathways can consist of one size of uniform conduits, or multi-sized conduits. The conduits may be in parallel or connected in any manner to form an internally conductive pathway. Although these models represent a dramatic simplification from reality, networks are useful because analytical solutions can often be derived for them.

In Figure 5, two nodes or junctions of a network within a porous medium are shown. The steady-state flows into and out of these junctions (Q_{ij} represents the flow from junction i to junction j) are shown along with the driving pressures at each junction. If the length (L_{ij}) and the radius of each cylindrical conduit (r_{ij}) between each junction is known, then the flow (neglecting entrance and exit effects) can be determined based upon the Hagen–Poiseuille equation:

$$Q_{ij} = \frac{\pi r_{ij}^4}{8\mu} \frac{\Delta P_{ij}}{L_{ij}} = K_{ij} \frac{\Delta P_{ij}}{L_{ij}} \tag{14}$$

At each node conservation of mass exists (inputs=outputs). Equations can be written for each node in terms of the dimensions of the conduits and the upstream and downstream pressures. At the boundaries of the tissue, constant pressure conditions exist. Therefore, when all of the equations are solved simultaneously, the pressure field in the porous medium (the pressure at the junctions) will be determined and all of the flows can be evaluated. The overall hydraulic conductivity of the medium

Figure 4

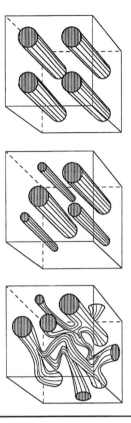

Networks for interstitial fluid transport

Three hypothetical sets of pathways which comprise networks for flow across interstitia are shown: the top schematic shows straight circular cylinders all of the same dimension; the middle schematic shows straight circular cylinders of different sizes; and the remaining depiction shows convoluted, tortuous and interconnected trans-interstitial pathways.

can therefore be determined as the sum of the flows at either boundary, times the length of the medium, divided by the overall pressure difference and the area [see eqn. (1)]. It is unlikely that sufficient information exists to describe nodes and connections for tissue interstitia sufficient for this type of calculation. However, for a tissue which displays significant heterogeneity which can be described or estimated, this analysis may prove useful.

It is generally known that this form of modelling is inappropriate for high-porosity media. In the case of low-porosity structures with clearly defined impermeable pathways, network modelling may represent a reasonable description of the actual situation. For example, in a skeletal muscle where much of the tissue space is occupied by cells and only a small fraction of the tissue is interstitium (the interstitium is defined as the extravascular and extracellular space), discrete pathways for fluid exchange may exist. These may be connected, based upon the spacing of the cells, to other pathways, thereby creating a network of equivalent

Figure 5

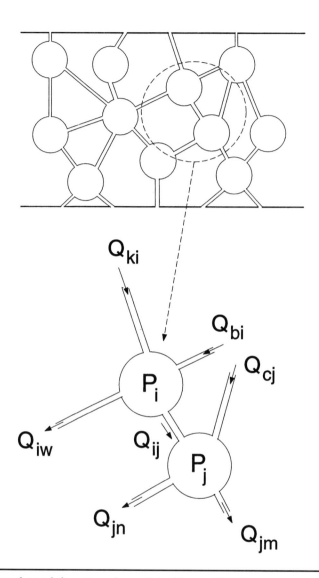

Node and conduit network model of interstitial transport
The top portion of this figure represents a series of nodes (circles) connected to each other and to the interstitial boundaries by filled conduits (parallel lines). The lower portion of the schematic is a blow-up of the dotted area in the upper portion and shows the flows (Q_{ij} — flow from node i to node j) and pressures (P_i is the pressure at node i) in the network. At steady state, all the flows into a node equal the sum of flows out of that node. Equations can be formulated which describe fluid exchange based on driving forces and geometry of the conduits. These can be solved simultaneously with appropriate boundary conditions to yield pressures in all nodes, from which all of the flows can be calculated.

conduits for mass exchange. Network modelling is also appropriate when heterogeneity exists within an interstitium. 'Free fluid channels' or 'rivulets' within an interstitium can form the fluid conductive pathways.

Percolation theory

A qualitatively different type of network model is considered by percolation theory. The theory has been extensively developed as a branch of statistical physics [15] and applied to diverse phenomena such as flow of fluid in a porous medium or the spread of disease in a population [16]. There have been several advances in the application of this theory to flow in porous media in which percolation models have been successfully applied to account for the transport properties in porous rock [15].

Just as in conduit network modelling, percolation theory describes flow in a porous medium to be through a connected lattice of junctions and conduits. To present the uniqueness of this concept, consider the symmetric lattice shown in Figure 6. At each point on the lattice junctions and conduits may be 'open' or 'closed' (this can be assessed statistically), either allowing or preventing flow at that point. The distribution of open or closed junctions or conduits can be independent of the behaviour of any of its neighbours. As shown in the upper panel of this figure, if all the junctions and conduits are open then there exists a large number of pathways from the top to bottom of the medium. These pathways are shown by the solid lines in the right-hand side of that figure. If we assign a probability (p) of only 75% of the junctions and conduits to be open (the middle panel of Figure 6), we see in the representative example that the fluid 'percolates' through a 'backbone' in the lattice. There are a large number of possibilities which satisfy the condition that $p=0.75$ for which a large number of different transmedium continuous pathways exist. What is also evident are a number of dangling and connected branches within the medium. These are analogous to dead-end pores, which may be filled but do not conduct fluid across the medium. In the lower panel, with a 25% probability of open junctions and conduits, for the representative example there exist no continuous pathways which traverse this particular lattice. Clearly, there must exist a statistically defined critical probability (p_c) below which 'no flow' conditions exist across the medium.

With this understanding of the network interconnectedness, it is now possible to consider how the overall hydraulic conductivity of the medium may be related to the probability of an open junction or conduit. Typically, it is suggested that the hydraulic conductivity is proportional to this probability in the following manner:

$$K \propto (p - p_c)^n \tag{15}$$

where n can be predicted using further refinements of percolation theory.

Percolation theory has been applied to blood flow through a geometrically well-defined microvascular network of muscle, in order to describe network resistance as a function of the decrease of capillary density: capillary rarefaction [17]. In order to apply a similar approach to fluid flow in interstitia, the geometry of the interstitium would have to

Figure 6

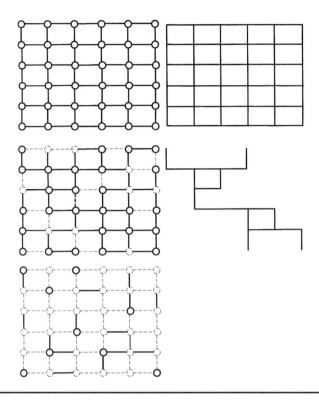

Percolation network

In the top left, a network of open junctions (open circles) and connected pathways (solid lines) is shown. To the right of that representation (which may correspond to the conditions in the interstitium) the pathways that exist from the top of the network to the bottom are shown as solid lines. There are many different routes available for transport across the porous medium described in this fashion. Middle panels: on the left is shown the same network for which only 75% of the junctions and connecting conduits are open for flow. The broken circles (closed junctions) and broken lines (closed conduits) do not support flow. The continuous pathway that exists between the top and the bottom of the middle figure is shown to its right. The pathway shown supports fluid exchange. For a probability of 75% that each junction and conduit is open, there are many such pathways. The schematic shown is only a representative example. For the figure shown in the lower left panel, the probability of supporting flow for each junction and conduit is 25%. For this probability the representative network has no continuous pathways across the medium.

be well characterized. This issue has been discussed previously. No attempts have yet been made to use percolation theory in this manner. Nonetheless, as we learn more about the architecture of the interstitium, the possibility of using this form of network analysis becomes greater. Percolation theory may be particularly useful to account for the heterogeneous nature of interstitia, which may also exhibit fractal characteristics.

Conclusion

Several different approaches to understanding quantitatively flow in the interstitium have been reviewed. Some speculation concerning the utility of these formulations has been offered. As a final point, it should be emphasized that there is a lack of data required for the formulation of many of the models of interstitial exchange. There is also a lack of accurate information required for validation. Under these conditions, the models, regardless of their complexity, can be considered to be no more than hypothetical. Validation of these models and of the approaches taken as part of their development requires comparison of model predictions with experimental observations.

We wish to thank Professor Norm Epstein for his editorial comments; and the Natural Science and Engineering Research Council of Canada, the British Columbia Health Research Foundation, and the Norwegian Council for Science and Humanities for their financial support.

References

1.   Greenkorn, R.A. (1986) Principles of flow through porous media. In *Encyclopedia of Fluid Mechanics* (Cheremisinoff, N.P., ed.), vol. 5, pp. 499–565, Gulf Publishing Company, Houston
2.   DeWiest, R.J.M. (1965) *Geohydrology*. Wiley, New York
3.   Levick, J.R. (1987) Flow through interstitium and other fibrous matrices. *Q. J. Exp. Physiol.* **72**, 409–438
4.   Tajaddini, A., Brown, L.V. and Lai Fook, S.J. (1994) Effect of hydration on lung interstitial permeability response to albumin and hyaluronidase. *J. Appl. Physiol.* **76**, 578–583
5.   Kim, A.C., Wang, M., Johnson, R. and Kamm, R. (1991) The specific hydraulic conductivity of bovine serum albumin. *Biorheology* **28**, 401–419
6.   Adler, P.M. (1992) *Porous Media: Geometry and Transports*, Butterworth–Heinemann, Boston
7.   Curry, F.E. and Michel, C.C. (1980) A fiber matrix model of capillary permeability. *Microvasc. Res.* **20**, 96–99
8.   Scheidegger, A.E. (1974) *The Physics of Flow Through Porous Media*, 3rd edn., University of Toronto Press, Toronto
9.   Bert, J. and Fatt, I. (1970) Relation of water transport content in swelling biological membranes. In *Surface Chemistry of Biological Systems* (Blank, M., ed.), pp. 287–294, Plenum Press, New York
10. Maroudas, A. (1979) Physiochemical properties of articular cartilage. In *Adult Articular Cartilage*, 2nd edn. (Freeman, M.A.R., ed.), pp. 215–290, Pitman Medical Publ. Co., Kent, U.K.
11. Fatt, I. and Weissman, B.A. (1992) *Physiology of the Eye. An Introduction to the Vegetative Functions*, 2nd edn., Butterworth–Heinemann, Boston
12. Ethier, C.R. (1991) Flow through mixed fibrous porous materials. *A. I. Ch. E. J.* **37**, 1227–1236
13. Tsay, R.Y. and Weinbaum, S.(1991) Viscous flow in a channel with periodic cross-bridging: exact solutions and Brinkman approximation. *J. Fluid Mech.* **226**, 125–148
14. Chen. V. and Hlacacek, M. (1994) Application of voroni tessellations for modeling randomly packed hollow-fiber bundles. *A. I. Ch. E. J.* **40**, 606–612
15. Berkowitz, B. and Balberg, I. (1993) Percolation theory and its application to groundwater hydrology. *Water Res.* **29**, 775–794
16. Zallen, R. (1983) Introduction to percolation: A model for all seasons. In *Percolation Structures and Processes* (Deutscher, G., Zallen, R. and Adler, J., eds.), pp. 3–16, Adam Higler Ltd., Bristol, U.K.
17. Hudetz, A.G. (1993) Percolation phenomena: The effect of capillary network rarefaction. *Microvasc. Res.* **45**, 1–10

9

Systems analysis and mathematical modelling of interstitial transport and microvascular exchange

David G. Taylor

Department of Chemical Engineering, University of Ottawa, 161 Louis Pasteur, Ottawa, Canada, K1N 6N5

Introduction

Because of its complex and fine structure, the microvascular exchange system poses many challenges to researchers seeking to better understand the forces and interactions governing its behaviour. In this regard, investigations of microvascular exchange are aided by mathematical models of the system. In particular, these models can be used to gain a better understanding of the system's operation by simulating its behaviour for a range of parameter values. Further, models prove useful in the interpretation of specific sets of experimental data.

Nomenclature: A_i, $i=1,2,3,...$, ith virial coefficient in interstitial osmotic pressure relationship (Pa·m^{3i}/kg^i); A^C, surface area of the blood capillary (m^2); A^L, lymphatic surface area per unit volume of lymphatic cuff (1/m); C, interstitial plasma protein concentration within the distribution volume (kg/m^3); $\hat{C}$, dimensionless concentration (C/C^{art}); C^C, capillary plasma protein concentration (kg/m^3); D_{eff}, plasma protein diffusivity within interstitial distribution volume (m^2/s); D^C, capillary permeability to plasma proteins (m/s); j_s, interstitial plasma protein flux vector (kg·m^{-2}·s^{-1}); $\hat{j}_s$, dimensionless interstitial plasma protein flux vector [$j_s L/(n^a D_{eff} C^{art})$]; j_s^C, transcapillary plasma protein flux (kg·m^{-2}·s^{-1}); j_w, interstitial fluid flux vector (m/s); $\hat{j}_w$, dimensionless interstitial fluid flux vector [$j_w L/(n^a D_{eff})$]; j_w^C, transcapillary fluid flux (m/s); J_s^L, interstitium–lymphatic plasma protein exchange rate per unit volume of lymphatic cuff (kg·m^{-3}·s^{-1}); $\hat{J}_s^L$, dimensionless protein exchange rate [$J_s^L L^2/(n^a D_{eff} C^{art})$]; J_w^L, interstitium–lymphatic volumetric fluid exchange rate per unit volume of lymphatic cuff (1/s); $\hat{J}_w^L$, dimensionless fluid exchange rate [$J_w^L L^2/(n^a D_{eff})$]; K, interstitial hydraulic conductivity (m^2·Pa^{-1}·s^{-1}); L, capillary length (m); L_p^C, average capillary hydraulic conductance (m·Pa^{-1}·s^{-1}); L_p^L, lymphatic hydraulic conductance (m·Pa^{-1}·s^{-1}); n^a, interstitial distribution volume fraction; n^t, interstitial mobile fluid volume fraction; P, interstitial hydrostatic fluid pressure (Pa); $\hat{P}$, dimensionless pressure (P/P^{art}); P^C, capillary hydrostatic fluid pressure (Pa); P^L, lymphatic hydrostatic fluid pressure (Pa); Pe, capillary Peclet number [$(1-\sigma^C) j_w^C/D^C$]; PS, capillary permeability–surface area product in whole organ (m^3/s·100 g); r, radial distance (m); R, radial dimension of tissue cylinder (m); R^C, capillary radius (m); R^L, radial position of lymphatic cuff (m); ΔR^L, radial thickness of lymphatic cuff (m); V^L, volume of lymphatic cuff (m^3); x, axial distance (m); x^L, axial position of lymphatic cuff (m); Δx^L, axial dimension of lymphatic cuff (m); β^L, fraction of total fluid entering lymphatic that contains protein; σ^C, capillary osmotic reflection coefficient; σ_f^C, capillary solvent drag reflection coefficient; σ^i, interstitial osmotic reflection coefficient; Π, interstitial protein osmotic pressure (Pa); $\hat{\Pi}$, dimensionless osmotic pressure (Π/P^{art}); Π^C, capillary protein osmotic pressure (Pa).

In the course of developing a mathematical description of the microvascular exchange system, the researcher must proceed through a series of stages: definition of modelling objectives; formation of the conceptual design upon which the model is based; mathematical formulation of the model; simulation and prediction; and finally, evaluation of model. This last stage may lead to further parameter estimation, model reformulation, or model acceptance. Together, these steps result in an iterative process whereby the conceptual design and model formulation may be re-evaluated in light of the study objectives, its principal assumptions, and new information concerning the system itself.

The following chapter provides a brief review of the various approaches to modelling microvascular exchange. Emphasis is placed on the general methodology rather than on model specifics. A more detailed examination of a specific model is then provided by way of example from the literature.

Modelling microvascular exchange

Models of the microvascular exchange system can be loosely grouped into two categories, depending on the general mathematical formulation: compartmental models of the system and those of the distributed form. We will briefly consider each of these separately.

Compartmental models of the microvascular exchange system

In compartmental modelling, the microvascular exchange system is reduced to a set of subsystems or compartments. Material is exchanged between compartments according to the driving forces present (such as differences in fluid chemical potential or solute concentrations) and the transport properties of the intervening boundaries. Each compartment is assumed to be homogeneous, thereby neglecting any spatial hetero-geneities in material properties that may exist in the physical counter-part. Further, the compartment is assumed to be well mixed, so that incoming material is instantaneously dispersed throughout its entire volume. It then follows that solute concentrations, fluid pressures and material properties associated with a given compartment are spatially averaged approximations to those found *in vivo*.

Because of the 'well mixed' assumption invoked in compartmental modelling, the driving forces for mass exchange between compartments will, in general, differ from the local driving forces found within the physical system. In some instances, this may limit the model's ability to simulate the behaviour of the microvascular exchange system, particularly under transient conditions. In addition, these models provide no information regarding mass transport within an individual com-partment or its effect on the overall behaviour of the system. How-ever, the assumptions of perfect mixing and homogeneity simplify the problem immensely, since they reduce the number of parameters needed to characterize the system and simplify its mathematical description. In addition, complex phenomena such as tissue swelling can be incor-porated with comparative ease in these models. For these reasons, com-partmental models are frequently used to simulate whole body fluid and solute exchange under normal and pathological states [1–7].

The complexity of these models increases with the number of compartments used to characterize the microvascular exchange system, which in turn depends on the specific model application. Consider, for example, Figure 1 illustrating the model of microvascular exchange following thermal injury proposed by Bert and co-workers [3]. In this case the body is divided into three interstitial compartments representing muscle, skin and injured skin, as well as a separate circulatory compartment. By way of comparison, Mazzoni and co-workers' [5] model of hyperosmotic resuscitation following haemorrhage considers both intracellular and extracellular fluid spaces, resulting in a total of five compartments.

Once the various compartments have been identified, mass balance equations are written to describe the exchange of fluid and solutes between them. These expressions are combined with auxiliary equations representing the characteristics of individual compartments relevant to exchange (such as a compliance relationship) and transport equations relating mass-exchange rates to the appropriate driving forces (e.g. Starling's Law).

Compartmental models of the microvascular exchange system have been applied to a number of tissues, including skin, muscle, lung, hindlimb and 'generalized tissues', and for various situations such as

Figure 1

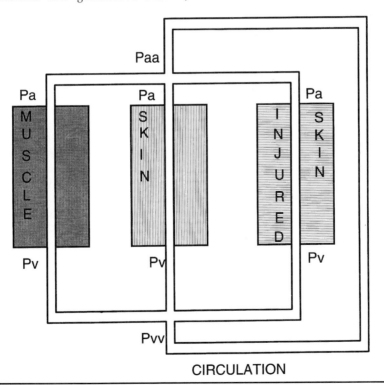

A compartmental model of the microvascular exchange system following thermal injury (after Bert et al. [3])
Abbreviations used: Pa, arterial capillary hydrostatic pressure; Paa, large artery hydrostatic pressure; Pv, venous capillary hydrostatic pressure; Pvv, large vein hydrostatic pressure.

hypertonic resuscitation, thermal injury and oedema formation (see Table 1 for a brief list). As such, this type of modelling remains a powerful tool for analysing the complex interactions that occur during exchange. However, to further investigate the influence of spatial heterogeneities and mass transport within individual compartments on microvascular exchange, we must turn to more complex models of the system.

Distributed models of the microvascular exchange system

Unlike their compartmental counterparts described above, distributed models of the microvascular exchange system can account for spatial heterogeneities within various compartments by lifting the 'well mixed' assumptions employed in the former method. Furthermore, the influence of fluid and solute transport on exchange is included to varying degrees in these models. For these reasons, distributed models provide a more accurate description of the system, at least in principle. However, the more realistic description has its costs: distributed models result in a larger number of system parameters that must be quantified and yield more complex mathematical formulations.

Whereas compartmental models are based on averaged properties of entire tissues or vascular compartments, distributed models are founded on local averaging procedures within a given compartment. Through the averaging procedure, the complex structure and interactions found at the microscopic level of the microvascular exchange system are replaced with a mathematical construct: the hypothetical continuum. This continuum displays certain characteristics and properties depicting the salient features of the physical system. Hence the interstitial space, for example, is replaced by a porous medium containing various volume fractions that represent the collagen, elastin, glycosaminoglycans, fluid regions accessible to interstitial plasma proteins and those regions from which the proteins are excluded. The fluid transport properties of the porous medium are described by its hydraulic conductivity, another mathematical construct which accounts for the tortuous fluid pathways characteristic of the real system. In a similar fashion, the hypothetical continuum is assigned other descriptive parameters and constitutive functions such as protein diffusivities, the convective hindrance, and the compliance relationship.

In developing the continuum representation described above, a representative elementary volume is centred about some point in the physical system (see Figure 2). The properties of this small volume are then averaged and assigned to that same point in the continuum. Following this, the representative elementary volume is moved a differential distance and the averaging procedure repeated. In this way the entire space is eventually converted into a continuum displaying local properties characteristic of small regions of the original system.

Once the volume averaging procedures have been applied to the system to yield its continuum representation, differential balances are carried out that provide equations describing the transport and exchange of fluid and solute species throughout the microvascular exchange system. This typically leads to a set of non-linear, coupled, partial differential equations that must be solved using numerical techniques.

Table 2 provides a brief list of some of the distributed models of

Table 1

Investigators [ref.]	Model application	Tissue	Transport species
Arturson et al. [1]	Burn model	Human whole body	Fluid, albumin
Bert et al. [2]	Hypothesis testing	Rat whole body	Fluid, albumin
Bert et al. [3]	Burn model	Rat whole body	Fluid, albumin
Chapple et al. [4]	Nephrosis	Human whole body	Fluid, albumin
Mazzoni et al. [5]	Hypertonic resuscitation	Rabbit whole body	Fluid, albumin, NaCl, Dextran 70
Riddle et al. [6]	Tracer analysis	Lung	Radiolabelled albumin
Thews and Hutten [7]	Haemodialysis	Human whole body	Fluid, small solutes

Some compartmental models of the microvascular exchange system

Figure 2

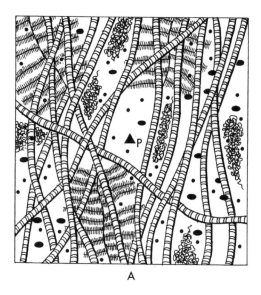

A

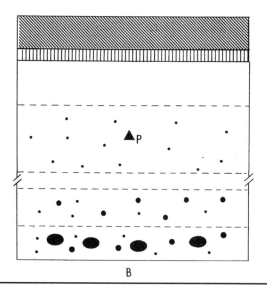

B

(A) A representative elementary volume of interstitial space centred about point p, over which volume averaging is performed, and (B) the resulting multiphase continuum (after Taylor et al. [26])

microvascular exchange found in the literature. These models take several different forms, depending on the study objectives. One such approach considers a single blood capillary, the surrounding interstitial space and, in some instances, draining lymphatics. Together, these components represent a basic functional unit of the microvascular exchange system which is assumed to operate independently of other neighbouring units. Such models have been used to study fluid, plasma

Table 2

Investigators [ref.]	Model application	Tissue	Transport species
Apelblat et al. [8]	Single capillary	Generalized tissue	Fluid
Bassingthwaite et al. [9]	Single capillary	Generalized tissue	Fluid, tracers
Baxter and Jain [23]	Regional averaged	Tumour	Fluid, trace macromolecules
Blake and Gross [16]	Single and multiple capillaries	Generalized tissue	Fluid, solute (in capillary only)
Fleischman et al. [17]	Single and multiple capillaries	Generalized tissue	Fluid
Flessner et al. [19]	Regional averaged	Peritoneum	Fluid, solutes
Fry [10]	Single capillary	Arterial wall	Macromolecules
Hsu and Secomb [18]	Multiple capillaries	Generalized tissue	Oxygen
Kim et al. [11]	Single capillary	Generalized tissue	Macromolecules
Levick [12]	Single capillary	Synovium	Fluid, macromolecules
Salathé and Xu [21]	Regional averaged	Skeletal muscle	Fluid, solutes
Seames et al. [20]	Regional averaged	Peritoneum	Fluid, solutes
Sharan et al. [13]	Single capillary	Generalized tissue	Oxygen
Taylor et al. [14]	Single capillary	Mesentery	Fluid, macromolecules
Taylor [24]	Single capillary	Generalized tissue	Fluid, macromolecules
Weerappuli and Popel [22]	Regional averaged	Generalized tissue	Oxygen

Some distributed models of the microvascular exchange system

protein and oxygen exchange (e.g. [8–15]), providing insights into the mechanisms governing exchange at the microscopic level.

In the next level of complexity, single capillary vessels are replaced by discrete capillary networks (see Figure 3); however, the representation of sets of distinct vessels embedded in an interstitial matrix increases the computational demands considerably. For this reason, such models have typically been limited to studies of fluid and oxygen exchange under idealized conditions (see, for example, [16–18]).

A third class of distributed models is designed to investigate entire capillary beds associated with a given tissue or organ. In this case the representative elementary volume used to carry out the volume averaging is expanded to include all major components of the tissue (i.e. capillaries, interstitium and lymphatics), so that these elements are present at all points within the hypothetical continuum. For example, the blood vessels are no longer considered discrete entities located at specific points within the microvascular exchange system, but rather are represented by a separate phase distributed throughout the system which is in contact with the other phases representing the interstitium and lymphatic vessels.

Regional averaging procedures have been applied to a number of tissues, including the peritoneum [19,20], skeletal muscle [21], hamster cheek pouch [22], and tumour [23]. While this type of averaging procedure forfeits, for example, a detailed description of the interstitial pressure and concentration gradients between adjacent blood vessels, it provides a more practical means of retaining regional heterogeneities in tissue properties and differences in mass exchange within a given tissue or organ when compared with discrete capillary models. The success of this modelling technique therefore depends, in part, on the validity of assuming that local gradients in fluid pressure and solute concentrations within the perivascular regions of the interstitium are negligible. This assumption may be appropriate in some vascular beds and not in others.

Figure 3

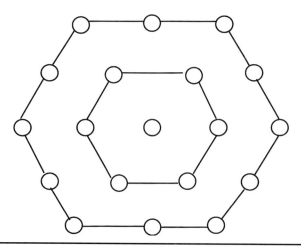

An axial view of a hexagonal capillary network (after Fleischman et al. [17])

As we have seen, each of the three modelling approaches discussed above offers certain advantages and is also hampered by certain limitations. In fact, our understanding of microvascular exchange is aided by all three forms of distributed models, as well as by the compartmental models described earlier. As an example of how these models can be applied to the physiological system, we will now consider a single capillary distributed model of fluid and protein exchange, the details of which can be found elsewhere [24].

A model study of exchange within a tissue functional unit

The mathematical model

Figure 4 is a schematic diagram of the basic functional unit of the microvascular exchange system modelled here, based on a modified version of the classic Krogh cylinder [25]. In this case the cylindrical domain, representing the interstitial space, extends indefinitely in the axial direction and to a distance R in the radial direction. A single permeable blood capillary of radius R^C, located along the central axis, extends for a distance $L/2$ on either side of the origin. The transport properties of the capillary wall and the hydrostatic pressure within the capillary lumen vary linearly in the axial direction from the arteriolar end of the vessel, located at $L/2$, to the venular end at $-L/2$. To maintain radial symmetry, the draining lymphatic vessel associated with the tissue segment is represented by an annular 'cuff' that behaves as a distributed sink for interstitial fluid and macromolecules. The cuff, located at some radial position R^L and beginning at the venular end of the capillary, is assumed to extend Δx^L in the axial direction and to be of finite, but small, thickness ΔR^L. No fluid or plasma proteins cross any of the outer boundaries of the tissue cylinder.

In developing equations to describe microvascular exchange within the tissue segment, we will assume that the interstitium behaves as a rigid, homogeneous, isotropic porous medium that displays membrane-like properties with respect to fluid and macromolecular movement. Hence, the effects of significant tissue swelling, as might arise in diseased states such as venous congestion or following thermal

Figure 4

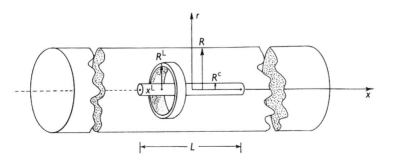

Schematic diagram of the tissue functional unit
Reproduced from [24] with permission.

injury, are not considered here. (The influence of tissue swelling on the interstitial transport equations is discussed elsewhere [26].) Further, the array of interstitial plasma protein species normally present within the interstitium is treated as a single aggregate species displaying transport properties similar to albumin. This assumption is based on the fact that albumin, the most abundant plasma protein, is also the principal contributor to the total colloidal osmotic pressure exerted by extra-cellular fluid such as serum [27]. This protein can therefore be expected to exert the greatest influence on microvascular fluid exchange.

Constitutive relationships for interstitial fluid and plasma protein transport

The exact nature of fluid and solute transport through the interstitial space remains uncertain. However, the interstitium does display some of the same characteristics that contribute to the overall transport properties of the capillary wall. For example, experimental measurements in model tissues consisting of hyaluronan solutions [28] support the notion that the interstitium, like the capillary wall, restricts the move-ment of interstitial plasma proteins. In addition, the excluding properties of the interstitium are well documented [29]. These similarities suggest a possible analogy between interstitial fluid and protein transport and transcapillary exchange that will be employed here (see also [12]). In particular, the membrane equations will be rewritten in differential form and used to quantify interstitial fluid and protein movement.

Applying the analogy between capillary exchange and interstitial transport, the local interstitial fluid flux, expressed in vector notation, is:

$$j_w = -K\nabla(P - \sigma^i \Pi) \qquad (1)$$

where j_w is the local fluid flux vector, K is the interstitial hydraulic conductivity, P is the local interstitial fluid pressure, σ^i is the interstitial reflection coefficient, and Π is the local colloid osmotic pressure generated by the interstitial macromolecules. A cubic relationship between this pressure and the local concentration of interstitial plasma proteins within the accessible regions of the interstitium, C, is assumed [24]:

$$\Pi = A_1 C + A_2 C^2 + A_3 C^3 \qquad (2)$$

where A_i is the ith virial coefficient of the osmotic relationship.

Eqn. (1) may be viewed as a modified form of Darcy's Law in which the driving force for fluid transport is the gradient in the effective fluid chemical potential, expressed in terms of hydrostatic and colloid osmotic pressures [24]. The degree to which protein osmotic pressures affect fluid movement is specified by the osmotic reflection coefficient, which varies from zero to one.

Applying a differential form of the capillary plasma protein transport equation to the interstitium gives:

$$j_s = (1 - \sigma^i) j_w C - n^a D_{eff} \nabla C \qquad (3)$$

D_{eff} being the solute's effective diffusivity within the regions of the interstitium accessible to the plasma proteins and where n^a is the interstitial volume fraction associated with that accessible space (i.e. the distribution volume fraction).

Differential fluid and protein mass balances

Given the assumptions of a rigid, homogeneous and isotropic system and eqn. (1) describing fluid transport, a steady-state mass balance on the fluid within a differential volume of interstitium yields:

$$K\nabla^2 (P - \sigma^i \Pi) - J_w^L = 0 \tag{4}$$

where J_w^L is the rate of fluid withdrawal by the lymphatic cuff, per unit volume of interstitium. J_w^L will be non-zero only in the interstitial space containing the cuff. A similar steady-state balance on the plasma proteins gives:

$$n^a D_{eff} \nabla^2 C - (1 - \sigma^i) j_w \cdot \nabla C - J_s^L = 0 \tag{5}$$

where J_s^L is the rate of plasma protein removal by the lymphatic vessel, per unit volume of interstitium. Again, J_s^L will be non-zero only in the region of the cuff.

Boundary conditions and lymphatic exchange

Eqns. (1) to (5) must be combined with the requisite boundary conditions and transport equations describing lymphatic exchange to fully specify the system. The radially directed fluid flux J_w^C entering the interstitium from the bloodstream, which is given by Starling's equation, is equal to the rate of interstitial fluid transport from the capillary wall:

$$-K \frac{\delta (P - \sigma^i \Pi)}{\delta r} \bigg|_{r=R^C} = L_P^C [P^C - P - \sigma^C (\Pi^C - \Pi)] \tag{6}$$

Meanwhile, the plasma protein flux j_s^C across this capillary membrane, given by the non-linear flux equation, is equated to the net rate of diffusive and convective transport of interstitial proteins from the wall:

$$\left[-n^a D_{eff} \frac{\delta C}{\delta r} + (1 - \sigma^i) j_w C \right]\bigg|_{r=R^C} = \frac{(1 - \sigma^C) j_w^C [C^C - C \exp(-Pe)]}{1 - \exp(-Pe)} \tag{7}$$

where Pe, the capillary Peclet number, is given by:

$$Pe = \frac{(1 - \sigma_f^C) j_w^C}{D^C} \tag{8}$$

Like the capillary wall, the wall of the initial lymphatics is formed of a single layer of thin endothelial cells; however, in the latter case a basal lamina is, at best, discontinuous and often absent [30]. As with the interstitium, the transport characteristics of the draining lymphatic vessels remain poorly defined. However, fluid transport across the lymphatic wall is thought to be initiated by both intrinsic factors (such as lymphatic pumping) and extrinsic ones (such as muscular massage) that generate a pressure difference across the wall, thereby providing the driving force for fluid withdrawal from the surrounding interstitial space. The presence of anchoring filaments maintains the vessel patent as interstitial pressure rises, while overlapping interendothelial junctions in the initial lymphatic wall and valves within the vessel interior prevent back flow of lymphatic fluid into the interstitium [30]. Experimental evidence also suggests that convection is the dominant mechanism for plasma protein transfer to the lymphatic vessel [27]. Given this, it is reasonable to assume, as a first approximation, that the fluid flux across the lymphatic wall is proportional to the pressure drop across it, i.e. $P - P^L$. Furthermore, since we have assumed that the lymphatic vessel behaves as a sink distributed throughout an annular cuff region of interstitium, we express lymphatic fluid exchange as an equivalent volumetric withdrawal rate per unit volume of annular cuff, J_w^L:

$$J_w^L = L_p^L A^L (P - P^L) \tag{9}$$

where L_p^L is the hydraulic conductance of the lymphatic wall and where A^L is the surface area of the lymphatic per unit volume of annular cuff.

Assuming that macromolecules cross the lymphatic wall by convection we have:

$$J_s^L = \beta^L J_w^L C \tag{10}$$

where J_s^L is the mass flow of macromolecules across the lymphatic wall per unit volume of lymphatic cuff. β^L represents the fraction of total fluid entering the lymphatic that carries with it macromolecules. Assuming, for example, a uniform flow of fluid throughout both the available volume fraction n^a and the total mobile fluid volume fraction, n^t, then:

$$\beta^L = \frac{n^a}{n^t} \tag{11}$$

The remaining boundary conditions stipulate that the gradients in interstitial plasma protein concentration and hydrostatic pressure drop to zero at the tissue segment's outer boundaries:

$$\frac{\delta P}{\delta x} = \frac{\delta C}{\delta x} = 0 \qquad x = \pm\infty, \forall r$$

$$\frac{\delta P}{\delta r} = \frac{\delta C}{\delta x} = 0 \qquad r = R, \forall x \tag{12}$$

which implies no fluid or plasma protein transport across the outer boundaries of the system. Alternatively, the pressures and concentrations at these outlying boundaries could be specified; however, simulations [24] revealed that the former boundary conditions are best suited to this problem. Together, eqns. (1) to (12) fully describe the system. Note that these equations were recast in dimensionless form before solving them.

Parameter evaluation and numerical simulations

Table 3 lists the values for the various system parameters assumed in the model study, which were taken, where available, from data typical of skin and skeletal muscle. Parameters associated with the lymphatic vessel, meanwhile, were selected to provide reasonable lymph flow rates for the tissue unit, based on the literature. For further discussion of, and justification for, the selected values, the reader is referred to the complete study [24].

Since the capillary hydraulic conductance typically increases towards its venular end, while the reflection coefficient decreases in that same direction, it is assumed here that σ^C, L_p^C and D^C all vary linearly from the arteriolar end of the capillary (denoted by a superscript art) to

Parameter	Assumed value	Table 3
A_1	$54.510 \ \text{Pa·m}^3 \cdot \text{kg}^{-1}$	
A_2	$-3.203 \times 10^{-1} \ \text{Pa·m}^6 \cdot \text{kg}^{-2}$	
A_3	$5.347 \times 10^{-2} \ \text{Pa·m}^9 \cdot \text{kg}^{-3}$	
C^C	$36 \ \text{kg·m}^{-3}$	
D^{art}	$2 \times 10^{-9} \ \text{m·s}^{-1}$	
D^{ven}	$6 \times 10^{-9} \ \text{m·s}^{-1}$	
D^{eff}	$1.47 \times 10^{-11} \ \text{m}^2 \cdot \text{s}^{-1}$	
K	$5.0 \times 10^{-15} \ \text{m}^2 \cdot \text{Pa}^{-1} \cdot \text{s}^{-1}$	
L	$7.5 \times 10^{-4} \ \text{m}$	
L_p^{art}	$1.00 \times 10^{-10} \ \text{m·Pa}^{-1} \cdot \text{s}^{-1}$	
L_p^{ven}	$2.00 \times 10^{-10} \ \text{m·Pa}^{-1} \cdot \text{s}^{-1}$	
$L_p^L A^L V^L$	Set equal to $L_p^C A^C$	
n^a	0.680	
n^t	0.789	
p^{art}	$3.270 \times 10^3 \ \text{Pa}$	
p^L	$-1.00 \times 10^3 \ \text{Pa}$	
p^{ven}	$0.790 \times 10^3 \ \text{Pa}$	
R	See text	
R^C	$2.5 \times 10^{-6} \ \text{m}$	
R^L	Set equal to R	
Δx^L	$7.5 \times 10^{-5} \ \text{m}$	
β^L	0.860	
σ^{art}	0.925	
σ^i	0.5	
σ^{ven}	0.825	
Π^C	$2.666 \times 10^3 \ \text{Pa}$	

Some compartmental models of the microvascular exchange system

the venular end of the blood vessel (denoted by a superscript ven). Likewise, the hydrostatic pressure, P^C, within the vessel is assumed to decrease linearly along its length. The osmotic pressure, Π^C, and the protein concentration, C^C, meanwhile, are not expected to change significantly from the arteriolar end of the vessel to its venular end, and so are held constant.

In the original study [24], a series of numerical simulations was performed to investigate the relative effects of various system parameters on fluid and plasma protein exchange within the model tissue. We will focus here on a single parameter: the cylinder radius R. In this case R is varied from a lower limit of 2.5×10^{-5} m (typical of capillary beds in some skeletal muscle tissue) to a maximum value of 2×10^{-4} m.

Because the field equations are coupled and include non-linearities associated, for example, with osmotic pressure terms, an analytical solution is not possible. The system of equations was therefore solved numerically using finite differences based on the control volume method of Patankar [31]. In particular, central differences were applied to the pressure field equation, while the power law scheme, which employs a variable degree of upwinding depending on local grid Peclet numbers, was used to solve for the interstitial plasma protein concentration distribution. The latter method provides a smooth transition from central differences applied in purely diffusive cases (e.g. when σ^1 equals 1) to convectively dominant cases in which full upwinding is required. The discretized equations were then solved using a line by line procedure and the Thomas algorithm; 2275 nodes were used in the finite difference grids.

Since the pressure and concentration equations are coupled, the system was solved iteratively. An initial estimate for the concentration distribution was used to calculate the interstitial pressure field. From this and the assumed concentration profile the interstitial fluid flow field was calculated and used to update the interstitial concentration distribution. The revised distribution was then applied to the pressure field equation to yield an improved estimate of the interstitial pressure distribution. This scheme was repeated until specific convergence criteria were met.

Results and discussion

Simulations reveal that the radial dimension, R, of the tissue cylinder influences both the total rate of exchange within the tissue segment and transcapillary flux distribution. For example, as the radius of the Krogh cylinder is increased from 2.5×10^{-5} m to 1×10^{-4} m, the total rate of fluid filtration (i.e. the total rate of fluid exchange from the capillary to the interstitium) increases approximately 2.8-fold. Increasing the radius further to 2×10^{-4} m results in a 4-fold increase in fluid filtration, compared with the base case in which R equals 2.5×10^{-5} m. This is in keeping with the general observations of Apelblat *et al.* [8] who modelled steady-state fluid exchange within a Krogh cylinder unit. These authors also predicted an increase in fluid filtration with larger cylinder radii, which was related to the tissue's capacity for fluid transport which, in turn, depends on the effective cross-sectional area for fluid flow. However, since their model neglected to account for lymphatic drainage, it always predicted fluid filtration at the arteriolar end of the capillary and an equal rate of fluid reabsorption along the venular portion of the vessel. The current study shows fluid filtration to depend strongly on the radial dimension of the tissue unit, even in the presence of a lymphatic vessel.

Of even greater significance here, however, is the variation in the transcapillary fluid flux distribution that arises when the combined influences of the lymphatic vessel and cylinder dimension are considered. In the absence of a lymphatic vessel, all fluid that filters from the capillary to the tissue space at the arteriolar end of the system is reabsorbed at the capillary's venular end. However, transcapillary fluid exchange is substantially different when the draining action of the lymphatic vessel is included in the model (see Figure 5). At the lowest value of R, fluid is filtered across the entire length of the capillary. Fluid crossing the arteriolar portion of the vessel must travel a distance through the interstitial space approximately equal to the entire length of the capillary before being taken up by the lymphatic vessel. The fluid filtering across the venular end of the capillary, meanwhile, travels a much shorter distance through the interstitium before reaching the lymphatic vessel.

As R increases, the effective cross-sectional area for flow from the arteriolar end of the system likewise increases while the pathlength through the interstitium for this fluid (and hence the resistance to flow) increases only marginally, so that exchange across this portion of the capillary also rises. In contrast, because the strength of the lymphatic sink is unchanged as the radius increases, and since the interstitial resistance to flow from the venular segment of the capillary to the lymphatic vessel is approximately proportional to R, exchange across the

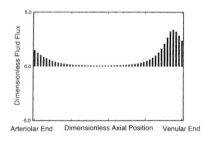
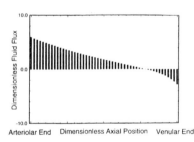
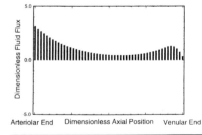
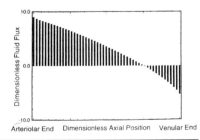

Figure 5

Dimensionless transcapillary fluid flux distributions as a function of R
Upper left-hand panel: R = 25 μm; lower left-hand panel: R = 50 μm; upper right-hand panel: R = 100 μm; lower right-hand panel: R = 250μm. Reproduced from [24] with permission.

venular end of the blood vessel decreases with increasing Krogh cylinder radius. However, given that the behaviour of the arteriolar end of the system dominates, the net effect is an overall increase in the rate of fluid filtration across the capillary with increasing R. In fact, at some point the rate of filtration exceeds the ability of the lymphatic vessel to drain the tissue segment, and the venular segment of the capillary shifts from a state of filtration to one of reabsorption. Hence, when R equals 1×10^{-4} m, for example, approximately 12% of the fluid filtered along the capillary is reabsorbed at its venular end; when R increases to 2×10^{-4} m, the rate of fluid reabsorption likewise increases to approximately 17% of the filtration rate.

Further investigation [24] revealed that fluid reabsorption is also influenced by the distribution of the lymphatic vessel within the model tissue, the magnitude of the interstitial hydraulic conductivity, and the relative degrees of transcapillary convection and diffusion of proteins which affect the protein distributions within the perivascular regions of the interstitial space. In general, the transcapillary fluid and protein flux distributions were found to be strong functions of both the system geometry and the properties and location of the draining lymphatic vessels. Hence, distributed models of the microvascular exchange system that neglect lymphatic action, or assume simply that the interstitium behaves as an unbounded sink for fluid and proteins, may be inadequate to describe transcapillary exchange in many tissues.

Concluding remarks

Our understanding of the functioning of the microvascular exchange system is enhanced, in part, through mathematical models of this system. These models take various forms, but can be loosely categorized into two general classes: compartmental and distributed types. The compartmental form offers certain advantages due to its simpler mathematical formulation and, for this reason, is well-suited to whole body simulations. Distributed models, on the other hand, are able to account for spatial heterogeneities in the system as well as local variations in fluid pressure and solute concentrations. However, because of their more complex nature, distributed models of microvascular exchange are best limited to single capillary models or, through regional averaging methods, individual tissues and organs.

Finally, modelling of microvascular exchange remains an evolutionary process. As we gain greater insight into the behaviour of the physiological system, we must review and, in some cases, rethink the premises upon which our models are based.

This work was supported by the Natural Sciences and Engineering Research Council of Canada.

References

1. Arturson, G., Groth, T., Hedlund, A. and Zaar, B. (1984) Scand. J. Plast. Reconstr. Surg. **18**, 39–48
2. Bert, J.L., Bowen, B.D. and Reed, R.K. (1988) Am. J. Physiol. **254**, H384–H399

3. Bert, J.L., Bowen, B.D., Reed, R.K. and Onarheim, H. (1991) *Circ. Shock* **34**, 285–297
4. Chapple, C., Bowen, B.D., Reed, R.K., Xie, S.L. and Bert, J.L. (1993) *Comput. Methods Programs Biomed*. **41**, 33–54
5. Mazzoni, M.C., Borgström, P., Arfors, K.-E. and Intaglietta, M. (1988) *Am. J. Physiol.* **255**, H629–H637
6. Riddle, W.R., Rosseli, R.J. and Pou, N.A. (1990) *J. Appl. Physiol.* **68**, 2434–2442
7. Thews, O. and Hutten, H. (1990) *Med. Prog. Technol.* **16**, 145–161
8. Apelblat, A., Katzir-Katchalsky, A. and Silberberg, A. (1974) *Biorheology* **11**, 1–49
9. Bassingthwaite, J.B., Chan, I.S.J. and Wang, C.Y. (1992) *Ann. Biomed. Eng.* **20**, 687–725
10. Fry, D.L. (1985) *Am. J. Physiol.* **248**, H240–H263
11. Kim, D., Armenante, P.M. and Durán, W.N. (1990) *Microvasc. Res.* **40**, 358–378
12. Levick, J.R. (1994) *Microvasc. Res.* **47**, 90–125
13. Sharan, M., Singh, B., Singh, M.P. and Kumar, P. (1991) *IMA J. Math. Appl. Med. Biol.* **8**, 107–123
14. Taylor, D.G., Bert, J.L. and Bowen, B.D. (1990) *Microvasc. Res.* **39**, 279–306
15. Taylor, D.G., Bert, J.L. and Bowen, B.D. (1991) *Microvasc. Res.* **42**, 209–216
16. Blake, T.R. and Gross, J.F. (1982) *Math. Biosci.* **59**, 173–206
17. Fleischman, G.J., Secomb, T.W. and Gross, J.F. (1986) *Math. Biosci.* **81**, 145–164
18. Hsu, R. and Secomb, T.W. (1992) *J. Biomech. Eng.* **114**, 227–231
19. Flessner, M.F., Dedrick, R.L. and Schultz, J.S. (1984) *Am. J. Physiol.* **246**, R597–R607
20. Seames, E.L., Moncrief, J.W. and Popovich, R.P. (1990) *Am. J. Physiol.* **258**, R958–R972
21. Salathé, E.P. and Xu, Y.-H. (1988) *Proc. R. Soc. London Ser. B* **234**, 303–318
22. Weerappuli, D.P.V. and Popel, A.S. (1989) *J. Biomech. Eng.* **111**, 24–31
23. Baxter, L.T. and Jain, R.K. (1989) *Microvasc. Res.* **37**, 77–104
24. Taylor, D.G. (1994) *Can. J. Chem. Eng.* **72**, 484–496
25. Bassingthwaite, J.B. and Goresky, C.A. (1984) in *Handbook of Physiology*, Vol. 4, The Cardiovascular System, Microcirculation Part 1 (Renkin, E. and Michel, C.C., eds.), pp. 549–626, Am. Physiol. Soc., Bethesda
26. Taylor, D.G., Bert, J.L. and Bowen, B.D. (1990) *Microvasc. Res.* **39**, 253–278
27. Aukland, K. and Reed, R.K. (1993) *Physiol. Rev.* **73**, 1–77
28. Laurent, T.C., Bjork, I., Pietruszkiewicz, A. and Persson, H. (1963) *Biochim. Biophys. Acta* **78**, 351–359
29. Bert, J.L. and Pearce, R.H. (1984) in *Handbook of Physiology*, Vol. 4, The Cardiovascular System, Microcirculation Part 1, (Renkin, E. and Michel, C.C., eds.), pp. 521–547, Am. Physiol. Soc., Bethesda
30. Gnepp, D. (1984) in *Edema* (Staub, N.C. and Taylor, A.E., eds.), pp. 263–298, Raven Press, New York
31. Patankar, S.V. (1981) *Numerical Heat Transfer and Fluid Flow*, pp. 25–108, Hemisphere, New York

10

The physiological functions of extracellular matrix macromolecules

C.P. Winlove* and K.H. Parker

Physiological Flow Studies Group, Centre for Biological and Medical Systems, Imperial College of Science, Technology and Medicine, London SW7 2BY, U.K.

Introduction

The extracellular matrix (ECM) is a ubiquitous component of biological tissues, composed of a network of the fibrous proteins collagen and elastin immersed in a highly hydrated gel containing proteoglycans (PGs) and other soluble glycoproteins [1]. It serves a range of physiological functions, defining the form of tissues and endowing them with their passive mechanical properties and influencing the distribution and rates of movement of water and solutes. At the cellular level it determines the nutrient composition of the cellular environment and transduces chemical and mechanical signals. These functions are fundamental to all tissues, but they assume particular importance in structures such as cartilage, intervertebral discs and the large blood vessels whose functions, which are primarily mechanical, are served directly by the ECM. Under pathological conditions, there is abundant evidence of involvement of the ECM in genetic abnormalities and diseases as diverse as atherosclerosis, arthritis and diabetes [2].

Our knowledge of the biochemistry and cell- and molecular-biology of the ECM has developed rapidly in recent years, but research on the biophysical properties both of the whole ECM and of its constituent macromolecules has lagged behind. It is therefore difficult to translate the wealth of biochemical information on the ECM into understanding of physiological function and pathological change. One of our aims in writing this chapter was to draw attention to this disparity in the hope of stimulating further work. Another aim was to attempt to summarize existing information and its relevance to physiology in the hope that the interstitium will no longer be regarded by many physiologists as a black box.

We will concentrate largely on the three major components of the ECM, the collagens, elastin and PGs. The ECM contains many other components which are present in such small quantities that their detection and characterization has been a major technical achievement of recent years. It has also become clear that many of these 'minor' components have functions which are far from minor, such as determining the assembly and organization of the ECM. However, the literature on the physicochemical properties of these molecules and on the biophysical basis of their functions is still too rudimentary to be

*To whom correspondence should be addressed.

amenable to review. This review may also fail to do justice to another important development in matrix biology, the realization that the ECM is a dynamic structure capable of remodelling in response to a wide variety of stimuli. Matrix molecules are continually being degraded and resynthesized, and homoeostasis is maintained by a complex mixture of chemical and mechanical signals regulating cellular and enzymic activities [3]. The biophysical processes involved in transducing signals between cells and matrix and in the assembly and organization of newly synthesized matrix have scarcely been addressed and must remain outside the scope of this review.

Proteoglycans

The ECM contains many species of glycoproteins, forming what the older histology texts referred to as the 'amorphous ground substance'. The proteoglycans (PGs) are the major subclass, the structure and tissue distribution of which are highly conserved between species. They are characterized by possessing an unbranched protein core to which is attached at least one glycosaminoglycan (GAG) side chain (Figure 1). The GAGs are a small family of unbranched heteropolymers composed of repeating disaccharide units each containing hexosamine and hexuronic acid or hexose. The large negative charge carried by these molecules, which is important to their physiological functions, arises from carboxyl and/or sulphate ester groups attached to the disaccharide units. Some PGs contain many more than the obligatory single GAG chain. The large PG aggrecan (molecular mass $\sim 3.5 \times 10^6$ Da), which constitutes up to 10% of the dry weight of cartilage, contains up to 150 side-chains of chondroitin sulphate and keratan sulphate, and these molecules are often found in tissue in the form of enormous multi-molecular aggregates. These aggregates are formed by a specific inter-action involving a globular domain on the protein core with hyaluronan, another long-chain GAG. Detailed discussions of the biochemistry of PGs are to be found in numerous review articles [4,5] (see also Chapter 2 by Hardingham *et al.* in this book).

The large PGs such as aggrecan are widely recognized as serving important physiological functions in controlling the hydration of the interstitium, determining its permeability to solutes and influencing its viscoelastic properties [6]. The view was advanced by both Ogston and Laurent that these functions are related to the 'general macromolecular and polyelectrolyte characteristics' of the molecules [6,7]. This is undoubtedly an adequate first approximation but it is difficult to believe that the elaborate structure of the PGs and the patterns of variation which occur between tissues and with age and disease do not have functional implications. Since this view was expressed, biochemists studying PGs have described many additional functions for these molecules, particularly the small PGs [8,9], in determining the structure and organization of the ECM. These functions involve specific inter-actions with other macromolecules such as cytokines, growth factors and enzymes. The explanation for the complexity and diversity of PG struc-ture may be found from a better understanding of the physio-chemical basis of these functions.

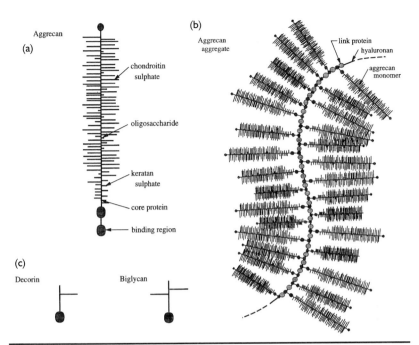

Figure 1

Schematical representations of aggrecan and other proteoglycan molecules

(a) A sketch of the structure of aggrecan, a large proteoglycan which accounts for approximately 10% of the dry weight of cartilage. Chondroitin sulphate (87%) and keratan sulphate (6%) glycosaminoglycans are attached to a core protein (7%). The large number of negatively charged side groups produce a high osmotic pressure which determines the hydration of tissues such as cartilage. Molecules such as aggrecan are also a major determinant of the permeability of the matrix to water and solutes. (b) An aggrecan aggregate. In tissues such as cartilage a large number of aggrecan monomers are attached via a specialized binding region on the protein core to a hyaluronan molecule. The attachment is stabilized by a small link protein. (c) Examples of small proteoglycans containing only a few glycosaminoglycan side chains. Decorin has a single chondroitin sulphate/dermatan sulphate side chain and biglycan has two. This family of proteoglycans binds with cells and other matrix components and is involved in matrix assembly and organization and with cell–matrix interactions.

There have been very detailed analyses of the conformation of GAGs using both theoretical molecular mechanics [10] and experimental measurements based on X-ray diffraction analyses of dried polymer films and n.m.r. spectroscopy [11]. Although some progress has been made in relating this very detailed molecular information to function [12], some difficulties remain in reconciling the information derived from the different techniques [13]. A major source of these difficulties has been taking into account the dramatic effects of water on polymer conformation, and for this reason some of the most valuable insights into the behaviour of GAGs and PGs under physiological conditions have been derived from rheological measurements.

Rheological properties

Measurements of the rheological properties of PGs and their constituent GAGs in solution fall into two groups. One group consists of experiments designed to characterize the conformations of the molecules in solution and the nature of intra- and inter-molecular interactions; these measurements are made in conditions close to the polymer scientist's ideal condition of 'infinite dilution'. The other group consists of experiments designed to understand molecular behaviour in the highly concentrated solutions which occur in tissue. In this section we will summarize information derived from a variety of techniques such as viscometry and static and dynamic light scattering. Measurements, particularly at physiological concentrations, are severely limited by the range of applicability of many of the techniques and are fraught with difficulties of interpretation which arise when measurements are made on very complex macromolecules. The reader interested or disturbed by these problems is urged to consult texts on experimental polymer science [14,15].

There have been a number of studies on the viscometric properties of hyaluronan [16–20]. Though many investigators have employed capillary viscometers which can provide only comparative data for these highly non-Newtonian solutions, the effects of polymer concentration, added salts, solution composition (e.g. hydrophobic solvents), temperature and shear rate have all been investigated. These data and results from static and dynamic light scattering measurements, which essentially provide equivalent information about molecular conformation and interactions, demonstrate the behaviour expected of an anionic polyelectrolyte, i.e. a decrease in molecular radius with increasing ionic strength and decreasing pH. The persistence length of hyaluronan is greater than that of a simple linear polyelectrolyte, which suggests a stiffening of the chains perhaps due to hydrogen bonding. Hyaluronan also aggregates readily *in vitro*, and this may be relevant to suggestions, based on ultrastructural evidence, that it forms multi-molecular assemblies in tissue [21,22].

The properties of chondroitin sulphate have been less extensively investigated, perhaps reflecting both the fact that it occurs in tissue only as a component of PGs and that, with a molecular mass of less than 20 kDa, its polymer properties are less rich than those of hyaluronan [23–25]. Viscometric and light scattering measurements on large PGs, such as those isolated from nasal, laryngeal or articular cartilage, suggest that in dilute solutions the molecules assume compact configurations [26–30]. This is particularly true of aggregates whose hydrodynamic radius is only 4–5-fold that of the monomer. Measurements on the temperature dependence of viscosity suggest that conformation may be influenced by hydrophobic interactions. The available data suggest that the isolated PG molecule can be represented as a 'wormlike cylinder' whose radius is determined by the root-mean-square length of the GAG chains. Viscometric measurements have also been made at concentrations comparable with those occurring in cartilage [31–33] (see also Chapter 2 by Hardingham *et al.* in this book). Under these conditions, rheological properties are highly non-linear and difficult to interpret at the molecular level, and complex phenomena such as the generation of a force orthogonal to the direction of shear are observed. The zero-shear viscosity of aggregates is more than five times that of monomers, indicating extensive intermolecular interactions which may be important in immobilizing the aggregates in tissue. The structure formed by aggregates also causes less energy dissipation than that of monomers and it is suggested that this is important in tissue viscoelasticity.

In tissue, GAGs and PGs are a major influence on the movement of water, as we discuss in the following section. Information on hydraulic permeability is implicit in dynamic viscosity measurements but has not, as far as we are aware, been analysed.

Hydraulic conductivity

The convective exchange of solutes with blood and lymph is important to the functioning of almost all physiological systems [34]. Convective transport is important as a means of nutrient transport within avascular tissues such as cartilage and the intervertebral disc [35]. The rate at which interstitial fluid is redistributed under the influence of mechanical loads is also a principal determinant of the viscoelastic properties of tissues [36]. Perhaps the first indication of the physiological importance of GAGs was the demonstration that they influence water movement [37]. This has been show both by the effects of enzymes such as hyaluronidase on the hydraulic conductivity of tissue and by analyses of the relationships between hydraulic conductivity and GAG content of different tissues (Figure 2). The current view is that GAGs are a major, but not the sole, determinant of hydraulic conductivity [38]. It is difficult, however, to draw quantitative conclusions because of uncertainties about the distribution and organization of GAGs in tissue and, particularly, because of the difficulty of measuring the hydraulic conductivity of GAG and PG solutions *in vitro*. Measurements have been based on ultracentrifugal sedimentation and direct measurements using a filter chamber [39–47]. Published estimates vary over two orders of magnitude which may, in part, be attributable to experimental difficulties. In direct measurements, where the polymer is contained within a flow cell by a semipermeable membrane on the downstream side, macromolecules tend to convect with the flow to form a 'filtercake' whose permeability dominates the measurements, and this was not corrected for in some experiments [48,49]. These experiments therefore underestimated permeability and their value now lies in reminding us of the unresolved question of how the macromolecules are constrained within the tissue matrix. Measurements based on ultracentrifugal sedimentation of the macromolecules are indirect and there is some concern that the large, flexible molecules assume unnatural configurations as they move under the large body forces they experience [14]. Hyaluronan, chondroitin sulphate and PG monomers and aggregates all have similar hydraulic conductivity and their flow resistance seems to be determined largely by the small, relatively rigid, hydrogen-bonded regions in their structure. Electrokinetic effects, which we discuss in the following section, also appear to have little influence on hydraulic conductivity.

Polyelectrolyte properties

One of the characteristic features of GAGs and PGs is their high content of anionic charges: the concentration of GAGs found in cartilage, for example, produces a charge density of 0.1 M. The mobile

Figure 2

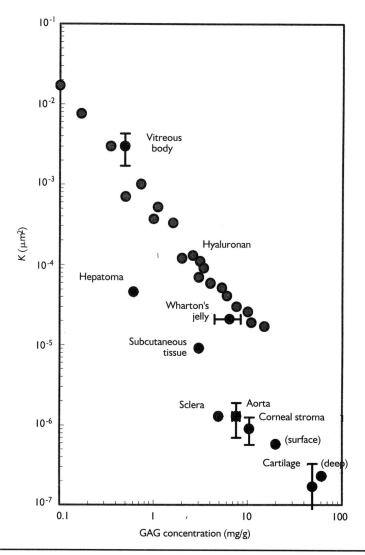

The relationship between the hydraulic conductivity of various tissues and their GAG content (note the logarithmic scales)
Hydraulic conductivity of different tissues is primarily dependent on the glycosaminoglycan content of the tissue; however, the much higher hydraulic conductivity measured for hyaluronan solutions suggests that other extracellular matrix components such as the collagen content are also important.

counterions which maintain electroneutrality generate an osmotic pressure which, in tissues such as cartilage, is central to their physiological role in supporting compressive loads [35]. The influence which PGs exert on the ionic composition of the interstitial fluid may affect cellular metabolism and thereby be involved in the transduction of information between cells and matrix [50]. The anionic character of the PGs is important in the calcification of the ECM as we discuss below and there is also evidence that electrical currents generated by the convection of ions through the interstitium are important in tissue growth, healing and homoeostasis [51]. More specialized and speculative uses of the electrical properties of GAGs include hair cell activity in the inner ear [52] and in the electric organs of fish [53]. Finally, it is hypothesized that negatively charged polymers may have been important during evolution in shielding tissues from attack by highly reactive hydrated electrons [54].

There is some evidence that the detailed structure of GAGs and PGs influence their polyelectrolyte properties. There are slight differences in the pK values of the charge groups on the various GAGs [53], and potentiometric titration of isolated molecules and fixed-charge titration on cartilage plugs both indicate that the pKs of PG monomers and particularly aggregates are less acidic than those of the constituent GAGs, perhaps indicating an effect of intramolecular charge repulsion (A. Maroudas, C.P. Winlove and K.H. Parker, unpublished work).

The effects of GAGs and PGs on the distributions of small ions have been extensively investigated [55–58]. The behaviour of calcium, sodium and chloride ions is, at physiological ionic strength, close to the predictions of the Donnan theory of ionic equilibrium. However, at low polymer and salt concentrations, where ionic interactions are less effectively shielded, an increase in the partition coefficient is observed. Measurements of the diffusivities of small ions show that under physiological conditions electrostatic interactions are well shielded and the reduction in diffusivity is comparable with that of small neutral solutes [58,59]. Only at low salt and polymer concentrations is a greater reduction observed, particularly for bivalent cations. This behaviour is in agreement with the predictions of polyelectrolyte theory [60]. For transition metals, complex ions and polyions, the formation of specific stereochemical complexes has been suggested [61] (D. O'Hare, I. Angel, C.P. Winlove and P.M. Gribbon, unpublished work), but these have not, as far as we are aware, been shown to have any biological significance. Specific binding of organic cations may be important in interactions with other matrix components and has been exploited to allow histochemical identification of particular GAGs [63].

Because of the importance of the osmotic pressures generated by the PGs to the function of tissues such as cartilage, and evidence that changes in the hydration and mechanical properties of cartilage occur in diseases such as osteoarthritis, there have been efforts to measure the osmotic pressures generated by GAGs and PGs *in vitro* and to correlate them with molecular structure [64–67]. There are some quantitative discrepancies between direct measurements and calculations from ultracentrifugal sedimentation data. However, both types of experiment show a non-linear increase in osmotic pressure with polymer concentration which, it has been noted, would have the effect of amplifying the contribution of osmotic forces to homoeostasis and only a weak dependence of osmotic pressure on biochemical composition. The osmotic pressure of GAGs and PGs tends to a non-zero value at high ionic strength (for chondroitin sulphate the osmotic pressure in 1.5 M NaCl is only about 40% of its osmotic pressure at physiological ionic strength), which indicates that there is a non-electrostatic contribution to osmotic pressure. The electrostatic contribution can be modelled qualitatively using polyelectrolyte theory, and with some 'fitting' of parameters such as polymer radius and charge density quantitative agreement between theory and experiment can by attained (S. Cohen, A. Maroudas, R. Schneiderman, K.H. Parker and C.P. Winlove, unpublished work; M.D. Buschmann and A.J. Grodzinsky, unpublished work).

The nature and concentration of the counterion strongly influences the conformation of GAGs and PGs, as is readily shown by viscometric, ultracentrifugation or light scattering measurements. In particular, the polymers assume a more compact configuration at high ionic strength and in the presence of bivalent cations. Bivalent cations do not cause charge reversal, which would be expected if the polymer were sufficiently rigid and the charges were too sparse to allow ion interaction with two fixed charges simultaneously [70]. It is suggested that ion-induced conformation changes may be involved in mechanochemical transduction [71].

It has been suggested that the anionic nature of GAGs plays a role in controlling the calcium content of tissues and in normal and pathological calcification [72–74]. In pathological situations, the preferential deposition of crystals such as sodium urate in distinct locations has been linked with the distribution of polyelectrolytes. However, no great differences have been observed in the interactions of calcium with particular GAGs and large PGs, even between those isolated from 'resting' and ossifying cartilage [75]; however, there is a suggestion that some small collagen-binding PGs have a particular affinity for calcium [76]. There have been a number of studies on the effects of PGs on the precipitation of calcium phosphates and although there are some conflicting reports, the consensus view appears to be that they are inhibitory, aggregates being more effective than monomers [77,78]. A number of mechanisms for this behaviour have been proposed [79].

Interactions with solutes
The PGs form the finest scale polymer network in the interstitium. In cartilage, for example, the size of the pores, estimated from structural analysis and partition coefficient data, is less than 3 nm in diameter [80]. They therefore influence the distribution and diffusivity of solutes. For neutral solutes the effect arises because the solutes are excluded from a space around the polymer, the volume of which depends on the combined radius of polymer and solute (Figure 3). The ratio between the accessible water volume and the total water volume of the matrix is often referred to as the partition coefficient of the solute. In cartilage it ranges from 0.92 for glucose to 0.01 for albumin and larger molecules [35]. Cartilage is one of the densest interstitia so these figures probably represent lower bounds, but in most tissues the partition coefficient of large molecules is probably sufficiently far from unity as to warrant more consideration than it customarily receives in discussions of the distribution of particular solutes in tissue. A simple, semi-empirical equation relating the partition coefficient to the radius and concentration of the polymer and the solute radius is widely used in the biological literature and gives an adequate description of the effects of GAGs and PGs [81]. More rigorous models have recently been developed which give closer agreement [82]. It has not yet proven possible, however, to

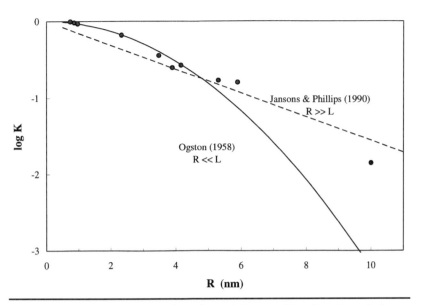

Figure 3

The available space, _K_, as a function of the combined radius of the solute and the fibre, _R_
The data are for various molecules in hyaluronan gels measured by exclusion chromatography [184]. Ogston's theory [81] assumes that the fibres are very long compared with the radius of the solvent and should be valid for small **R** _values. The theory of Jansons and Phillips [82] assumes that the fibres can be approximated by a Brownian path and should be more valid for large R values._

derive models which faithfully represent the complex geometry of the PGs. Experimentally, however, the most important parameter determining the distribution of solutes appears to be the total chain length of polymer per unit volume, perhaps because there is so much overlap and entanglement of molecules that their conformation is obscured. It may be, of course, that in tissue the ECM has a much more ordered organization than can be reproduced in model systems _in vitro_.

In addition to influencing the distribution of solutes, the PGs also affect their mobility. Steric exclusion and the tortuosity of pathways through the polymer network both reduce solute diffusivity. These effects increase rapidly with the size of the solute (Figure 4) and also depend on the nature of the polymer. Hyaluronan causes a greater reduction in diffusivity than chondroitin sulphate at the same concentration, probably because the chondroitin sulphate molecules are too small to form extensive entanglements. Laryngeal PGs also have a smaller effect than hyaluronan, particularly if the comparison is made at the same fixed charge density rather than at the same concentration. There have been a number of measurements of the diffusivity of GAGs and PGs themselves [29,83,84] These measurements are important in understanding the balance between synthesis, degradation and migration out of the tissue, which determines the concentration of PG in the tissue. A variety of methods have been used with sometimes contra-

Figure 4

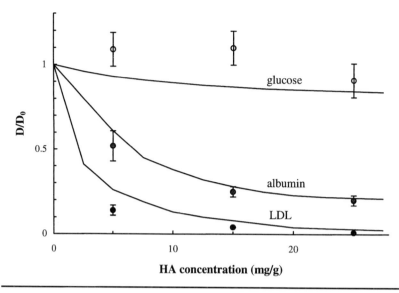

The effects of hyaluronan (HA) concentration on the diffusivities of solutes of different sizes

Small solutes such as glucose suffer almost no retardation, but larger molecules are significantly retarded. The effects of proteoglycans are qualitatively similar. Data such as these and those in Figure 3 indicate that the extracellular matrix acts as a dispersive filter, determining the composition of the extracellular fluid and the rate at which solutes can be exchanged.

dictory results, particularly concerning the concentration dependence, at least some of which is attributable to confusion between self- and mutual diffusion coefficients. Measured by light scattering, the free diffusivity of bovine nasal cartilage PG monomer in water was 2.5 μm^2/s at very low PG concentrations, and this fell to 0.4 μm^2/s as the PG concentration increased to 3 mg/ml. The same measurements at physiological ionic strength gave a free diffusivity of 5.7 μm^2/s which increased very slightly as the PG concentration was increased [29].

Measurements of diffusivity have generally used solutes which are convenient 'molecular probes' rather than of direct interest in their own right and so there is a dearth of literature on biologically important molecules. It is therefore difficult to make general statements or predictions because the presence of a polymer network can have a variety of effects on macromolecule diffusion. For example, the rotation of asymmetrical molecules is impeded by the polymer and so they migrate as though their equivalent hydrodynamic radius is reduced, and flexible, long-chain molecules can tunnel or 'reptate' through channels inaccessible to more rigid molecules giving a higher than expected diffusivity [86]. Where, as in many biological systems, transport occurs under the combined influences of convection and diffusion, the matrix may exhibit 'exclusion chromatography' behaviour in which large molecules migrate more rapidly than small ones [87]. This arises because the large molecules are sterically confined to large channels where convection is rapid while small molecules are able to diffuse into regions of tissue with smaller pores and therefore smaller convective velocities and are thereby retarded. Enhanced transport has also been observed where concentration gradients of polymer exist which may generate convective flows [88]. The physiological significance of all these effects remains to be demonstrated.

It is becoming increasingly clear that the ability of PGs to bind to other molecules is important in connective-tissue physiology and pathology. A discussion of the interactions between PGs and other matrix molecules which are involved in growth and development is outside the scope of this review and, indeed, the underlying physical chemistry has hardly been investigated. The ability of PGs to bind cytokines, growth factors and degradative enzymes has only recently been recognized [89], but is probably very important in modulating the effects of these agents, and further work in this area is clearly required. It has been appreciated for rather longer that the GAGs have anti-coagulant activity similar to that of heparin, to which they are closely related structurally. This property may be important for PGs on the endothelial cell surface (see below). Its role within the tissue is less clear, though the concentration of plasma proteins in the interstitium can be quite high. In the large blood vessels it is observed that both the interstitial concentration of proteins and the concentration of GAGs with high anticoagulant activity increase with age [90]. The interaction of PGs with plasma lipoproteins has attracted the attention of vascular biologists as a potential source of lipid accumulation in atherosclerosis [91–93]. This interaction is initiated by electrostatic forces, perhaps facilitated by bivalent cations, but is thought to be stabilized by hydrophobic protein–protein interactions. Various specificities with regard to both PG and lipoprotein are reported and the interactions are believed not only to trap lipoproteins within the interstitium but also to modify their interactions with cells.

Interfacial properties

Most of the above discussion has concentrated on the properties of GAGs and PGs in bulk solution, primarily because this represents most of the available biophysical literature. PGs are, however, found both on the surface of cells, where they are a major component of the glycocalyx, and coating collagen and elastin fibres. The PGs associated with collagen and elastin are generally small, containing only one or two GAG chains, and bind via their protein core leaving the polysaccharides free [94–97]. As we discuss in the following section, the surface molecules appear to influence collagen fibre assembly, the size of fibrils and interfibrillar spacing which is important, for example, in maintaining the transparency of the cornea. A variety of cell-surface PGs have been identified, some with hydrophobic tails to the protein cores which can be inserted directly into the lipid bilayer of the plasma membranes and others which bind to membrane proteins via either their protein or GAG moieties. These molecules may act as chemo- or mechano-receptors either directly or in conjunction with other membrane components [95]. Cell-surface PGs are therefore likely to be involved in the control of cell metabolism, adhesion and migration. The molecules covering the luminal surface of endothelium may have additional roles in providing a non-thrombogenic interface with blood, regulating the movement of water and solutes across the endothelium and, perhaps, acting as a 'flow transducer' to communicate information about flow conditions to the underlying tissue [96]. Both cell- and fibril-associated PGs are likely to be particularly important during development and remodelling, and understanding of the biophysical basis of their functions is expected to assume increasing importance.

Collagens

The collagens are the primary structural proteins of tissue and in vertebrates constitute approximately one-third of the total protein. Eighteen different collagens have now been identified, coded by 30 genes distributed over more than a dozen chromosomes. All the collagens contain a characteristic triple-chain helix with varying amounts of non-helical domains. The chains themselves are characterized by a repeating triplet amino acid sequence, Gly-Xaa-Yaa, where Xaa and Yaa are frequently proline and hydroxyproline. The major fibrillar collagens are types I and III and, in cartilaginous tissues, type II. These three collagens have been extensively characterized biochemically and structurally, have well-defined mechanical functions and will receive most of our attention in this review. Type-IV collagen is also widely distributed and has well-defined physiological functions in determining the permeability and, perhaps, the mechanical properties of basement membranes. It has, however, a rather different structure with a high proportion of non-helical domains and forms tetravalent cross-links only at its ends. Instead of forming fibrils, therefore, it produces a three-dimensional 'chicken wire' network which acts as a skeleton of basement membrane structure. The other collagens are often referred to as the 'minor collagens' because they are present only in small quantities in most tissues. Their biological functions are often not clear but their importance is indicated by the degree to which structure has been conserved during evolution. Some collagens, for example types V and XI, are intimately associated with fibrillar collagen and it is suggested that they regulate fibril diameter and/or serve as a core for fibril formation. Other collagens, such as types IX and XII, are hybrid molecules containing GAG side-chains and have been demonstrated to bind to both collagen and other matrix constituents. They are therefore likely to be involved in interactions between fibrils or between fibrils and other matrix molecules. Further details of the biochemistry and molecular biology of the collagens are to be found in many excellent reviews [97,98].

Central to the functions of type I, II and III collagens is their ability to form almost inextensible fibres of great tensile strength. The molecular organization of fibrils and the process of fibril formation has been extensively investigated [99]. Certain steps such as the conversion of procollagen (the secreted form of collagen, containing non-helical domains at either end of the triple helix which are cleaved by extracellular enzymes) into collagen and the oxidation of lysine and hydroxylysine to aldehydes to form intermolecular cross-links have been characterized. There is, however, uncertainty concerning the factors controlling the assembly of molecules at the appropriate place and time and the extent of cellular involvement in the process. *In vitro*, preparations of soluble collagen will, under suitable conditions, reform fibrils closely resembling those found in tissue. This process, too, has been extensively studied using a range of physicochemical techniques.

The physiological functions of collagen depend not only on the properties of the fibrils but on the ways in which these are assembled into higher-order structures. As we will discuss below, the mechanical properties of collagenous tissues depend not only on the properties of the individual fibrils but also on their organization. Many of the other physiological functions of collagen also depend on its ability to form ordered structures. For example, networks of collagen type IV have pores approximately 400 nm in size which can be filled with other matrix macromolecules to form membranes of any required size- or charge-selectivity and this is exploited in the renal glomerulus. The regular size and spacing of type-I collagen in the cornea are essential to its transparency. The regularity of collagen matrices may also be important in the epitatic nucleation of bone mineral.

Mechanical properties

The most obvious biological functions of collagen are mechanical. It is the major structural element in both hard and soft tissues. Fine networks of collagen fibres define the shape of organs and provide a framework for cellular attachment and for the transmission of cell-generated forces. In ligaments and tendons the collagen assumes a primary role and cells play the secondary role of maintaining and repairing the collagen network. In bone the mechanical properties of collagen are supplemented by mineral deposited around the collagen matrix. It is not surprising, therefore, that there exists an extensive literature on collagen mechanics which has been reviewed by many authors [100]. We will consider first the intrinsic mechanical properties of the collagen molecule itself. Analyses of the rheological, ultracentrifugal sedimentation and light-scattering properties of suspensions of collagen molecules all indicate that the isolated molecule behaves as a rigid rod. Analyses of Brillouin scattering suggest that the longitudinal stiffness of the molecule is twice as high as that measured in tissue [101]. It is difficult, however, in measurements on collagen networks isolated from tissue to distinguish intrinsic fibril properties from those of the whole network. In addition, it is not clear how the extraction procedures necessary to separate collagen from cells and other matrix constituents affect mechanical properties. The least equivocal data on collagen mechanics come from studies on type-I collagen from tendons such as that of the rat tail. Tendons contain a very high proportion of type-I collagen, which minimizes the problem of isolation and purification, and the fibrils are aligned in the direction of *in vivo* stresses which simplifies the geometrical problems. Even in these specimens, however, the fibres follow an undulating course, referred to as 'crimp', which complicates the interpretation of mechanical tests. Force–extension curves (Figure 5) are non-linear and comprise three regions: an initial 'toe' portion in which the collagen is relatively compliant, a linear region in which force is proportional to extension, and a third region of falling slope.

Figure 5

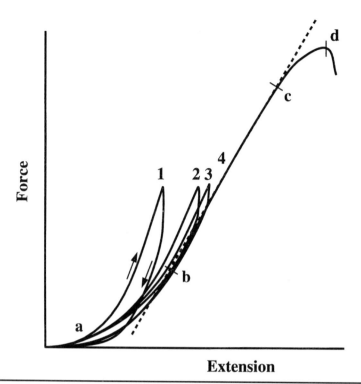

A sketch of data from a typical experiment measuring the force need to extend the collagen in a tendon

In this experiment the tendon was exposed to three loading–unloading cycles (1, 2, and 3) before it was loaded to rupture. The difference between cycles is typical of most tissues and is termed 'conditioning'. Even when the tissue is conditioned, it still exhibits different behaviour as it is loaded and unloaded, a consequence of the viscoelastic nature of tissue. The magnitude of this hysteresis depends upon the strain rate which is applied to the tissue. The final loading curve exhibits three distinct regions: a 'toe' (a–b) where the force increases exponentially with extension, a linear region (b–c) where the tissue behaves like an elastic material, and a highly non-linear (and relatively irreproducible) region (c–d) leading to rupture. The physiological range is generally between a and the lower regions of the linear portion of the curve. The ultimate strain of human tendon (corresponding to point d) can be as high as 1000 MPa.

Morphological evidence indicates that the 'toe' region is associated with straightening of the crimp and it is suggested that the physiological function of crimp is to introduce compliance into the structure to absorb initial shocks or to allow the fibres to follow a tortuous path. How the crimp is formed is still unknown [102]. In the linear portion, electron microscopy shows that 90% of the strain arises from an increase in the head to tail spacing of the molecules and only 10% arises from straightening of the fibre [103]. The effects of biochemical parameters such as the amino acid sequence and the density of cross-links on the conformation of fibrils and their mechanical properties have been described. The final non-linear portion of the force–extension curve represents yield of the fibril which is associated with the breakdown of its regular repeating structure.

An aspect of collagen mechanics which has received less analysis than the quasi-static force–extension characteristics is its viscoelasticity. This is shown by the difference between the loading and unloading curves in Figure 5, but its molecular basis is unknown. Some authors suggest that the rate of redistribution of water in the small intrafibrillar spaces is a contributory factor [104].

Type-II collagen is found only in hyaline cartilage and the intervertebral disc, where it is the main structural component. It forms finer fibrils than type I and the individual molecules are more widely spaced. In hyaline cartilage the fibrils are assembled into an elaborate three-dimensional network spanning the whole depth of the tissue and the alignment of fibres has been correlated with the direction of prevailing loads at different depths [105]. Biomechanically, the unique feature of type-II-containing tissues is that they support compressive loads. These loads are opposed by the osmotic pressure generated by the PGs which we have discussed above, and the imbalance between these forces is sufficient to generate tension within the collagen meshwork. Its mechanical functions are thus somewhat different to those of type I, but whether certain features of its structure make it suitable for its task has not been established. It is interesting, however, that when tissues, such as blood vessels, which normally experience tensile loads are subject to compression they are capable of synthesizing type II [106]. Type IX is another cartilage-specific collagen which bonds covalently to the surface of type-II fibrils and some authors feel that it has a mechanical role, either directly through the formation of interfibrillar links or indirectly by increasing interactions with other molecules [107].

There is no quantitative information on the mechanical properties of the other principal fibrillar collagens, types III and V, and there are no tissues in which they are thought to be the major structural elements. Fibrils of type III are generally finer than type I and it is found in higher proportion in the more distensible tissues such as large blood vessels. This suggests that it does have a particular mechanical function, which some authors believe to be involved in forming attachments between cells and matrix [108]. In conditions such as Ehlers Danlos syndrome where weakening of collagenous tissues occurs there is a reduction in the content of type III [109].

Type-IV collagen is normally considered to be more important in regulating tissue permeability than mechanics, but there is some evidence that in delicate structures such as capillaries and lung alveoli, in which it is quantitatively a major component of the interstitium, it makes a contribution to mechanical properties [110]. The small scale of the networks of type IV has made it something of a challenge to measure their mechanical properties directly, though some results have been presented [111,112].

Interactions with other molecules

Since collagen networks are large-scale structures their influence on the distribution and mobility of solutes in the interstitium is often ignored.

This may not be valid. First, in many tissues the 'excluded volume' of collagen fibres may not be negligible and needs to be considered in calculating the interstitial concentrations of solutes and of matrix molecules themselves [38]. Secondly, by providing a framework within which soluble molecules are enmeshed, the collagen fibres probably influence the organization and hence the permeability of the matrix. This may be particularly important in the function of basement membranes [113]. Some authors also suggest that the charge associated with the type-IV collagen in basement membranes is sufficient to contribute to the charge-selective filtration properties of the glomerulus [114].

Interactions between collagen and other tissue components are important in many contexts. One example which has already been noted is the binding to PGs, which is important in matrix assembly. There is also evidence that interactions with cells are important in intercellular communication and cell migration, particularly in developing tissue [115]. The charge properties of collagen fibrils have been characterized [116] and are important to both their organization and interactions with other charged macromolecules. Interactions with small ions are important in both the normal and the pathological calcification of connective tissue [117]. It was demonstrated many years ago that reconstituted collagen fibres could, unlike soluble collagen, act as a catalyst for the heterogeneous nucleation of apatite crystals from metastable solutions of calcium and phosphate. The nucleation site has been variously identified with the 64 nm banding period or the features of the intrafibrillar space. The importance of intracellular processing of minerals in the calcification process is becoming increasingly evident and a number of hypotheses have been advanced linking collagen with the deposition of cell-secreted mineral rather than *ab initio* nucleation [118]. Most studies of calcification have used type-I collagen since it is found in both calcifying and non-calcifying tissues. The regulation of calcification must be due to molecules other than collagen itself and, as we discussed in the previous section, the PGs are likely to be important in this connection.

Recent research has shown that the rate of collagen synthesis in mature tissue is higher than was previously thought and a number of enzymes capable of degrading collagen have been identified [119]. A number of physicochemical and mechanical factors affecting the rate of collagen synthesis [50,120] and collagenase activity [121] have already been identified and this is an active field of research pertinent to diseases as diverse as pulmonary fibrosis, hypertension and osteoarthritis. Nevertheless, collagen is a relatively long-lived protein and this means that it is susceptible to modification by slow chemical reactions. These may be important in normal ageing and in connective-tissue diseases. Amino acids, particularly the ε-amino group of lycine, undergo very slow reactions with sugars through a process known as non-enzymic glycosylation [122]. These reactions modify the organization [123] and mechanical properties of collagen [124] and alter its reactivity towards other molecules [125]. It is suggested that these modifications may be responsible for some of the microvascular and connective-tissue changes which are long-term complications of diabetes mellitus [126]. Collagen also binds lipids and lipoproteins [127] and these interactions may be important both in determining the fate of lipid vesicles containing calcium [128] and in the deposition of lipids in the arterial wall in atherosclerosis [129].

A slightly different aspect of collagen reactivity is that towards cells. We have already alluded to the importance of collagen in cell migration and differentiation during development [115]. The interactions of collagen types I and III in the blood vessel wall with blood platelets is also important in haemostasis. This is obviously beneficial in the case of injury, but it may also lead to thrombosis if rupture of an athero-sclerotic plaque (either spontaneously or during angioplasty) exposes collagen to blood. Adhesion and activation both require collagen to be in triple-helical form and the physical dimensions of the fibrils also appear to be important [130]. The specific amino acid sequences on collagen molecules and the platelet integrins involved in the interactions have been identified [131].

Electrical properties
We have already discussed the importance of electrostatic forces in the interactions between collagen and other molecules. Electrostatic inter-actions also influence the dimensions and conformation of collagenous structures themselves. It has been suggested that changes in the ionic environment in cartilage may, through this effect, alter the mechanical properties of cartilage [132]. This and the possibility of chemo-mechanical or electromechanical transduction which collagen and similar synthetic polymers afford have been used to develop 'intelligent' filtration membranes [133] and even collagen 'motors' [134].

Dehydrated collagen fibres are piezoelectric and it has been suggested that this is important in determining the organization of bone with respect to prevailing mechanical loads [135]. However, under physiological conditions collagen fibres are highly hydrated and it now seems more plausible that streaming currents generated by the convective movement of ions are the signals responsible for determining the growth and organization of the bone matrix [136] although research in this area is continuing [137]. Collagen also displays the properties of pyroelectricity and optical anisotropy and there are suggestions that these properties are of biological importance [138].

Elastin

Elastin is widely distributed throughout the vertebrate body and is found in the lung, dermis, blood vessels and ligaments but, with the exception of the large arteries and some specialized ligaments (notably the ligamentum nuchae of grazing animals), it is present in smaller quantities than collagen. Its most important function is generally considered to be that of endowing tissues with the properties of elasticity and elastic recoil and it therefore serves as the biomechanical complement of collagen.

Elastin, unlike collagen, is a single-gene-copy protein, though multiple isoforms may be produced by alternative splicing of its pre-mRNA [139]. The biochemistry and molecular biology of elastin are summarized in a number of review articles [140–142]. Just two features of its biochemistry are central to its biophysical properties and physiological functions. The first is the existence of frequent repeats of two highly non-polar peptide sequences, the pentapeptide Val-Gly-Val-Pro-Gly and the hexapeptide Val-Gly-Val-Ala-Pro-Gly. These sequences form folded structures (β-spirals) not known to occur in any other mammalian proteins, which possess a high degree of distensibility and whose hydrophobicity is a major factor in the elasticity of the protein and in the assembly of supramolecular structures. The second feature, also involved in the formation of supramolecular assemblies, is the existence of desmosine and isodesmosine. These amino acids, unique to elastin, are formed by the covalent cross-linking between molecules of four lysyl residues and allow the construction of extended cross-linked networks which are remarkably resistant to degradation [143] (Figure 6).

The network structure of elastin is central to its physiological functions. Molecules of elastin have the capacity to self-assemble *in vitro*, largely under the influence of interactions between hydrophobic domains but, unlike most fibrillar proteins, form disordered aggregates [144]. During development, however, elastin appears to accrete on to a skeleton of microfibrillar glycoproteins and the intimate association between elastin and other proteins to form 'elastic tissue' has been a recurring source of confusion [145], only clearing as the biochemistry of the microfibrils is better understood [146]. Although the physical chemistry of matrix assembly *in vivo* is still unclear, elastin forms a wide variety of structures ranging from the sparse network of fine fibrils found in tissues such as the intervertebral disc [147] and skin [148] to the lamellar structures which constitute more than 50% of the dry weight of the thoracic aorta. Even within blood vessels many different patterns of elastin organization are found [149]. These appear to be related to the haemodynamic forces to which the tissue is exposed, though the mechanisms by which physical forces influence the large-scale organization of the network have not yet been established.

Very few diseases are associated with defects in elastin, in contrast to collagen where a number of developmental defects are known, perhaps because elastin formation is a relatively simple process and defects are lethal to the organism [140]. Variations and abnormalities in elastic tissue therefore tend to be associated with degradation or ageing. These effects are exacerbated by the fact that elastin has the lowest rate of turnover of all the matrix macromolecules with a half-life of years or even decades [150]. With the exception of the pregnant uterus, synthesis is almost unmeasurably small under normal conditions. Many cells do, however, retain a latent capacity to synthesize elastin as is demonstrated by the synthesis of elastin, albeit frequently with impaired functional properties, after injury or in response to changing biomechanical conditions such as hypertension.

Mechanical properties

Like collagen, the most obvious function of elastin is mechanical. The manner in which parallel networks of elastin and collagen give rise to the non-linear mechanical properties of blood vessels which are essential to their functions was described semi-quantitatively in the 1950s [151]. In skin, too, elastin has an obvious role in providing distensibility [152, 152a], but in many other tissues, such as the intervertebral disc, elastin

(b)

Figure 6

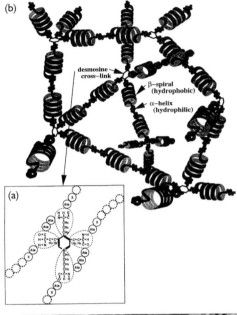

(a)

(c)

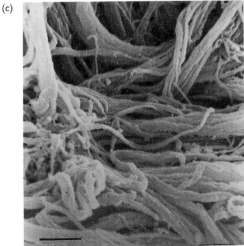

Elastin structure

The desmosine cross-links (a) are unique to elastin and enable it to form into complex three-dimensional structures (b). The regions shown rather speculatively as β-spirals are hydrophobic and it is thought that some of the remarkable elasticity of elastin is the result of hydrophobic interactions when the elastin is stretched. From both biochemical and mechanical evidence, there are an average of about 70 amino acid residues between each cross-link. Elastin exhibits rubber-like elasticity which means that its elasticity is predominantly derived from changes in its entropy as it is deformed and, as a result, it becomes stiffer when it is heated. In tissue a variety of fibrillar and lamellar structures are produced as seen in (c) which is a scanning electron micrograph of the outer media of porcine thoracic aorta after alkali digestion. The scale bar represents 10 μm.

is present in much smaller amounts. It is not clear whether it contributes directly to the load-bearing properties of the tissue or is involved only in coupling together of other primary mechanical elements to maintain their alignment under different loading conditions.

The molecular basis of elastin elasticity has been investigated extensively. The most common experimental approach has been measurement of the thermomechanical properties of elastin networks coupled with a theoretical analysis based on the theory of rubber-like elasticity [153]. Neither experiment nor theory is straightforward when applied to a multiphase, anisotropic network but the consensus view is that the dominant contribution to elasticity is entropic and internal energy changes contribute no more than 10–20% to the isometric force. A number of static, two-phase models of the elastin molecule such as the 'liquid drop' and the 'oiled coil' have been proposed, but have subsequently been found to be incompatible with the experimental observations [154]. There is evidence from other techniques such as n.m.r. that the elastin molecule is a dynamic structure containing regions of α-helix and β-coil and, while the mechanical measurements are consistent with these structures, they do not provide conclusive evidence of their existence. Analyses of the mechanical behaviour of fibrils using the theory of polymer elasticity indicate that the amount of elastin between cross-links is 6–7 kDa [155] but, though this value appears reasonable on the basis of biochemistry, some authors have expressed reservations about the accuracy of the theory [156].

A source of difficulty in interpreting measurements on the mechanical properties of elastin networks, which we have already mentioned in connection with collagen, is that of separating intrinsic mechanical properties of individual fibres from the effects of their geometrical organization. There have been a limited number of measurements on individual elastin fibres teased from ligamentum nuchae which give an elastic modulus of 1.2 MPa and a breaking strain of 100–200%. Both values, as was found for collagen, are substantially higher than those measured for networks [155].

Most mechanical testing has been performed on ligamentum nuchae elastin but, while this is a convenient source of material, there is greater physiological interest in measurements on tissues such as blood vessels. The available data fall into two groups, one consisting of direct measurements on 'pure' elastin isolated by acid, alkali, cyanogen bromide or enzyme digestion and the other of correlations between the mechanical properties of intact tissues and their biochemical composition. Both approaches suffer methodological problems [153], so that although the suggestion that elastin is the major determinant of the small-strain modulus of blood vessels has stood the test of time it has not yet proven possible to relate the mechanical properties of elastin networks from different vessels to their geometry and organization. We therefore do not know whether there are differences in the intrinsic mechanical properties of elastin from different vessels or what the functional consequences of the variations of elastin architecture are. Similarly it is not certain how the fragmentation of the elastic lamellae and the accumulation of polar glycoproteins, minerals and lipids which occurs with age and disease affect the mechanical function of elastin.

A subject which has received remarkably little attention considering its physiological importance is the dynamic mechanical properties of elastin. *In vivo* vascular elastin experiences oscillating loads at frequencies of up to 10 Hz and its elastic recoil is essential to the efficient functioning of the circulation. The resilience of elastin falls rapidly at high frequencies because, it is suggested, the elastin chains are insufficiently mobile to change conformation in response to the applied load [157]. The frequency dependence of the elasticity is extremely sensitive to the degree of hydration of the elastin and the hydration has been shown to affect the rate of stress relaxation in elastin networks [158]. It has been suggested that the rate of redistribution of intra-fibrillar water is important to elastin dynamics [158,159]. Both lines of evidence indicate that changes in the hydration of elastin, perhaps by binding of other molecules or changes in the composition or osmotic properties of the surrounding interstitium could modify the mechanical properties of the tissue.

Chemical reactivity
Having been regarded for many years as the most inert and unreactive of matrix molecules, it is becoming increasingly clear that elastin does play a very active role in matrix biology, interacting both with matrix molecules and with cells. Its interactions with microfibrillar glyco-proteins are important in developing tissues and its strong binding to PGs [160] may, as in the case of collagen, be involved in fibril organization and growth although the physicochemical basis of these interactions has not been established. Receptors both for fibrous elastin and for elastin-derived peptides have been found on the surfaces of many cells and have been shown to influence intracellular ion balances, chemotaxis and adhesion [161]. It is suggested that these receptors are involved in development and wound healing as well as pathological processes such as atherosclerosis, emphysema and tumorigenesis [162].

Elastin is also implicated in arterial disease through its capacity to bind both minerals [163] and lipids [164], and the literature on the physical chemistry of both processes is summarized in [153]. Diffuse crystalline deposits of mineral appear in the elastic lamellae of arteries to an extent which increases with age. Elastin calcification occurs focally in atherosclerotic plaques and more extensively in rarer conditions such as Monkenberg's sclerosis. There have been *in vitro* experiments demonstrating the deposition of apatite crystals in the elastic lamellae of blood vessels [165] and the binding of calcium phosphate to purified elastin [166]. There is still, however, some controversy about the mechanism of calcium binding to elastin. Because of its predilection for calcium binding yet relative paucity of anionic groups, it has been suggested that elastin also contains a neutral site for calcium binding, and a conformation of acyl oxygen groups within the β-turn structure has been proposed as a possible candidate [167]. Several lines of evidence indicate that neutral site binding is very sensitive to the conformation of the elastin so that, although electrostatic binding to carboxyl groups is the dominant mechanism in alkali-extracted elastin in physiological salt solutions [168,169], the possibility exists that neutral site binding is important, particularly if the elastin structure is degenerate. Elastin calcification is generally regarded as a deleterious process associated with loss of elasticity. Direct experimental evidence of changes in mechanical properties has been obtained only at very high calcium concentrations [170] though a number of mechanisms, such as loss of hydrophobicity due to the presence of calcium within the domain, have been suggested. An alternative view of the effects of calcification has also been advanced, suggesting that the complex is a unique cationic hydrophobic polymer which contrasts with the hydrophilic anionic character of other matrix molecules and may be important, for example, in directing the inter- actions of elastin with enzymes and similar molecules [167].

Arterial elastin normally contains 1–2% (dry weight) of lipid, but in elastin isolated from atherosclerotic plaques this may rise to 40% [171]. Cholesterol esters are the major component but phospholipids and triacylglycerols are also present. The individual roles of elastin and its associated glycoproteins in lipid binding *in vivo* have not been distinguished but there have been a number of studies on the binding of lipids and lipoproteins to purified elastin *in vitro* [171–174]. High-density lipoprotein (HDL), low-density lipoprotein (LDL) and very-low-density lipoprotein (VLDL) all interact with elastin and both LDL and VLDL are able to transfer lipid without measurable apoprotein binding. There is evidence that particular subfractions of both elastin and lipoprotein bind preferentially and that the network structure of arterial elastin imposes steric constraints on the interaction. There have been a number of studies on the mechanisms of interaction of lipids with elastin. Hydrophobic interactions are important and may be associated with conformational changes in the elastin [175]. These conformational changes on binding of fatty acids or similar amphoric molecules introduce new anionic binding sites and may make the elastin more susceptible to enzyme attack [176]. The sensitization of elastin to elastase or other cationic species is believed to be important in atherosclerosis [177]. Conversely, it is reported that calcium-induced changes in elastin conformation can enhance lipid binding and it is suggested that this process may underlie the correlation between lipid accumulation and calcification which is observed in pathological conditions [178].

In most tissues elastin is present only in small quantities and so its effect on the permeability of the tissue to water and solutes is negligible. This is not true in large blood vessels where elastin constitutes a major proportion of the interstitium. Both the internal elastic lamella (the first continuous layer of elastin, defining the border between intima and media) and the underlying lamellae are believed to be barriers to solute transport [179]. The internal elastic lamella has attracted particular attention as a barrier which may be responsible for the accumulation of lipids and other blood-derived solutes in atherosclerosis [180]. The exact nature of the barrier, its solute selectivity and the contributions of elastin itself and of the other macromolecules which make up the lamella have not been established. One problem in addressing these questions is that the elastic lamellae themselves have quite a complex internal structure. Although the lamellae appear amorphous in transmission electron micrographs pre- pared using conventional stains, certain negative staining procedures reveal fibrils within the lamellae [181] and scanning electron microscopy reveals a variety of structures: plane sheets perforated with holes and assemblies of fibrils approximately 1 μm in diameter [149]. Mechanical disruption of both arterial and ligament elastin reduces it to fibrils of these dimensions and we would suggest that they form a basic structural unit. The fibrils themselves have an internal structure which is permeable to water and solutes with molecular masses of less than approx. 1 kDa [182]. It is possible in principle, therefore, for water and solutes to pass through or around the fibrils, or through larger channels in the lamellae. In isolated elastin a number of pathways depending on the size and charge of the solute have been identified [183], but the situation *in vivo* is difficult to investigate experimentally and will obviously depend on the presence of other macromolecules which could block some of the pathways.

Conclusions

We have attempted in this review to summarize some of the available information on the physical properties and physiological functions of the major classes of matrix macromolecules. We felt it important to cover the three major species rather than, as in many excellent reviews in the past, concentrating on a particular class in order to emphasize the similarities and differences in their individual properties and to draw attention to the co-operativity between them. While there is still much to be done on the characterization of the properties of the individual molecules, it is these interactions which will undoubtedly attract greater attention in the future. We have excluded many molecules from this review, not because we consider them to be unimportant but because too little is known about their physical properties. Another very important subject which we have not considered is the physicochemical basis of the interactions between cells and matrix. Though this is important to many aspects of cellular physiology and to the maintenance and remodelling of the matrix itself, it is again an area of research still in its infancy.

Our understanding of the physical properties of the connective tissues, which is, after all, their principal function, has not kept pace with the extraordinary developments in our understanding of the biochemistry and genetics of the matrix macromolecules. We hope that this review might stimulate further research to redress this imbalance of understanding.

We are grateful to the Wellcome Trust, the Arthritis and Rheumatism Council, the Clothworkers' Foundation, the British Heart Foundation, the SERC and the MRC for their support of the original work cited herein.

References

1. Ayad, S., Boot-Handford, R.P., Humphries, M.J., Kadler, K.E. and Shuttleworth, C.A. (eds.) (1994) *Extracellular Matrix Protein FactsBook*, Academic Press, London
2. Uitto, J. and Perejda, A. (eds.) (1987) *Connective Tissue Disease: Molecular Pathology of the Extracellular Matrix*, Dekker, New York
3. Tyler, J.A., Bolis, S., Dingle, J.T. and Middleton, J.F.S. (1992) Mediators of matrix catabolism. In: Articular Cartilage and Osteoarthritis (Kuettner, K.E., Schleyerbach, R., Peyron, J.G. and Hascall, V.C., eds.), pp. 251–262, Raven Press, New York
4. Carney, S.L. and Muir, H. (1988) The structure and function of cartilage proteoglycans. *Physiol. Rev.* **68**, 858–910
5. Forsang, M. and Hardingham, T.E. (1992) Proteoglycans — many forms, many functions. *FASEB J.* **6**, 861–870
6. Comper, W.D. and Laurent, T.C. (1978) Physiological function of connective tissue polysaccharides. *Physiol. Rev.* **58**, 255–315

7. Ogston, A.G. (1970) The biological functions of the glycosaminoglycans. In *Chemistry and Molecular Biology of the Extracellular Matrix* (Balazs, E.A., ed.), pp. 1231–1240, Academic Press, London

8. Greiling, H. and Scott, J.E. (eds.) (1989) *Keratan Sulphate*, Biochemical Society, London

9. Scott, J.E. (ed.) (1993) *Dermatan Sulphate Proteoglycans*, Portland Press, London

10. Augé, J. and David, S. (1984) Hexopyranose sugar conformation revised. *Tetrahedron* **40**, 2101–2106

11. Atkins, E.D.T., Isaac, K.D., Nieduszynski, I.A., Phelps, C.F. and Sheehan, J.K. (1974) The polyuronides: their molecular architecture. *Polymer* **15**, 263–271

12. Casu, B., Petitoum, M., Provasoli, M. and Sinay, P. (1988) Conformational flexibility: a new concept for explaining binding and biological properties of iduronic acid-containing glycosaminoglycans. *Trends Biochem. Sci.* **13**, 221–225

13. Rees, D.A., Morris, E.R., Stoddart, J.F. and Stevens, E.S. (1985) Controversial glycosaminoglycan conformations. *Nature (London)* **317**, 480

14. Spragg, S.P. (1980) *The Physical Behaviour of Macromolecules with Biological Funtions*, Wiley, Chichester

15. Tanford, C. (1961) *Physical Chemistry of Macromolecules*, Wiley, New York

16. Balazs, E.A. and Laurent, T.C. (1951) Viscosity function of hyaluronic acid as a polyelectrolyte. *J. Polymer Sci.* **6**, 665–667

17. Cleland, R.L. and Wang, J.L. (1970) Ionic polysaccharides III. Dilute solution properties of hyaluronic acid solutions. *Biopolymers* **9**, 799–810

18. Cleland, R.L. (1984) Viscometry and sedimentation equilibrium of partially hydrolysed hyaluronate: comparison with theoretical models of wormlike chains. *Biopolymers* **23**, 647–666

19. Webb, E.F., Rees, D.A., Morris, E.R. and Madden, J.K. (1980) Competitive inhibition evidence for specific intermolecular interactions in hyaluronate solutions. *J. Mol. Biol.* **138**, 375–382

20. Matthews, M.B. and Decker, L.V. (1977) Conformations of hyaluronate in neutral and alkaline solutions. *Biochim. Biophys. Acta* **498**, 259–263

21. Gibbs, D.A., Merrill, E.W. and Smith, K.A. (1968) Rheology of hyaluronic acid. *Biopolymers* **6**, 777–791

22. Scott, J.E. (1992) Supramolecular organisation of extracellular matrix glycosaminoglycans, *in vitro* and in the tissue. *FASEB J.* **6**, 2639–2645

23. Matthews, M.B. (1953) Chondroitin sulfuric acid - a linear polyelectrolyte. *Arch. Biochem. Biophys.* **43**, 181–193

24. Mathews, M.B. (1959) Macromolecular properties of isomeric chondroitin sulphates. *Biochim. Biophys. Acta* **35**, 9–17

25. Panov, B.P., Osipov, S.A., Lukina, I.V., Kiryanov, N.A. and Vasyukov, S.E. (1989) Macromolecular characteristics of chondroitin sulfates. *Khimiko Farmatsevticheskii Zhurnal* **23**, 508–512

26. Shogren, R.L., Jamieson, A.M., Blackwell, J., Carrino, D.A. and Caplan, A.I. (1982) Light-scattering studies of chick limb bud proteoglycans. *J. Biol. Chem.* **257**, 8627–8629

27. Shogren, R.L., Blackwell, J., Jamieson, A.M., Carrino, D.A., Peckak, D. and Caplan, A.I. (1993) Light-scattering-studies of chick limb bud proteoglycan aggregate. *J. Biol. Chem.* **268**, 14741–14744

28. Harper, G.S. and Preston, B.N. (1987) Molecular shrinkage of proteoglycans. *J. Biol. Chem.* **262**, 8088–8095

29. Li, X. and Reed, W.F. (1991) Polyelectrolyte properties of proteoglycan monomers. *J. Chem. Phys.* **94**, 4568–4580

30. Gribbon, P.M., David, L., Parker, K.H. and Winlove, C.P. (1994) The physicochemical properties of cartilage proteoglycans. Proc. 40th Meet. ORS. *J. Bone Joint Surg.*, in the press

31. Mow, V.C., Mak, A.F., Lai, W.M., Rosenberg, L.C. and Tang, L.H. (1984) Viscoelastic properties of proteoglycan monomers and aggregates in varying solution concentration. *J. Biomech.* **17**, 325–338

32. Hardingham, T.E., Muir, H., Kwan, M.K., Lai, W.M. and Mow, V.C. (1987) Viscoelastic properties of proteoglycan solutions with varying proportions present as aggregates. *J. Orthopaedic Res.* **5**, 36–46

33. Soby, L., Jamieson, A.M., Blackwell, J., Choi, H.U. and Rosenberg, L.C. (1990) Viscoelastic and rheological properties of concentrated solutions of proteoglycan subunit and proteoglycan aggregate. *Biopolymers* **29**, 1587–1592

34. Bert, J.L. and Pearce, R.H. (1984) The interstitium and microvascular exchange. In *Handbook of Physiology*, Cardiovascular System, Vol. VI - Microcirculation (Renkin, E.M. and Michel, C.C., eds.), chapt. 12, American Physiological Society, Bethesda, MD

35. Maroudas, A. (1980) Physical chemistry of articular cartilage and the intervertebral disc. In *The Joints and Synovial Fluid* (Sokoloff, L., ed.), pp. 239–291, Academic Press, New York

36. Mow, V.C., Holmes, M.H. and Lai, W.M. (1984) Fluid transport and mechanical properties of articular cartilage: a review. *J. Biomech.* **17**, 377–394

37. Day, T.D. (1952) The permeability of interstitial connective tissue and the nature of the interfibrillar substance. *J. Physiol. (London)* **117**, 1–8

38. Levick, J.R. (1987) Flow through interstitium and other fibrous matrices. *Q. J. Exp. Physiol.* **72**, 409–438

39. Ogston, A.G. and Sherman, T.F. (1961) Effects of hyaluronic acid upon diffusion of solutes and flow of solvent. *J. Physiol. (London)* **156**, 67–74

40. Preston, B.N., Davies, M. and Ogston, A.G. (1965) The composition and physicochemical properties of hyaluronic acids prepared from ox synovial fluid and from a case of mesothelioma. *Biochem. J.* **96**, 449–474

41. Adamson, R.H. and Curry, F.E. (1982) Water flow through a fibre matrix of hyaluronic acid. *Microvasc. Res.* **23**, 239

42. Jackson, G.W. and James, D.F. (1982) The hydrodynamic resistance of hyaluronic acid and its contribution to tissue permeability. *Biorheology* **19**, 317–330

43. Carr, M.E. and Hadler, N.M. (1980) Permeability of hyaluronic acid solutions. *Arthritis Rheum.* **23**, 1371–1375

44. Ethier, C.R. (1986) The hydrodynamic resistance of hyaluronic acid. Estimates from sedimentation studies. *Biorheology* **23**, 99–113

45. Comper, W.D. and Williams, R.P.W. (1987) Hydrodynamics of concentrated proteoglycan solutions. *J. Biol. Chem.* **262**, 13464–13471

46. Zamparo, O. and Comper, W.D. (1989) Hydraulic conductivity of chondroitin sulphate proteoglycan solutions. *Arch. Biochem. Biophys.* **274**, 259–269

47. Comper, W.D. and Lyons, K.C. (1993) Non-electrostatic factors govern the hydrodynamic properties of articular cartilage proteoglycans. *Biochem. J.* **289**, 543–547

48. Parker, K.H. and Winlove, C.P. (1984) The macromolecular basis of the hydraulic conductivity of the arterial wall. *Biorheology* **21**, 181–196

49. Johnson, M., Kamm, R., Ethier, C.R. and Pedley, T.J. (1987) Scaling laws and the effects of concentration polarisation on the permeability of hyaluronic acid. *Physicochem. Hydrodynamics* **9**, 427–441

50. Urban, J.P.G. and Hall, A. (1992) Physical modifiers of cartilage metabolism. In *Articular Cartilage and Osteoarthritis* (Kuettner, K., Schleyerbach, R., Peyron, J.G. and Hascall, V.C., eds.), pp. 393–405, Raven Press, New York

51. Grodzinsky, A.J. and Frank, E.H. (1990) Electromechanical and physicochemical regulation of cartilage strength and metabolism. In *Connective Tissue Matrix*, Part 2 (Hukins, D.W.L., ed.), pp. 91–126, MacMillan, London

52. Christiansen, J.A. (1964) On hyaluronate molecules in the labyrinth as mechano-electrical transucers and as molecular motors acting as resonators. *Acta Oto-Laryngol.* **57**, 33–49

53. Mathews, M.B. (1975) *Connective Tissue Macromolecular Structure and Evolution.* Springer, Berlin

54. Scott, J.E. (1988) How did biopolymers evolve before life began? *TREE* **3**, 340–342

55. Dunstone, J.R. (1962) Ion-exchange reactions between acid mucopolysaccharides and various cations. *Biochem. J.* **85**, 336–351

56. Preston, B.N., Snowden, J.McK. and Houghton, K.T. (1972) Model connective tissue systems. The effect of proteoglycans on the distribution of small non-electrolytes and microions. *Biopolymers* **11**, 1645–1659

57. Matthews, M.B. (1970) Binding of calcium by proteoglycans and chondroitin sulphate. In *Chemistry and Molecular Biology of the Intercellular Matrix* (Balazs E.A., ed.), Academic Press, New York

58. Maroudas, A., Weinberg, P.D., Parker, K.H. and Winlove, C.P. (1988) The distributions and diffusivities of small ions in chondroitin sulphate, hyaluronate and some proteoglycan solutions. *Biophys. Chem.* **32**, 257–270

59. Magdelenat, M., Turq, P. and Chemla, M. (1974) Study of the self diffusion coefficients of cations in the presence of acid polysaccharides. *Biopolymers* **13**, 1535–1548

60. Parker, K.H., Winlove, C.P. and Maroudas, A. (1988) The theoretical distributions and diffusivities of small ions in chondroitin sulphate and hyaluronate. *Biophys. Chem.* **32**, 271–281

61. Mathews, M.B. (1964) Structural factors in cation binding to anionic polysaccharides of connective tissue. *Arch. Biochem. Biophys.* **61**, 367–377

62. Reference deleted.

63. Scott, J.E. (1968) Patterns of specificity in the binding of organic cations with acid mucopolysaccharides. In *The Chemical Physiology of Mucopolysaccharides* (Quintarelli, G., ed.), Littlejohn, Boston, MA

64. Comper, W.D. and Preston, B.N. (1974) A study of polyion-mobile ion and of excluded volume interactions of proteoglycans. *Biochem. J.* **143**, 1–9

65. Urban, J.P.G., Maroudas, A., Bayliss, M.T. and Dillon, J. (1979) Swelling pressures of proteoglycans at the concentrations found in cartilaginous tissues. *Biorheology* **16**, 447–464

66. Comper, W.D. and Zamparo, O. (1990) Hydrodynamic properties of connective tissue polysaccharides. *Biochem. J.* **269**, 561–566

67. Pietzch, R.M. and Reed, W.F. (1992) High osmotic stress behaviour of hyaluronate and heparin. *Biopolymers* **32**, 219–238

68. Reference deleted.

69. Reference deleted.

70. Gribbon, P.M. (1994) Biophysical properties of glycosaminoglycans, proteoglycans and cartilage. PhD Thesis, University of London

71. Katchalsky, A. (1954) Polyelectrolyte gels. In: *Progress in Biophysics and Biophysical Chemistry* (Butler, J.A.V. and Randall, J.T., eds.), pp. 1–59, Pergamon, London

72. Safford, R.E. and Bassingthwaite, J.B. (1977) Calcium diffusion in transient and steady states in muscle. *Biophys. J.* **20**, 113–136

73. Byers, P.D. and Brown, R.A. (1990) Reflections on the repair of articular cartilage. In *Methods in Cartilage Research* (Maroudas, A. and Kuettner, K., eds.), pp. 318–321, Academic Press, London

74. Boskey, A.L. (1992) Mineral-matrix interactions in bone and cartilage. *Clin. Orthop. Relat. Res.* **281**, 244–274

75. Smith, Q.T. and Lindenbaum, A. (1971) Composition and calcium binding of protein polysaccharides of calf nasal septum and scapula. *Calc. Tissue Res.* **7**, 290–298

76. MacGregor, E.A. and Bowness, J.M. (1971) Interactions of proteoglycans and chondroitin sulphate with calcium or phosphate ions. *Can. J. Biochem.* **49**, 417–425

77. Boskey, A.L., Maresca, M., Wikstrom, B. and Hjerpe, A. (1991) Hydroxyapatite formation in the presence of proteoglycans of reduced sulfur content: Studies in the brachymorphic mouse. *Calc. Tissue Int.* **49**, 389–393

78. Cuervo, L.A., Pita, J.C. and Howel, D.S. (1973) Inhibition of calcium phosphate mineral growth by proteoglycan aggregate fractions in a synthetic lymph. *Calc. Tissue Res.* **13**, 1–10

79. Hunter, G.K. (1987) An ion-exchange mechanism of cartilage calcification. *Connect. Tissue Res.* **16**, 111–120

80. Byers, P.D., Bayliss, M.T., Maroudas, A., Urban, J.P.G. and Weightmann, B. (1983) Hypothesising about joints. In *Studies in Joint Disease II* (Maroudas, A. and Holborow, E.J., eds.), pp. 241–276, Pitman, London

81. Ogston, A.G. (1958) The spaces in a uniform random suspension of fibres. *Trans. Faraday Soc.* **54**, 1754–1757

82. Jansons, K.M. and Phillips, C.G. (1990) On the application of geometric probability theory to polymer networks and suspension. *J. Collagen. Int. Sci.* **137**, 75–91

83. Harper, G.S., Comper, W.D., Preston, B.N. and Davis, P. (1985) Concentration dependence of proteoglycan diffusion. *Biopolymers* **24**, 2165–2173

84. Reihanian, H., Jamieson, A.M., Tang, L.H. and Rosenberg, L. (1979) Hydrodynamic properties of proteoglycan subunit from bovine nasal cartilage. *Biopolymers* **18**, 1727–1747

85. Reference deleted.

86. Doi, M. and Edwards, S.F. (1986) *The Theory of Polymer Dynamics*. Oxford University Press, Oxford

87. Laurent, T.C. (1970) The structure and function of the intercellular polysaccharides in connective tissue. In *Capillary Permeability* (Crone, C. and Lassen, N.A., eds.), pp. 261–277, Academic Press, New York

88. Preston, B.N., Laurent, T.C. and Comper, W.D. (1984) Transport of molecules in connective tissue polysaccharide solutions. In *Molecular Biophysics of the Extracellular Matrix* (Arnott, S., Rees, D.A. and Morris, E.R., eds.), pp. 119–162, Humana Press, Clifton, NJ

89. Ruoslahti, E. and Yamaguchi, V. (1991) Proteoglycans as modulates of growth factor activity. *Cell* **64**, 867–869

90. Wight, T. (1980) Vessel proteoglycans and thrombogenesis. *Prog. Thromb.* **5**, 1–39

91. Camejo, G. (1982) The interaction of lipids and lipoproteins with the intercellular matrix of arterial tissue: its possible role in atherogenesis. *Adv. Lipid Res.* **19**, 1–53

92. Vijayagopal, P., Srinivasan, S.R., Radhakrishnamurthy, B. and Berenson, G.S. (1983) Hemostatic properties and serum lipoprotein binding of a heparan sulphate proteoglycan from bovine aorta. *Biochim. Biophys. Acta* **758**, 70–83

93. Bihari-Varga, M., Gruber, E., Rotheneder, M., Zechner, R. and Kostner, G.M. (1988) Interactions of lipoprotein Lp(a) and low density lipoprotein with glycosaminoglycans from human aorta. *Arteriosclerosis* **8**, 851–857

94. Scott, J.E. (1988) Proteoglycan-fibrillar collagen interactions. *Biochem. J.* **252**, 313–323

95. Hook, M., Woods, A., Johansson, S., Kjellan, L. and Couchman, J.R. (1986) Functions of proteoglycans at the cell surface. *CIBA Found. Symp.* **124**, 143–157

96. Haldenby, K.A., Chappell, D.C., Winlove, C.P., Parker, K.H. and Firth, J.A. (1994) Focal and regional variations in the composition of the glycocalyx of large vessel endothelium. *J. Vasc. Res.* **31**, 2–10

97. Armstrong, C.G., O'Connor, P. and Gardner, D.L. (1992) Mechanical basis of connective tissue disease. In *Pathological Basis of the Connective Tissue Diseases* (Gardiner, D.L., ed.), Chap. 6, Edward Arnold, London

98. Kielty, C.M., Hopkinson, I. and Grant, M.E. (1993) Collagen: The collagen family: Structure, assembly, and organization of the extracellular matrix. In *Connective Tissue and Its Inheritable Disorders* (Royce, P.M. and Steinman, B., eds.), pp. 103–147, Wiley-Liss, New York

99. Piez, K.A. (1984) Molecular and aggregate structures of the collagens. In *Extracellular Matrix Biochemistry* (Piez, K.A. and Reddi, A.H., eds.), pp. 1–40, Elsevier, New York

100. Silver, F.H. (1987) *Biological Materials: Structure, Mechanical Properties, and Modeling of Soft Tissues*, New York University Press, New York

101. Baer, E., Cassidy, J.J. and Hiltner, A. (1988) Hierarchical structure of collagen and its relationship to the physical properties of tendon. In: *Collagen, Vol. II, Biochemistry and Biomechanics* (Nimni, M.E., ed.), chap. 9, CRC Press, Boca Raton

102. Gathercole, L.J. and Keller, A. (1978) Early development of crimping in tail tendon collagen: a polarising optical and SEM study. *Micron* **9**, 83–89

103. Cowan, P.M., North, A.C.T. and Randall, J.T. (1955) X-ray diffraction studies of collagen fibres. *Symp. Soc. Exp. Biol.* **9**, 115–126

104. Lanir, Y., Salant, E.L. and Foux, A. (1988) Physicochemical and microstructural changes in collagen fibre bundles following stretch *in vitro*. *Biorheology* **25**, 591–603

105. Kempson, G.E. (1980) The mechanical properties of articular cartilage. In *The Joints and Synovial Fluid*, (Sokoloff, L., ed.), pp. 140–176, Academic Press, New York

106. Kinoshita, Y. and Robard, S. (1981) Aneurism pressure-volume relationships of a physical model. *Cardiology* **67**, 193–205
107. van der Rest, M. and Mayne, R. (1987) Type IX collagen. In *Structure and Function of Collagen Types* (Mayne, R. and Burgeson, R.E., eds.), pp. 195–221, Academic Press, London
108. Boucek, R.J. (1988) Contributions of elastin and collagen organisation to passive mechanical properties of arterial tissue. In *Collagen, Vol. II, Biochemistry and Biomechanics* (Nimni, M.E., ed.), chap. 10, CRC Press, Boca Raton
109. Byers, P.H., Barsh, G.S. and Holbrook, K.A. (1981) Molecular mechanisms of connective tissue abnormalities in the Ehlers-Danlos syndrome. *Collagen Relat. Res.* **1**, 475–489
110. West, J.B. and Mathieu-Costello, O. (1992) Stress failure of pulmonary capillaries: role in lung and heart disease. *Lancet* **340**, 762–767
111. Fisher, R.F. and Wakely, J. (1976) The elastic constants and ultrastructural organisation of a basement membrane (lens capsule). *Proc. R. Soc. London Ser. B* **193**, 335–358
112. Welling, L.W. and Grantham, J.J. (1972) Physical properties of isolated perfused renal tubules and tubular basement membranes. *J. Clin. Invest.* **51**, 1063–1075
113. Deen, W.M., Bridges, C.R. and Brenner, B.M. (1983) Biophysical basis of glomerular filtration. *J. Membr. Biol.* **71**, 1–10
114. Bray, J. and Robinson, G.B. (1984) Influence of charge on filtration across renal basement membrane films *in vitro*. *Kidney Int.* **25**, 527–533
115. Bard, J.B.L. (1990) The role of extracellular matrix in development. In *Connective Tissue Matrix* (Hukins, D.W.L., ed.), vol. II, pp. 11–43, Macmillan, London
116. Li, S.-T. and Katz, E.P. (1979) Electrostatic properties of reconstituted collagen fibrils. In *Electrical Properties of Bone and Cartilage* (Brighton, C.T., Black, J. and Pollack, S.R., eds.), p. 119, Grune and Stratton, New York
117. Glimcher, M.J. (1976) Composition, structure and organisation of bone and other mineralised tissues and the mechanisms of calcification. In: *Handbook of Physiology, Section 7, Endocrinology VII* (Greep, R.O. and Astwood, E.B., eds.), pp. 25–116, Williams and Wilkins, Baltimore
118. Howell, D.S. (1971) Current concepts of calcification. *J. Bone Joint Surg.* **53a**, 250–258
119. Laurent, G.J. (1987) Dynamic state of collagen, pathways of collagen degradation *in vivo* and their possible role in regulation of collagen mass. *Am J. Physiol.* **252**, C1–9
120. Banes, A.J. (1994)) Mechanical strain and the mammalian cell. In *Physical Forces and the Mammalian Cell* (Frangos, J.A., ed.), pp. 81–124, Academic Press, San Diego
121. Wooley, D.E. (1984) Mammalian collagenases. In *Extracellular Matrix Biochemistry* (Piez, D.A. and Reddi, A.H., eds.), pp. 119–158, Elsevier, New York
122. Trueb, B., Holenstein, C.G., Fisher, R.W. and Winterhalter, K.H. (1980) Non-enzymatic glycosylation of proteins. *J. Biol. Chem.* **255**, 6717–6720
123. Bai, B., Phua, K., Hardt, T., Cernadas, M. and Brodsky, B. (1992) Glycation alters collagen fibril organisation. *Connect. Tissue Res.* **28**, 1–12
124. Andreassen, T.T., Seyerhansen, K. and Bailey, A.J. (1981) Thermal stability, mechanical properties and reducible cross-links of rat tail tendons in experimental diabetes. *Biochim. Biophys. Acta* **677**, 313–317
125. Guitton, J.D., Le Pape, A. and Muh, J.P. (1984) Influence of *in vitro* non-enzymatic glycosylation on the physicochemical parameters of type I collagen. *Collagen Relat. Res.* **4**, 253–264
126. Kennedy, L. and Baynes, J.W. (1984) Non-enzymatic glycosylation and the chronic complications of diabetes: an overview. *Diabetologia* **26**, 93–98
127. LeLous, L., Boudin, D., Salmon, S. and Polonovski, J. (1982) The affinity of type I collagen for lipid *in vitro*. *Biochim. Biophys. Acta* **708**, 26–32
128. Ali, S.Y. (1980) Mechanisms of calcification. In: *Scientific Foundations of Orthopaedics and Traumatology* (Owen, R., Goodfellow, J. and Bullough, P., eds.), pp. 175–184, W.B. Saunders, Philadelphia
129. Dmitrovsky, E. and Boskey, A.L. (1985) Calcium-acidic phospholipid-phosphate complexes in human atherosclerotic aortas. *Calcified Tissue Int.* **37**, 121–125
130. Meyer, F.A. (1982) Adhesion-induced platelet aggregation on collagen fibers. *Int. J. Microcirc.* **1**, 247
131. Morton, L.F., Zijenah, L.S., Coller, B.S., Humphries, M.J. and Barnes, M.J. (1991) Collagen-platelet interactions: $\alpha_2\beta_1$ integrin dependent and other mechanisms. *Thromb. Haemostasis* **65**, 679
132. Grodzinsky, A.J., Roth, V., Myers, E., Grossman, W.D. and Mow, V.C. (1981) The significance of electromechanical and osmotic forces in the non-equilibrium swelling behaviour of articular cartilage in tension. *J. Biomech.* Eng. **103**, 221–231
133. Grodzinsky, A.J. and Melcher, J.R. (1976) Electromechanical transduction with charged polyelectrolyte membranes. *IEEE Trans. Biomed. Eng. MBE* **23**, 421–433
134. Steinberg, I.Z., Oplatka, A. and Katchalsky, A. (1966) Mechanochemical engines. *Nature (London)* **210**, 568–571
135. Fakuda, E. and Yasuda, I. (1957) On the piezoelectric effect of bone. *J. Phys. Soc. Jpn.* **12**, 1158–1169
136. Pienkowski, D. and Pollack, S. (1983) The origin of stress-generated potentials in fluid-saturated bone. *J. Orthopaed. Res.* **1**, 30–41
137. Scott, G.C. and Korostoff, E. (1990) Oscillatory and step response electromechanical phenomena in human and bovine bone. *J. Biomech.* **23**, 127–143
138. Roth, S. and Freund, I. (1981) Optical second harmonic scattering in rat-tail tendon. *Biopolymers*

20, 1271–1290

139. Bashir, M., Indik, Z., Yeh, H., Abrams, W., Ornstein-Goldstein, N., Rosenbloom, J.C., Fazio, M., Uitto, J., Mecham, R., Parks, W. and Rosenbloom, J. (1990) Elastin gene structure and mRNA alternative splicing. In: *Elastin: Chemical and Biological Aspects* (Tamburro, A.M. and Davidson, J.M., eds.), pp. 45–70, Congedo Editore, Galatina

140. Sandberg, L.B., Soskel, N.T. and Leslie, J.G. (1987) Elastin structure, biosynthesis and relation to disease states. *N. Engl. J. Med.* **304**, 566–577

141. Gosline, J.M. and Rosenbloom, J. (1984) Elastin. In *Extracellular Matrix Biochemistry* (Piez, D.A. and Reddi, A.H., eds.), pp. 191–228, Elsevier, New York

142. Rosenbloom, J., Abrams, W.R. and Mecham, R. (1993) Extracellular-matrix. 4. The elastic fiber. *FASEB J.* **7**, 1208–1218

143. Partridge, S.M. (1980) The lability of elastin structure and its probable form under physiological conditions. *Frontiers Matrix Biology* **8**, 3–32

144. Bressan, G.M., Castellani, I., Giro, M.G., Volpin, D., Fornieri, C. and Pasquali-Ronchetti, I. (1983) Banded fibers in tropoelastin coacervates at physiological temperatures. *J. Ultrastruct. Res.* **82**, 335–340

145. Urry, D.W. (1983) What is elastin; what is not? *Ultrastruct. Pathol.* **4**, 227–251

146. Cleary, E.G., Gibson, M.A., Kumaratilake, J.S. and Fanning, J.C. (1990) The microfibrillar component of elastic fibres. In *Elastin: Chemical and Biological Aspects* (Tamburro, A.M. and Davidson, J.M., eds.), pp. 189–203, Congedo Editore, Galatina

147. Hickey, D.S. and Hukins, D.W.L. (1981) Collagen fibril diameter and elastic fibres in the annulus fibrosis of the human fetal intervertebral disc. *J. Anat.* **133**, 351–357

148. Crossman, R.S. and Cannas, M.F. (1990) The elastic fibre system in the papillary system of human dermis: a scanning electron microscopic study. In: *Elastin: Chemical and Biological Aspects* (Tamburro, A.M. and Davidson, J.M., eds.), pp. 207–212, Congedo Editore, Galatina

149. Nestaiko, G.V. and Shekhter, A.B. (1982) The collagen-elastic framework of major arteries. In: *Vessel Wall in Athero- and Thrombogenesis* (Chazov, E.I. and Smirnov, V.N., eds.), pp. 63–79, Springer-Verlag, Berlin

150. Davidson, J.M. and Giro, M.G. (1986) Regulation of elastin production. In *Biology of the Extracellular Matrix* (Mecham, R.P., ed.), pp. 177–216, Academic Press, New York

151. Dobrin, P.B. (1983) Vascular mechanics. In *Handbook of Physiology*, Section 2, vol. 3, Cardiovascular System (Shephard, J.T. and Abboud, F.M., eds.), pp. 65–102, Am. Physiol. Soc., Washington, DC

152. Lanir, Y. and Fung, Y.C. (1974) Two-dimensional mechanical properties of rabbit skin. *J. Biomech.* **7**, 29–34

152a. Lanir, Y. and Fung, Y.C. (1974) *J. Biomech.* **7**, 171–182

153. Winlove, C.P. and Parker, K.H. (1990) Physicochemical properties of vascular elastin. In *Connective Tissue Matrix* (Hukins, D.W.L., ed.), vol.2, pp. 167–198, Macmillan Press, London

154. Gray, W.R. (1977) Molecular models for elastin structure and function (discussion). *Adv. Exp. Med. Biol.* **79**, 743–757

155. Aaron, B.B. and Gosline, J.M. (1981) Elastin as a random-network elastomer: a mechanical and optical analysis of single elastin fibres. *Biopolymers* **20**, 1247–1260

156. Hoeve, C.A.J. (1977) Elastin elasticity in the presence of diluents. *Adv. Exp. Med. Biol.* **79**, 607–620

157. Gosline, J.M. and French, C.J. (1979) Dynamic mechanical properties of elastin. *Biopolymers* **18**, 2091–2103

158. Winlove, C.P. and Parker, K.H. (1990) Influence of solvent composition on the mechanical properties of arterial elastin. *Biopolymers* **29**, 729–735

159. Dorrington, K.L. (1980) The theory of viscoelasticity of biomaterials. *Symp. Soc. Exp. Biol.* **34**, 289–314

160. Vijayagopal, P., Srinivasan, S.R., Radnakrishnamurthy, B. and Berenson, G.S. (1983) Hemostatic properties and serum lipoprotein binding of a heparan-sulfate proteoglycan from bovine aorta. *Biochim. Biophys. Acta* **758**, 70–83

161. Fulop, T.J., Jacob, M.P., Varga, Z., Foris, G., Leavey, A. and Robert, L. (1986) Effect of elastin peptides on human monocytes: Ca^{2+} mobilisation, stimulation of respiratory burst and enzyme secretion. *Biochem. Biophys. Res. Commun.* **141**, 92–98

162. Hunninghake, G.W., Davidson, J.M., Rennard, S., Szapiel, S., Gadk, J.E. and Crystal, R.G. (1981) Elastin fragments attract macrophage precursors to diseased sites in pulmonary emphysema. *Science* **212**, 925–927

163. Urry, D.W. (1978) Molecular perspectives of vascular wall structure and disease: the elastic component. *Perspectives Biol. Med.* **21**, 265–295

164. Hornebeck, W. and Robert, L. (1987) Elastin-lipid interactions in atherogenesis. In *Atherosclerosis. Biology and Clinical Science* (Olsson, A.G., ed.), pp. 147–149, Churchill Livingstone, Edinburgh

165. Martin, G.R., Schiffman, E., Bladen, H.A. and Nylen, M. (1963) Chemical and morphological studies on *in vitro* calcification of aorta. *J. Cell Biol.* **16**, 243–252

166. Eisenstein, R., Ayer, J.P., Papajiannis, S., Haas, G.M. and Ellis, H. (1964) Mineral binding by human arterial elastic tissue. *Lab. Invest.* **13**, 1198–1204

167. Urry, D.W. (1980) Sequential polypeptides of elastin; structural properties and molecular pathologies. In *Frontiers of Matrix Biology* (Robert, A.M. and Robert, L., eds.), vol. 8, pp. 78–103, Karger, Basel

168. Winlove, C.P., Parker, K.H., Ewins, A.R. and Birchler, N. (1992) The polyelectrolyte properties of elastin. *J. Biomech. Eng.* **114**, 293–300

169. Winlove, C.P. and Parker, K.H. (1994) Microcalorimetric investigations of the interactions of small ions and elastin. *Biopolymers* **34**, 393–401

170. Minns, R.J. and Stevens, F.S. (1977) The effect of calcium on the mechanical behaviour of aorta media elastin and collagen. *Br. J. Exp. Pathol.* **58**, 572–579

171. Kramsch, D.M. and Hollander, W. (1973) The interaction of serum and arterial lipoproteins with elastin of the arterial intima and its role in the lipid accumulation in the atherosclerotic plaque. *J. Clin. Invest.* **52**, 236–247

172. Tokita, K., Kanno, K. and Ikeda, K. (1977) Elastin subfractions as binding site for lipids. *Atherosclerosis* **28**, 111–119

173. Noma, A., Hirayama, T. and Yachi, A. (1983) Studies on the binding of plasma low density lipoproteins to arterial elastin. *Connect. Tissue Res.* **11**, 123–133

174. Winlove, C.P., Parker, K.H. and Ewins, A.R. (1988) Some factors influencing the interactions of plasma lipoproteins with arterial elastin. *Artery* **15**, 292–303

175. Jacob, M.P., Hornebeck, W. and Robert, L. (1983) Studies on the interactions of cholesterol with soluble and insoluble elastin. *Int. J. Macromol.* **5**, 275–278

176. Jordan, R.E., Hewitt, N., Wis, W.L., Kagan, H. and Franzblau, C. (1974) Regulation of elastase-catalyzed hydrolysis of insoluble elastin by synthetic and naturally occurring hydrophobic ligands. *Biochemistry* **13**, 3497–3503

177. Robert, L. and Robert, A.M. (1980) Elastin, elastase and arteriosclerosis. In *Frontiers of Matrix Biology* (Robert, A.M. and Robert, L., eds.), vol. 8, pp. 130–173, Karger, Basel

178. Hornebeck, W. and Partridge, S.M. (1975) Conformational changes in fibrous elastin due to calcium ions. *Eur. J. Biochem.* **51**, 73–78

179. Penn, M.S., Saidel, G.M. and Chisolm, G.M. (1994) Relative significance of endothelium and internal elastic lamella in regulating the entry of macromolecules into arteries *in vivo*. *Circ. Res.* **74**, 74–82

180. Smith, E.B. and Staples, E.M. (1982) Plasma protein concentrations in interstitial fluid from human aorta. *Proc. R. Soc. London Ser. B* **217**, 59–75

181. Cleary, E.G. and Cliff, W.J. (1978) Substructure of elastin. *Exp. Mol. Pathol.* **28**, 227–246

182. Partridge, S.M. (1967) Diffusion of solutes in elastin fibres. *Biochim. Biophys. Acta* **140**, 132–141

183. Winlove, C.P. and Parker, K.H. (1987) The influence of the elastin lamellae on mass transport in the arterial wall. *Adv. Microcirc.* **13**, 74–81

184. Laurent, T.C. (1964) The interaction between polysaccharides and other macromolecules. The exclusion of molecules from hyaluronic acid gels and solutions. *Biochem. J.* **93**, 106–112

11

Interrelationships among interstitial fluid volume, interstitial fluid pressure, interstitial fluid protein concentration and lymph flow

Arthur C. Guyton

University of Mississippi Medical Center, Department of Physiology and Biophysics, 2500 N. State Street, Jackson, MS 39216-4505, U.S.A.

Introduction

The purpose of this chapter is to present as quantitatively as possible the interrelationships between the different physical conditions of the interstitial fluids such as interstitial fluid volume, interstitial fluid pressure, interstitial fluid protein concentration and others. To help in this quantitative understanding, a simplified mathematical computer model will be presented showing how each of the interstitial fluid variables interacts with the others. The model will emphasize especially how certain of the variables are very precisely controlled, while other variables function as 'operators' in the control process.

Because this chapter presents a 'synthesis' type of discussion, it calls on data from numerous research studies that cannot be discussed here. However, these studies have been presented in detail in previous reviews [1,2].

Interstitial fluid volume is the most tightly controlled variable of the interstitial fluid compartment

The interstitial fluid volume is a very tightly controlled variable, averaging in the average adult very near to 12 litres under virtually all normal conditions, and near to this value in many abnormal conditions even though many other variables change drastically.

Why is it important for the interstitial fluid volume to remain so constant? The answer appears to be that when the volume is too small, the spaces between the cells become tightly compacted. Therefore, diffusion of substances from the capillaries to distant cells, requiring that the substances diffuse through tightly packed tissues, becomes restricted. At the other extreme, when the interstitial fluid volume is too great, the distance from the capillaries to outlying cells becomes correspondingly increased. Therefore, again, transfer of substances between the capillaries and the cells becomes compromised. Thus, from very basic logic, one can see that there is an optimal interstitial fluid volume for maximum transfer of nutrients, such as oxygen, from the capillaries to the cells or of cellular excreta, such as carbon dioxide, back to capillaries.

Two basic relationships dominate control of the interstitial fluid: (1) the effect of increasing interstitial fluid volume on interstitial fluid pressure, and (2) the effect of increasing interstitial fluid pressure on rate of lymph flow

Two specific relationships have proved to have by far the most important effects on overall control of the interstitial fluids. These are: (1) the relationship between interstitial fluid volume and interstitial fluid pressure; and (2) the relationship between interstitial fluid pressure and lymph flow.

Figure 1 illustrates the effect on interstitial fluid pressure when the interstitial fluid volume increases [3]. The curve in this figure is made up of two separate segments. The first segment is very steep and vertical, and it lies entirely in the negative interstitial fluid pressure range (less than atmospheric pressure). The second segment is quite flat and lies horizontal in the positive pressure range (above atmospheric pressure).

It is on the steep portion of the curve in Figure 1 that the interstitial fluid control system normally operates. Because of this steepness, even an extremely slight decrease in interstitial fluid volume below normal will cause the interstitial fluid pressure to fall drastically towards extremely negative values. Conversely, a very small increase in

Figure 1

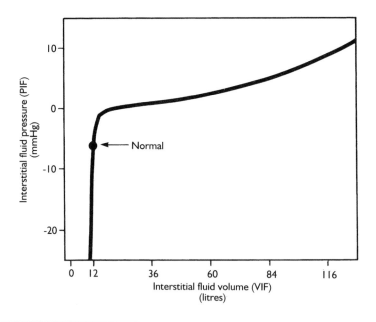

Relationship between interstitial fluid volume (VIF) and interstitial fluid pressure (PIF)
Results are extrapolated from measurements in dog legs.

interstitial fluid volume will cause the interstitial fluid pressure to rise from its normal negative value up towards atmospheric pressure (0 mmHg).

The cause of the steep portion of the curve in Figure 1 is compaction of the tissues. That is, in the normal state, the interstitial fluid volume is small enough that cells, intercellular fibrils and tissue gel are all compacted against each other. Therefore, it is difficult for additional amounts of fluid to be removed from the interstitial fluid spaces. For this reason, the interstitial fluid pressure can vary widely from very negative values as low as -30 to -50 mmHg all the way up to atmospheric pressure (0 mmHg) with very little change in interstitial fluid volume.

The horizontal portion of the curve in Figure 1 demonstrates that in most tissues even a slight rise of the interstitial fluid pressure into the positive pressure range (that is, above atmospheric pressure) can cause extreme expansion of the interstitial fluid spaces. In this portion of the curve, very slight further increases in interstitial fluid pressure push the cells apart, and excess fluid accumulates extremely rapidly. This is the state known clinically as 'extracellular fluid oedema'. The reason for this extreme expansion of the interstitial fluid spaces is that in most tissues, especially the subcutaneous tissues, the fibrils holding the cells together are very weak. Therefore, even the slightest increase in interstitial fluid pressure above 0 (above atmospheric pressure) can push the cells and other tissue elements apart. Once this occurs, the limiting factor against developing still more oedema is not tensional elements within the tissues themselves but instead is the tensional strength of the outer covering of each respective tissue. For instance, for the subcutaneous tissues of the body, the limit becomes the tensional elements of the skin.

Therefore, from a functional point of view, it is important for the interstitial fluid control system to operate on the steep portion of the curve in Figure 1, operating usually near the point illustrated in the Figure labelled 'Normal'.

Figure 2 illustrates the second crucial relationship for control of the interstitial fluid [4]. This is the effect on lymph flow caused by increasing interstitial fluid pressure. Note that lymph flow is normally very small. However, also note that an increase in interstitial fluid pressure above the normal level causes a drastic increase in the flow. Quantitatively, this relationship between interstitial fluid pressure and lymph flow differs in different organs of the body. The curve shown in Figure 2 is representative of the hindlegs of dogs, showing a 20- to 25-fold increase in lymph flow as the interstitial fluid pressure rises from the normal negative value of about -6 mmHg up to $+1$–2 mmHg above atmospheric pressure. During the phase of rapidly rising interstitial fluid pressure, the lymphatics become progressively more filled with fluid, thereby stretching the walls of the lymphatics and also increasing the activity of the lymphatic pump. However, once the interstitial fluid pressure rises above atmospheric pressure, oedema fluid collecting in the interstitial spaces also begins to compress the outer walls of the lymphatic vessels, and this compression generally prevents further increases in lymph flow. Therefore, the important increase in lymph flow occurs mainly in the negative or very slightly positive

Figure 2

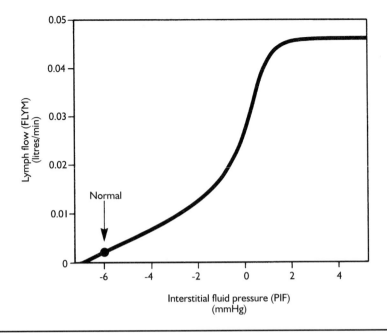

Relationship between interstitial fluid pressure (PIF) and lymph flow (FLYM)
Results are based on studies of lymph flow in dog legs.

interstitial fluid pressure range before clinical oedema occurs, thus helping tremendously to allay the development of oedema.

Why are the two relationships of Figures 1 and 2 so important for interstitial fluid control?

A moment's thought will explain why the relationships of Figures 1 and 2 are so important in interstitial fluid control. The following four steps give the reasons: (1) a very, very slight increase in interstitial fluid volume (only a few percent increase) above the normal level of 12 l causes a very, very rapid increase in interstitial fluid pressure above the normal negative value of -6 mmHg (Figure 1); (2) the increase in interstitial fluid pressure causes a marked increase in lymph flow (Figure 2); (3) the increase in lymph flow causes rapid drainage of fluid from the interstitial spaces through the lymphatics into the circulating blood; and (4) this drainage of fluid from the interstitial spaces returns the interstitial fluid volume back towards normal.

Thus, the above four steps demonstrate a negative feedback control system with extremely high feedback gain. That is, within wide limits, if ever the interstitial fluid volume rises even slightly above normal, rapid changes occur in both interstitial fluid pressure and lymph flow until the interstitial fluid volume is returned very, very nearly back to normal, hopefully to prevent the oedema state from ever being reached.

However, to understand the quantitative importance of each factor in this control system, it is necessary to put the two relationships in Figures 1 and 2 together with still other operational factors of the interstitial fluid system. This can be done using the mathematical computer model presented in the following section.

A simple mathematical computer model of interstitial fluid dynamics

This section describes the details of a mathematical computer model of interstitial fluid dynamics. These details are presented for those persons who might wish to go more deeply into the model or perhaps even operate the model on their own computers. For those who do not have this interest, they may proceed to the following sections of the paper which give examples of the manner in which the computer model quantifies important changes in fluid dynamics during specific abnormalities of the interstitial fluid system.

Figure 3 illustrates a block diagram of the simple mathematical computer model of interstitial fluid dynamics. The numbers on the lines are normal values for the respective variables. A description of the blocks in the model and meanings of the variables is given below. Block 1: this block mathematically integrates the rate of change of interstitial fluid volume (DVIF) to give interstitial fluid volume (VIF). Block 2: this block corrects VIF for factors that have physically stretched the interstitial fluid spaces (IFSTRTCH). Block 3: this is the relationship between interstitial fluid volume after correction for stretch (VIFN) and interstitial fluid pressure (PIF). This block is the same as Figure 1. Block 4: the effect of PIF on lymph flow when resistance to lymph flow is normal (FLYMN). This block is the same as Figure 2. Block 5: correction of the lymph flow (FLYMN) for changes in resistance to flow in the lymph system (RSLYMF) to give the true value of lymph flow (FLYM). Block 6: calculation of flow of protein in the lymph (FLYMPR) by multiplying lymph flow (FLYM) by the concentration of protein in the interstitial fluid from which the lymph is derived (CPRIF). Block 7: the input to Block 7 is capillary pressure (PC), and the output is the square of capillary pressure (PCSQ). The reason for this square effect is that much of the leakage of protein through capillary pores of the body increases almost in proportion to the square of capillary pressure. Block 8: multiplication of PCSQ by a leak factor for protein through the capillary pores (LKPRP) gives rate of leak of protein from all the capillaries in the total body caused by increasing capillary pressure (LKPRPK). Block 9: basic leak of protein per unit difference in protein concentration inside the capillary versus that outside (LKPRK) equals leak of protein caused by increasing capillary pressure (LKPRPK) plus leak of protein caused by other factors besides pressure (LKPRBK). Block 10: multiplication of basic leak of protein per unit protein concentration gradient across the capillary membranes

Figure 3

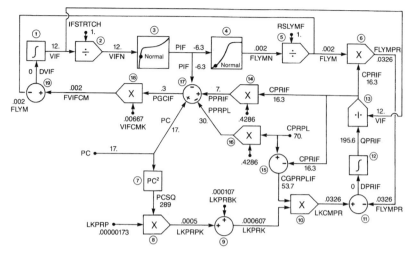

INTERSTITIAL FLUID DYNAMICS

Control system diagram for interstitial fluid dynamics, illustrating interrelationships for control of interstitial fluid volume (VIF), interstitial fluid pressure (PIF), lymph flow (FLYM), interstitial fluid protein concentration (CPRIF) and other variables of interstitial fluid function

The meanings of the different variables are given in the text. The normal quantitative value for each variable is given on the respective line in this Figure.

(LKPRK) by the protein concentration gradient from the plasma to the interstitial fluid (CGPRPLIF) gives the total leak rate of protein through all capillary membranes per minute (LKCMPR). Block 11: rate of change of protein in the interstitial fluid (DPRIF) equals rate of leakage of protein into the interstitial spaces (LKCMPR) minus rate of flow of protein out of the interstitial spaces into the lymph (FLYMPR). Block 12: integration of the rate of change of protein in the interstitial spaces (DPRIF) gives the actual quantity of protein in the interstitial volume at any given instant (QPRIF). Block 13: quantity of protein in the interstitial fluid (QPRIF) divided by interstitial fluid volume (VIF) gives concentration of protein in the interstitial fluid (CPRIF). Block 14: concentration of interstitial fluid protein (CPRIF) multiplied by the factor 0.4286 gives the colloid osmotic pressure of the interstitial fluid (PPRIF). Block 15: the concentration gradient of protein between the plasma and the interstitial fluid (CGPRPLIF) equals concentration of protein in the plasma (CPRPL) minus concentration of protein in the interstitial fluid (CPRIF). Block 16: colloid osmotic pressure of the protein in the plasma (PPRPL) equals concentration of protein in the plasma (CPRPL) multiplied by the factor 0.4286. Block 17: the summated pressure gradient that causes fluid flow from the capillaries into the interstitial fluid (PGCIF) equals capillary pressure (PC) plus colloid osmotic pressure of the interstitial fluid (PPRIF) minus colloid osmotic pressure of the plasma (PPRPL) minus interstitial fluid pressure (PIF). Block 18: the net rate of fluid flow from the capillaries into the interstitial spaces through the capillary membranes (FVIFCM) is equal to the net pressure gradient across the capillary membrane (PGCIF) multiplied by the capillary volume filtration coefficient per minute into the interstitial fluid (VIFCMK). Block 19: the rate of change of interstitial fluid volume (DVIF) is equal to the rate of filtration of fluid through the capillary membranes (FVIFCM) minus the rate of lymph flow (FLYM).

Thus, we return to the input of Block 1, the beginning of the interstitial fluid system control diagram. We can now use this mathematical computer model to understand more clearly the quantification of interstitial fluid control. From the diagram itself, one can already see that important input factors controlling interstitial fluid dynamics are the following: (1) capillary pressure (PC); (2) protein concentration of the plasma (CPRPL); (3) resistance to lymph flow (RSLYMF); (4) stretch of the interstitial fluid spaces (IFSTRTCH); (5) volume filtration coefficient per minute from capillaries into the interstitial fluid (VIFCMK); and (6) protein leakage through capillary pores caused by pressure-stretch of capillaries (LKPRP).

Important outputs of the model are: (1) volume of interstitial fluid (VIF); (2) pressure of the interstitial fluid (PIF); (3) total lymph flow (FLYM); (4) total flow of protein in the lymph (FLYMPR); (5) quantity of protein in all the interstitial fluid (QPRIF); and (6) concentration of protein in the interstitial fluid (CPRIF).

Changes in interstitial fluid dynamics caused by increased capillary pressure

Figure 4 illustrates the computer model predictions for changes in interstitial fluid volume and other important interstitial fluid variables caused by increasing the capillary pressure from its normal value of 17 mmHg up to 36 mmHg. The following points should be noted:

The interstitial fluid volume (VIF) increases hardly at all for the first 10 mmHg rise in capillary pressure above the normal value of 17 mmHg. In fact, clinical oedema appears only after the capillary pressure (PC) rises still higher, to about 13 mmHg above normal, because the interstitial fluid volume can normally increase this much without significant evidence of oedema developing. Therefore, one can state that the interstitial fluid volume remains very near to the normal level despite an increase of up to 50–70% in capillary pressure.

On the other hand, note that all the other variables displayed in Figure 4 change rapidly as capillary pressure increases. Each one of these other variables plays its individual role as an 'operator' in helping to keep the interstitial fluid volume constant as follows. (1) The interstitial fluid pressure (PIF) rises along with the rising capillary pressure. This increasing interstitial fluid pressure causes back pressure on the outsides of the capillary membranes with a resultant decrease in filtration of fluid through the capillary membranes into the interstitial spaces, thus helping to prevent further increase in interstitial fluid volume. (2) Also, as the capillary pressure rises, lymph flow (FLYM) increases from the normal value of 1.0 up to about 22 times normal levels as the capillary pressure

Figure 4

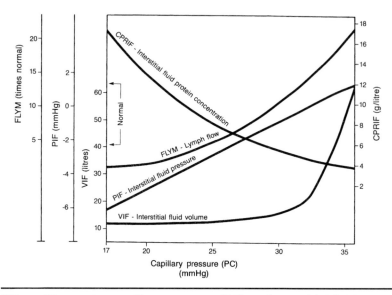

Effect of increasing capillary pressure (PC) on interstitial fluid volume (VIF) and other interstitial fluid variables (PIF, FLYM and CPRIF)

Note the excellent control of VIF up to capillary pressures of 25–30 mmHg.

approaches 36 mmHg. Here again, this extreme flow of lymph from the tissues helps to prevent any further increase in interstitial fluid volume. (3) Now note the top curve in the Figure, representing the concentration of protein in the interstitial fluid (CPRIF). This protein concentration decreases from its normal value of almost 18 g of protein per litre in normal interstitial fluid down to less than one-quarter of the normal level by the time the capillary pressure rises to 36 mmHg. This decreases the colloid osmotic pressure of the protein in the interstitium and therefore removes much of the normal effect of this osmotic pressure to oppose fluid reabsorption by the capillaries. Thus, one sees that the decrease in interstitial fluid protein concentration that occurs when the capillary pressure rises is still another important effect to prevent excess increase in interstitial fluid volume.

In toto, therefore, Figure 4 illustrates that interstitial fluid volume remains very tightly regulated near to the normal value despite pathological increases in capillary pressure to far above normal levels (up to almost double normal). On the other hand, the other three variables illustrated in Figure 4 change markedly from the outset and play definitive, quantitatively highly important, roles in preventing a significant increase in interstitial fluid volume. Therefore, the interstitial fluid volume is said to be the principal controlled variable while the other variables of the Figure [interstitial fluid pressure (PIF), lymph flow (FLYM), and interstitial fluid protein concentration (CPRIF)] are all 'operators' in the system. They all change drastically, and each in its own way plays an exceedingly important role in maintaining very tight control of the interstitial fluid volume.

Decreasing the plasma protein concentration: effect on interstitial fluid volume and other interstitial fluid variables

A decrease in the plasma protein concentration (CPRPL) decreases the plasma colloid osmotic pressure, and this decrease in plasma osmotic pressure allows greatly increased fluid volume filtration out of the capillaries through the capillary membranes into the interstitial fluid. To oppose this, the control mechanisms of the interstitial fluid system exert powerful influences to maintain the interstitial fluid volume (VIF) very near to normal. Thus, in Figure 5, one sees that the interstitial fluid volume is controlled very near to normal levels despite a decrease of the plasma protein concentration from 100 g/l (far above normal) down to 70 g/l (normal value) and then even down to 35 g/l (only one-half of normal). But, just as soon as the plasma protein falls below the 35 g/l level, an extreme increase in interstitial fluid volume occurs, with development of very marked peripheral oedema. Therefore, Figure 5 illustrates once again that interstitial fluid volume (VIF) is tightly controlled despite a very pathological change of plasma protein concentration to either 45% above normal or 50% below normal.

By contrast, note the other three curves in Figure 5, illustrating that: (a) interstitial fluid pressure (PIF) rises, which helps to prevent leakage of fluid into the interstitial fluid because of increasing back pressure on the capillary membranes; (b) lymph flow (FLYM) increases, which carries excess interstitial fluid volume back into the circulating blood volume; and, (c) the interstitial protein concentration (CPRIF)

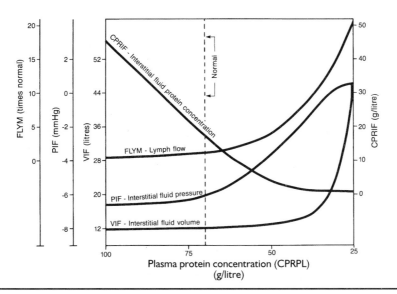

Figure 5

Effect of decreasing plasma protein concentration (CPRPL) on interstitial fluid volume (VIF) and other interstitial fluid variables (PIF, FLYM and CPRIF)

Note the excellent control of VIF between plasma protein concentrations as high as 100 g/l and as low as 40 g/l.

falls markedly because the increased lymph flow carries away tissue protein and also because of the decreased concentration of protein in the plasma fluid that leaks into the interstitium. If the reader will stop for a moment and think about each one of these changing factors, he/she will see that they all change in the appropriate direction to keep the interstitial fluid volume as near to normal as possible. Therefore, once again the changing interstitial fluid pressure, lymph flow, and interstitial fluid protein concentration are all 'operators' for the purpose of maintaining interstitial fluid volume near to normal.

Increased resistance to lymph flow in the lymph vessels: effect on interstitial fluid volume and other interstitial fluid factors

In Figure 6, the resistance to lymph flow in the lymph vessels (RSLYMF) is increased from the normal value of 1 up to 50 times normal. Shown by the top curve in the Figure, lymph flow (FLYM) itself decreases only 3–4-fold, but much more drastic changes occur for other variables. For instance, note in the Figure that interstitial fluid pressure (PIF) rises rapidly because (a) the diminished lymph flow carries much less fluid than normal away from the interstitium, and (b) the quantity of protein in the interstitium increases markedly, thus increasing the colloid osmotic pressure of the interstitial fluid. This in turn pulls fluid outward through the capillary membranes.

Note that interstitial fluid volume (VIF) tends to rise more rapidly in Figure 6 than it did in Figures 4 and 5. This occurs because

Figure 6

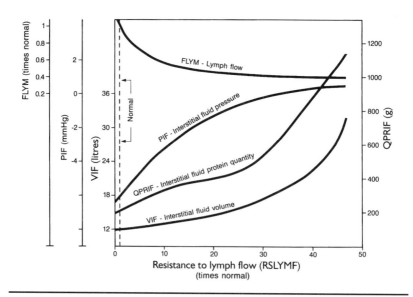

Effect of increasing lymph flow resistance (RSLYMF) on interstitial fluid volume (VIF) and other important interstitial fluid variables
Note that control of VIF is only moderately good in this abnormality.

only one of the usual control system operator factors (rising interstitial fluid pressure) functions to prevent a further increase in interstitial fluid volume. Therefore, control of interstitial fluid volume is much poorer in lymphatic drainage abnormalities than in most other abnormalities of fluid control.

Some of the clinical conditions that increase resistance to lymph flow are (1) blockage of lymph nodes by filariasis infection, (2) cancer cells blocking lymphatics, (3) blockage when proteins coagulate in the lymphatics, (4) congenital absence of, or abnormalities of, the lymphatics, and (5) blockage of lymphatic drainage following surgical procedures that remove lymph nodes, especially operations for preventing the spread of cancer. Unfortunately, in many of these instances, the lymph flow blockage is so severe that no type of treatment for the resulting oedema is truly satisfactory.

Effect of increased coefficient for volume filtration through capillaries

Figure 7 illustrates the effect on interstitial fluid volume and other interstitial fluid dynamic factors caused by increasing the coefficient for volume filtration of water through capillaries (VIFCMK) up to 70 times its normal level. Figure 7 is quite surprising. Actually, it illustrates the importance of making mathematical models for the following reason: even when there is greatly increased volume filtration through the capillaries, with water molecules moving through the capillary pores one

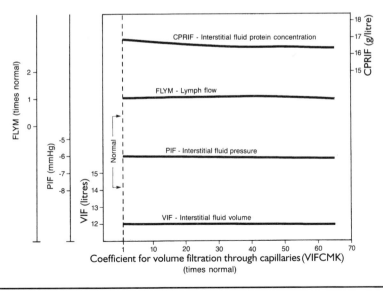

Figure 7

Effect of increasing coefficient for volume filtration through the capillary membrane (VIFCMK), showing surprisingly minor changes in the steady-state values of interstitial fluid volume (VIF) and other interstitial fluid variables (PIF, FLYM and CPRIF)

molecule at a time, the direction of movement of the molecules is still controlled by the Starling forces at the capillary membranes. These forces are (1) colloid osmotic pressure of the plasma, (2) colloid osmotic pressure of the interstitial fluid, (3) capillary hydrostatic pressure, and (4) interstitial fluid hydrostatic pressure. Therefore, Starling's equilibrium at the capillaries still applies. (In the case of Figure 7, it is assumed that protein filtration through the capillary membrane is no greater than normal.) Consequently, the increase in filtration coefficient for volume exchange of water molecules through the capillary membranes merely changes the rapidity with which capillary membrane equilibrium takes place, not quantitatively how much net volume will have to exchange to maintain equilibrium. Because normal capillary equilibria are still in effect, the various volumes and pressures on the two sides of the capillary membrane, as well as the protein concentrations on the two sides of the membrane, remain roughly normal despite extreme increases in the coefficient for volume filtration.

Figure 7 is presented for the purpose of showing that intuition (which in this case makes one believe that an increased volume filtration coefficient would vastly increase leakage of fluid into the tissues) is not always correct. However, if the capillary pores are also leaky to protein along with the water leakage, then the results are markedly different, as discussed in the following section.

Increasing capillary protein leakage: effect on interstitial fluid volume and other interstitial fluid factors

Figure 8 illustrates the effect of increasing capillary protein leakage in response to increasing capillary pressure (LKPRP) from the normal value of 1 up to values as high as 80 times normal.

Note that the interstitial fluid volume is moderately well controlled up to increases in capillary protein leakage as high as 30–40 times normal. However, it is less well controlled than in Figure 4 where capillary pressure was changed markedly and in Figure 5 where plasma protein concentration was changed markedly. The reason for this difference is that in Figure 8 one of the usual operator factors for preventing interstitial fluid volume change now operates in the wrong direction. That is, capillary protein leakage increases the concentration of protein in the interstitial fluid rather than decreasing the concentration, and this causes interstitial fluid colloid osmotic pressure to rise. This increasing tissue fluid colloid osmotic pressure pulls more fluid out of the capillaries into the interstitial spaces. On the other hand, the other two important operator factors for preventing a rise in interstitial fluid volume are still active to prevent interstitial volume increase; these are (1) increasing interstitial fluid pressure, which pushes fluid backwards against the capillary membranes to prevent further volume leakage, and (2) increasing lymph flow which carries increasing fluid back to the blood. These two operator factors, functioning without the usual third operator, still allow as much as a 20–30 times increase in capillary protein leakage without increasing the interstitial fluid volume to serious levels of oedema.

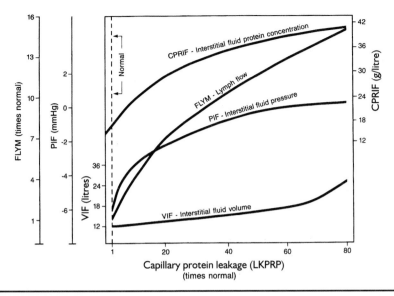

Effect of increasing capillary protein leakage (LKPRP) on interstitial fluid volume (VIF) and other interstitial fluid variables (PIF, FLYM and CPRIF)

Note that control of VIF is only moderately good because rising interstitial fluid protein concentration opposes the control benefits of other parts of the system.

Thus, the analysis in Figure 8 illustrates that the interstitial fluid control system has moderate safety factors for maintaining interstitial fluid volume very near to normal despite serious capillary protein leakage. Even so, there still are many clinical conditions that increase capillary protein leakage beyond these limits and lead to the development of serious peripheral oedema.

Conclusions

From a qualitative point of view, most of the findings in this study are not at all surprising. However, quantitatively, the mathematical model predicts that most interstitial fluid abnormalities must be very severe before interstitial fluid volume will change significantly from normal. The reason for this is that, within wide limits, multiple feedback elements in the system converge to give extremely stable control of the interstitial fluid volume. These feedbacks are as follows. (1) Rapidly increasing interstitial fluid pressure, which occurs in virtually all conditions of increased interstitial fluid volume, has a backward pressure effect to oppose capillary membrane filtration of fluid. (2) Increasing interstitial fluid pressure can increase lymph flow as much as 20–25-fold; this carries away large amounts of interstitial fluid volume, thus further opposing an increase of interstitial fluid volume above normal. (3) The increasing lymph flow decreases the concentration of protein in the interstitial fluid because of rapid return of protein to the blood; the decreased interstitial fluid protein, in turn, decreases interstitial fluid colloid osmotic pressure, thereby allowing the plasma colloid osmotic pressure to hold far greater quantities of fluid in the capillaries and thus help to prevent a rising interstitial fluid volume.

Overall, the controlling mechanisms of the interstitial fluid system provide an excellent example of a very powerful feedback physiological controller, especially for very tight control of the interstitial fluid volume within wide limits of functional disorders of the system. Let us remember the discussion at the start of this chapter describing the role of interstitial fluid in the transport of nutrients such as oxygen from the blood capillaries to the tissues and of excreta such as carbon dioxide away from the tissues. These transport processes are diminished when there is either (1) too little interstitial fluid, because diminishing space widths between the cells and other tissue elements of the interstitial spaces limit transport of the metabolic substances, or (2) when the fluid becomes excessive in volume, this time because the metabolic substances must be transported greater distances and also because blood and lymph capillaries are often compressed by the excess volume. Thus there is definitely an optimum interstitial fluid volume for proper survival of the tissues. The body has gone to great lengths to provide very tight control of this optimum interstitial fluid volume.

This study was supported in part by the National Heart, Lung, and Blood Institute Grant HL-11678.

References

1. Guyton, A.C., Granger, H.J. and Taylor, A.E. (1971) Interstitial fluid pressure. *Physiol. Rev.* **51**, 527–563
2. Guyton, A.C., Taylor, A.E. and Granger, H.J. (1975) *Circulatory Physiology II: Dynamics and Control of the Body Fluids*, pp. 1–385, W. B. Saunders Co., Philadelphia
3. Guyton, A.C. (1965) Interstitial fluid pressure. II. Pressure-volume curves of interstitial space. *Circ. Res.* **16**, 452–460
4. Taylor, A.E., Gibson, W.H., Granger, H.J. and Guyton A.C. (1973) The interaction between intracapillary forces in the overall regulation of interstitial fluid volume. *Lymphology* **6**, 192–208

12

Regulation of lymphatic pumping

Miles G. Johnston

Trauma Research Program and Department of Pathology,
Sunnybrook Health Science Centre, University of Toronto,
2075 Bayview Avenue, Toronto, Ontario M4N 3M5, Canada

Introduction

Contractile activity has been observed in each anatomically distinct element within the lymphatic system including initial lymphatics [1,2], prenodal ducts [3–6], lymph nodes [7] and postnodal vessels [8–10]. The contractile ability of lymphatic collecting vessels (intrinsic lymph pump) is due to the smooth muscle in the duct wall. However, the role of the lymph pump in lymph propulsion remains controversial. It has been very difficult to separate the intrinsic from the extrinsic factors that may influence lymph flow. The latter include arteriolar vasomotion, skeletal muscle and visceral smooth muscle contractions. Few experimental studies have assessed directly the relative importance of lymphatic contractions and tissue compression forces and as a consequence, this debate will probably continue for many years. The possibility that extrinsic forces play a role in lymph formation and propulsion has been reviewed by Schmid-Schönbein [11].

The two important issues that relate to lymph flow are the entry of interstitial fluid into the initial lymphatics (lymph formation) and the transport of fluid in the collecting ducts back to the venous circulation. The process of lymph formation is poorly understood [11,12]. While uncertainty also exists with regards to the mechanisms responsible for lymph transport through the collecting vessels, an increasing body of evidence points to an important role for lymphatic contractions in this process. Lymphatics in several tissue compartments have been studied extensively. It is clear that these vessels adjust their contractile activity in response to physical, neurogenic and humoral factors. This brief review will focus on the physical and humoral factors that may play a role in modulating lymphatic pumping in the larger collecting ducts. Neurogenic regulatory mechanisms are discussed in another chapter in this volume.

Pressure–flow relationships in lymphatic collecting ducts

The lymphatic vessel is composed of individual pumping units termed lymphangions each bordered by one-way valves. Lymphangions are arranged in series in converging parallel networks. In most species, these networks empty into the thoracic and right lymph ducts which drain into the venous circulation. Spontaneous contractile activity can be induced by distension of the duct wall through increases in transmural pressure. There is little information on how contractions of lymphangions in different locations along the lymphatic system relate to one another. It would appear that the inherent contraction frequency of a segment is not determined by its position in the lymphatic tree [13]. Contraction waves are propagated both in the direction of flow and retrogradely and the volume pumped is not significantly affected by the direction of propagation [13,14].

In describing lymphangion pumping, several groups introduced terminology that is analogous to that used in the heart [8,9,15]. The contraction cycle can be divided into several phases of systole and diastole. The ejection fraction appears to be in the range 45 to 67% for rat and bovine lymphangions [9,15]. When lymph formation was increased with plasma dilution, the elevated lymph flow was attributed to enhanced stroke volume and contraction frequency resulting from intrinsic stretch-dependent mechanisms [15].

In living animals the most convincing evidence that lymphatic vessels are capable of pumping in the absence of extrinsic compression forces comes from studies in which vessels were isolated from lymph input (but with blood and nerve supply intact). Lymphatic segments were cannulated in the direction of flow and provided with input from a reservoir. Outflow was monitored at a downstream location from another catheter inserted against the direction of flow [16–20]. In this model, filtration changes have no impact on lymph pump output. In addition, potential extrinsic forces have been demonstrated to have no temporal relationship with the pulsatile flow through the vessels. An increase in transmural pressure results in an elevation of flow (pumping) until a peak pressure is reached, beyond which flow declines. Even more impressive is the pumping activity measured from lymphatic vessels suspended in an organ bath. In these preparations there can be no question of any extrinsic factors affecting the flow through the vessels. The transmural pressure that induces maximum pumping activity is between 6 and $10\,cmH_2O$ for bovine or sheep postnodal mesenteric vessels [8,19] and between 18 and $26\,cmH_2O$ for sheep prenodal ducts [6]. An example of a transmural pressure-pumping curve for a postnodal bovine vessel is illustrated in Figure 1.

Lymphatic vessels also appear to increase their contractile activity when challenged with an elevation in outflow pressure. Studies carried out *in vivo* suggest that outflow pressure–lymph flow relationships in some species are non-linear [21,22]. Lymph flow rates in these preparations remain relatively constant as outflow pressures are increased. This may be due to the lymph pump, which appears to increase pumping activity under these conditions [21]. However, a point is reached when it is presumed that the lymph pump fails and flows decline.

The conclusion that the outflow pressure–flow relationships observed *in vivo* are due, at least in part, to the activity of the lymph pump is supported by studies carried out in an organ bath preparation [6,23]. In this model there are no passive factors contributing to flow. All output from the ducts is due to contractions of the isolated segments. Under these conditions, contractions of the lymphatics are able to maintain flow against an outflow pressure challenge. However, this ability is dependent on the initial level of distension of the duct. If the vessels are operating at the peak of the transmural pressure–pumping relationship or beyond, their ability to maintain flow is compromised. It

Inflow Reservoir   Figure 1

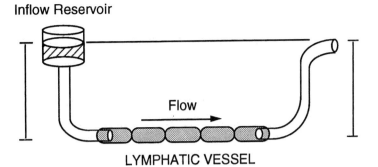

Flow

LYMPHATIC VESSEL

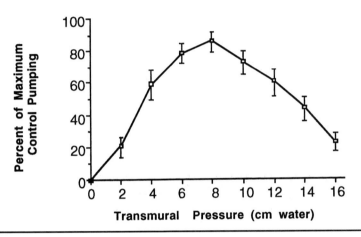

Transmural   Pressure (cm water)

**Effect of transmural pressure on flows through isolated bovine
mesenteric lymphatic vessels suspended in an organ bath**
*Flows at each transmural pressure were expressed as a percentage of the
maximum flow obtained at peak pressure.*

will be of interest to determine whether the increased pumping is
restricted to the outflow end of the system or whether upstream
lymphangions are mobilized to maintain flow.

Dissociation of lymph flow and lymphatic pumping

Under resting conditions, the most important factors that regulate
contractions of the lymphatic vessels appear to be the physical forces
that lead to the development of tension in the vessel wall (myogenic mechanisms). However, in pathophysiological conditions, other
regulatory factors appear to modulate the pressure–flow relationship by
depressing or facilitating the pumping response to a given distending
pressure.

    The systemic administration of endotoxin in sheep suppressed
fluid propulsion in an *in vivo* isolated mesenteric duct preparation but,

Figure 2   (a)

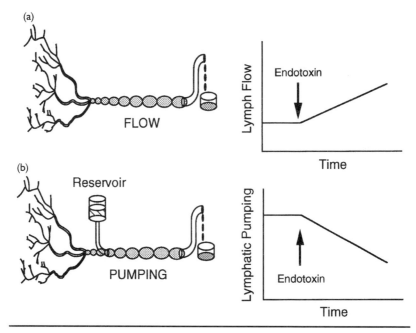

Schematic illustrating the effects of the systemic administration of endotoxin on lymph flow and lymphatic pumping in sheep

In (a) lymph flow was measured from an indwelling catheter in a mesenteric vessel. In (b) a similar vessel was isolated from lymph input and provided with fluid from a reservoir. A fixed transmural pressure was applied to the vessel to induce pumping activity. All flow in this preparation was due to the contractions of the lymphatic vessel.

at the same time, increased lymph flow rates from similar vessels that had lymph input intact [19,20]. These results are illustrated schematically in Figure 2. It is well established that endotoxin increases vascular permeability and elevates lymph flow rates in many tissue compartments. However, in the vessel receiving input from a reservoir, pumping was inhibited. If contractions of the lymphatic vessel are important in regulating lymph flow, how can flows increase as lymph pump activity declines?

The answer to this paradox may reside in changes in the pressure sensitivity of the duct. In the aforementioned endotoxin experiments, a fixed transmural pressure was applied to the isolated duct. Following endotoxin infusion, pumping declined. This depression of pumping activity could be reversed by elevating the transmural pressure above the level originally chosen for the experiment. This approach yielded a new peak pressure that induced maximum pumping and this transmural pressure was 5–6 cmH$_2$O greater than the value determined before the endotoxin was administered. These data demonstrated that the transmural pressure–pumping relationship was shifted to the right. These experiments also indicated that this curve shift was due to the formation of a host-derived factor that was not endotoxin itself [20].

One might predict that oedema occurs when the accumulation of tissue water simply overwhelms the ability of the lymph pump to remove this fluid. However, since the operational pressure range of the lymphatics does not appear to be fixed but, rather, is a variable that can be controlled by the host, lymphatic vessels may play a more active role in inflammatory oedema formation. If the lymph pump becomes 'desensitized', one might speculate that the lymphatic vessels will pump only when enough liquid has accumulated in the interstitium to create a new (higher) threshold pressure that is capable of initiating contractions. Another way of looking at this problem is to consider the shift in the transmural pressure–pumping curve as a method to enable the lymph pump to operate at pressures that would have been originally on the descending portion of the curve. A 'desensitization' of the duct may enable the lymphatic system to pump more effectively in situations in which tissue water is markedly increased and distension of the vessel is such that the pump cannot operate effectively in its originally programmed pressure range. These concepts are, of course, highly speculative. Whether a reduction in the pumping of downstream collectors could have an impact at the upstream end of the system, and on the interstitial space, awaits further investigation.

The importance of dissociating lymphatic pumping from lymph flow is further illustrated in another pathophysiological condition, hypovolaemia. Using the isolated duct model in sheep, Hayashi et al. [18] and Boulanger et al. [24] demonstrated that lymphatic pumping was significantly increased after haemorrhage in both anaesthetized and non-anaesthetized sheep. It is tempting to speculate that a stimulated lymph pump may play a role in mobilizing tissue protein and returning it to a diminished vascular space. The mechanisms that mediate the increase in lymphatic pumping following blood loss are unknown. Since haemorrhage is associated with a rapid increase in sympathetic activity, and since a significant increase in lymphatic pumping was not demonstrated within the first hour after haemorrhage, neurogenic mechanisms are unlikely to be solely responsible.

Using a similar model in sheep, McHale and Adair [25] demonstrated that a cerebral ischaemic response, produced by injecting air into the carotid artery, resulted in an increase in lymphatic pumping activity. In this case, the response was reduced with phentolamine pretreatment or adrenalectomy, indicating that reflex activation of the sympathetic nervous system and circulating catecholamines played a role in regulating the response.

Humoral regulation of the lymph pump

Table 1 illustrates some of the factors that have been tested for effects on lymphatics or have been implicated in the regulation of the contractile response. These studies are not limited to animal models but also include experiments on human vessels. For example, noradrenaline and thromboxane can alter the contractility of human lymphatics [26,27]. While most studies have focused on the pharmacology of postnodal ducts, there is some evidence that prenodal vessels also

Table 1	Humoral factor	References
	Noradrenaline	[26,27,43–49]
	Acetylcholine	[34,38]
	Arachidonic acid metabolites	[10,26,29–33,40,50,52]
	Bradykinin, histamine, 5-hydroxytryptamine	[50,51,53]
	Interleukin 1α,β	[40]
	EDRF/NO	[34]
	Endothelin	[39]
	Oxyhaemoglobin/oxymyoglobin	[35–37]
	Reactive oxygen metabolites, H_2O_2	[54,55]
	Atrial natriuretic peptide	[56]
	Vasoactive intestinal peptide	[57]

A selection of humoral factors/chemical agents that have been tested for effects on lymphatic vessels

respond to selected agents [28]. Clearly, lymphatic vessels respond to a wide variety of humoral factors. However, very little information is available on the role of these agents in modulating contractile activity in the living animal.

The catecholamines have perhaps received the most attention, due to their importance in the vascular system (reviewed by McHale elsewhere in this volume). Arachidonic acid metabolites also appear to warrant further investigation. Inhibitors of arachidonate metabolism depress lymphatic contractile acitivity, suggesting that prostaglandins or leukotrienes produced within the lymphatic vessel have a role in regulating spontaneous activity [29–31]. These agents may provide a background excitability which facilitates the vessel's response to stretch or to chemical agents [31]. Several of the cyclo-oxygenase and lip-oxygenase products are potent stimulators or inhibitors of lymphatic contractions [10,32,33]. Since various agonist-induced responses can be inhibited with known blockers of endothelium-derived relaxing factor (EDRF)/nitric oxide (NO), including oxyhaemoglobin, Methylene Blue and N^G-monomethyl-L-arginine [34–38], it is possible that NO or a related compound is released by the lymphatic endothelium or smooth muscle and plays a role in regulating the contractile responses. Since many of the inhibitors of NO are not particularly specific and as there is no definitive evidence as yet that the lymphatic system produces NO, this hypothesis needs to be explored further. In addition, another endothelium-derived factor, endothelin, has been demonstrated to be a potent constrictor of lymphatic smooth muscle [39], although to the best of our knowledge there is no evidence to suggest that lymphatic endothelial cells can generate this peptide.

That host-derived factors can directly target the lymphatic vessel has been demonstrated in sheep studies using a modification of the isolated duct model [20]. The isolated duct in one animal was provided with lymph from an indwelling catheter in a second donor sheep. Endotoxin was injected into the donor animal and the pumping activity in the second sheep declined. A factor (or factors) from the donor (not endotoxin itself) desensitized the lymphatic vessel to transmural pressure as described earlier. The identity of this factor is unknown.

Some of the inflammatory mediators that would probably be formed in response to endotoxin, have been tested on lymphatics. All mediators tested depressed lymphatic pumping with little evidence of any shift to the right of the transmural pressure–pumping relationship. These included a thromboxane–endoperoxide analogue [10], interleukins 1α and 1β, and prostaglandin E_2 [40]. However, red blood cells and erythrolysate consistently appeared in lymph following endotoxin administration. Surprisingly, when tested on isolated lymphatics, erythrolysate produced effects on the lymph pump similar to those of the endotoxin-induced factor(s) [35]. Under some circumstances, erythrolysate shifted the transmural pressure–pumping curve to the right. Oxyhaemoglobin (but not methaemoglobin) appeared to be the active principle [37].

There are many situations in which red blood cells and erythrolysate would be expected to enter lymph, including tissue injury, surgery, inflammation, etc. The possibility that oxyhaem proteins depress the sensitivity of the intrinsic lymph pump and contribute to oedema formation would appear to warrant further investigation.

Role of the lymphatic endothelial cells in regulating pumping activity

Hanley et al. [41] compared pressure–flow curves in endothelium-intact and endothelium-denuded bovine mesenteric lymphatics. The endothelial cells were removed physically with preservation of the smooth muscle responses to KCl. Transmission electron microscopy, as well as silver staining techniques, confirmed that all of the endothelium had been removed leaving the subendothelium and smooth muscle cells undamaged. These studies demonstrated that the pumping activity in response to changes in transmural pressure did not depend on an intact endothelium.

However, there is evidence that the endothelium may be important in modifying responses to chemical agents. Dog thoracic ducts precontracted with noradrenaline (norepinephrine) relaxed in response to acetylcholine. The relaxation was inhibited with endothelial denudation [34]. Similarly, acetylcholine has negative chronotropic and inotropic effects on the spontaneous contractions of bovine mesenteric lymphatics and these effects were abolished with removal of the endothelium [38]. In porcine tracheobronchial lymphatic rings, endothelial removal abolished acetylcholine- and bradykinin-induced relaxation in histamine-precontracted vessels [42].

Studies by Hanley et al. [41] suggested that, in bovine mesenteric lymphatics, the endothelium may not play a role in the transduction of a pressure signal to the vessel. However, this may not be true of the 'desensitization' of the lymphatics that occurs with oxyhaem proteins. One of the unique pharmacological properties of oxyhaemoglobin is that it is capable of shifting the transmural pressure–pumping curve to the right. Once pumping was inhibited with oxyhaemoglobin in a vessel stimulated with a fixed transmural pressure, further stimulation of the duct, with elevations in transmural pressure, partially restored pumping activity. This was true only when endothelial cells were present. In the absence of endothelium, pumping decreased with increases in distending pressures [36]. These results suggested that oxyhaemoglobin had a direct inhibitory effect on lymphatic smooth muscle. However, the ability of oxyhaemoglobin to alter the pressure range over which the lymph pump operates appeared to be dependent on an intact endothelium. Therefore lymphatic pressure sensitivity may involve endothelium-dependent and endothelium-independent mechanisms.

Summary

The ability to separate flow from lymphatic pumping activity in several experimental model systems has provided new insights into the regulation of lymphatic contractile activity. In several pathophysiological states, it would appear that the intrinsic lymph pump is controlled in ways that cannot be predicted from the associated changes in filtration. The sensitivity of this pump, as defined by the transmural pressure–pumping relationship, is not an immutable property of the lymphatic vessel, at least in bovine and sheep postnodal mesenteric vessels. It remains to be seen whether this concept applies to other lymphatic vessels in other tissues and whether the alterations in pumping activity in a lymphatic collecting vessel have a significant impact on the interstitial space.

References

1. Hogan, R.D. and Unthank, J.L. (1986) Mechanical control of initial lymphatic contractile behavior in bat's wing. *Am. J. Physiol.* **251**, H357–H363
2. Hogan, R.D. and Unthank, J.L. (1986) The initial lymphatics as sensors of interstitial fluid volume. *Microvasc. Res.* **31**, 317–324
3. Zweifach, B.W. and Prather, J.W. (1975) Micromanipulation of pressure in terminal lymphatics in the mesentery. *Am. J. Physiol.* **228**, 1326–1335
4. Hargens, A.R. and Zweifach, B.W. (1977) Contractile stimuli in collecting lymph vessels. *Am. J. Physiol.* **233**, H57–H65
5. Olszewski, W.L. and Engeset, A. (1980) Intrinsic contractility of prenodal lymph vessels and lymph flow in human leg. *Am. J. Physiol.* **239**, H775–H783
6. Eisenhoffer, J., Lee, S. and Johnston, M.G. (1994) Pressure–flow relationships in isolated sheep prenodal lymphatic vessels. *Am. J. Physiol.* **267**, H938–H943
7. Thornbury, K.D., McHale, N.G., Allen, J.M. and Hughes, G. (1990) Nerve-mediated contractions of sheep mesenteric lymph node capsules. *J. Physiol. (London)* **422**, 513–522
8. McHale, N.G. and Roddie, I.C. (1976) The effect of transmural pressure on pumping activity in isolated bovine lymphatic vessels. *J. Physiol. (London)* **261**, 255–269
9. Ohhashi, T., Azuma, T. and Sakaguchi, M. (1980) Active and passive mechanical characteristics of bovine mesenteric lymphatics. *Am. J. Physiol.* **239**, H88–H95
10. Elias, R. and Johnston, M.G. (1988) Modulation of fluid pumping in isolated bovine mesenteric lymphatics by a thromboxane/endoperoxide analogue. *Prostaglandins* **36**, 97–106
11. Schmid-Schönbein, G.W. (1990) Microlymphatics and lymph flow. *Physiol. Rev.* **70**, 987–1028
12. Adair, T.H. and Guyton, A.C. (1985) Lymph formation and its modification in the lymphatic system. In *Experimental Biology of the Lymphatic Circulation* (Johnston, M.G., ed.), pp. 13–44, Elsevier, Amsterdam
13. McHale, N.G. and Meharg, M.K. (1992) Co-ordination of pumping in isolated bovine lymphatic vessels. *J. Physiol. (London)* **450**, 503–512
14. Zawieja, D.C., Davis, K.L., Schuster, W.M., Hinds, W.M. and Granger, H.J. (1993) Distribution, propagation, and coordination of contractile activity in lymphatics. *Am. J. Physiol.* **264**, H1283–H1291
15. Benoit, J.N., Zawieja, D.C., Goodman, A.H. and Granger, H.J. (1989) Characterization of intact mesenteric lymphatic pump and its responsiveness to acute edemagenic stress. *Am. J. Physiol.* **257**,

H2059–H2069

16. Reddy, N.P. and Staub, N.C. (1981) Intrinsic propulsive activity of thoracic duct perfused in anesthetized dogs. *Microvasc. Res.* **21**, 183–192

17. McHale, N.G. and Thornbury, K. (1986) A method for studying lymphatic pumping activity in conscious and anaesthetized sheep. *J. Physiol. (London)* **378**, 109–118

18. Hayashi, A., Johnston, M.G., Nelson, W., Hamilton, S. and McHale, N.G. (1987) Increased intrinsic pumping of intestinal lymphatics following hemorrhage in anesthetized sheep. *Circ. Res.* **60**, 265–272

19. Elias, R.M., Johnston, M.G., Hayashi, A. and Nelson, W. (1987) Decreased lymphatic pumping after intravenous endotoxin administration in sheep. *Am. J. Physiol.* **253**, H1349–H1357

20. Elias, R. and Johnston, M.G. (1990) Modulation of lymphatic pumping by lymph-borne factors following intravenous endotoxin administration in sheep. *J. Appl. Physiol.* **68**, 199–208

21. McGeown, J.G., McHale, N.G., Roddie, I.C. and Thornbury, K. (1987) Peripheral lymphatic responses to outflow pressure in anaesthetized sheep. *J. Physiol. (London)* **383**, 527–536

22. Drake, R.E., Weiss, D. and Gabel, J.C. (1991) Active lymphatic pumping and sheep lung lymph flow. *J. Appl. Physiol.* **71**, 99–103

23. Eisenhoffer, J., Elias, R.M. and Johnston, M.G. (1993) Effect of outflow pressure on lymphatic pumping *in vitro*. *Am. J. Physiol.* **265**, R97–R102

24. Boulanger, B.R., Lloyd, S.J., Walker, M. and Johnston, M.G. (1994) The intrinsic pumping of mesenteric lymphatics is increased after hemorrhage in awake sheep. *Circ. Shock* **43**, 95–101

25. McHale, N.G. and Adair, T.H. (1989) Reflex modulation of lymphatic pumping in sheep. *Circ. Res.* **64**, 1165–1171

26. Sjoberg, T. and Steen, S. (1991) In vitro effects of a thromboxane A2-analogue U46619 and noradrenaline on contractions of the human thoracic duct. *Lymphology* **24**, 113–115

27. Sjoberg, T. and Steen, S. (1991) Contractile properties of lymphatics from the human lower leg. *Lymphology* **24**, 16–21

28. Dobbins, D.E., Buehn, M.J. and Dabney, J.M. (1987) Constriction of canine prenodal lymphatic vessels following the intra-arterial injection of vasoactive agents and hemorrhage. *Microcirc. Endoth. Lymphatics* **3**, 297–310

29. Johnston, M.G. and Gordon, J.L. (1981) Regulation of lymphatic vessel contractility by arachidonate metabolites. *Nature (London)* **293**, 294–297

30. Johnston, M.G. and Feuer, C. (1983) Suppression of lymphatic vessel contractility with inhibitors of arachidonic acid metabolism. *J. Pharmacol. Exp. Ther.* **226**, 603–607

31. Allen, J.M., Burke, E.P., Johnston, M.G. and McHale, N.G. (1984) The inhibitory effect of aspirin on lymphatic contractility. *Br. J. Pharmacol.* **82**, 509–514

32. Johnston, M.G., Kanalec, A. and Gordon, J.L. (1983) Effects of arachidonic acid and its cyclo-oxygenase and lipoxygenase products on lymphatic vessel contractility *in vitro*. *Prostaglandins* **25**, 85–98

33. Ohhashi, T. and Azuma, T. (1984) Variegated effects of prostaglandins on spontaneous activity in bovine mesenteric lymphatics. *Microvasc. Res.* **27**, 71–80

34. Ohhashi, T. and Takahashi, N. (1991) Acetylcholine-induced release of endothelium-derived relaxing factor from lymphatic endothelial cells. *Am. J. Physiol.* **260**, H1172–H1178

35. Elias, R., Eisenhoffer, J., Wandolo, G., Ranadive, N.S. and Johnston, M.G. (1990) Lymphatic pumping in response to changes in transmural pressure is modulated by erythrolysate/hemoglobin. *Circ. Res.* **67**, 1097–1106

36. Elias, R.M., Eisenhoffer, J. and Johnston, M.G. (1992) Role of endothelial cells in regulating hemoglobin-induced changes in lymphatic pumping. *Am. J. Physiol.* **263**, H1880–H1887

37. Wandolo, G., Elias, R.M., Ranadive, N.S. and Johnston, M.G. (1992) Heme-containing proteins suppress lymphatic pumping. *J. Vasc. Res.* **29**, 248–255

38. Yokoyama, S. and Ohhashi, T. (1993) Effects of acetylcholine on spontaneous contractions in isolated bovine mesenteric lymphatics. *Am. J. Physiol.* **264**, H1460–H1464

39. Fortes, Z.B., Scivoletto, R. and Garcia-Leme, J. (1989) Endothelin-1 induces potent constriction of lymphatic vessels *in situ*. *Eur. J. Pharmacol.* **170**, 69–73

40. Hanley, C., Elias R., Movat, H.Z. and Johnston, M.G. (1989) Suppression of fluid pumping in isolated bovine mesenteric lymphatics by interleukin-1: Interaction with prostaglandin E2. *Microvasc. Res.* **37**, 218–229

41. Hanley, C., Elias, R. and Johnston, M.G. (1992) Is endothelium necessary for transmural pressure-induced contractions of bovine truncal lymphatics? *Microvasc. Res.* **43**, 134–146

42. Ferguson, M.K. (1992) Modulation of lymphatic smooth muscle contractile responses by the endothelium. *J. Surg. Res.* **52**, 359–363

43. McHale, N.G. and Roddie, I.C. (1983) The effect of intravenous adrenaline and noradrenaline infusion on peripheral lymph flow in the sheep. *J. Physiol. (London)* **341**, 517–526

44. McHale, N.G., Allen, J.M. and Iggulden, H.L.A. (1987) Mechanism of α-adrenergic excitation in bovine lymphatic smooth muscle. *Am. J. Physiol.* **252**, H873–H878

45. McHale, N.G., Allen, J.M. and McCarron, J.G. (1988) Transient excitatory responses to sustained stimulation of intramural nerves in isolated bovine lymphatic vessels. *Q. J. Exp. Physiol.* **73**, 175–182

46. McHale, N.G., Roddie, I.C. and Thornbury, K.D. (1980) Nervous modulation of spontaneous contractions in bovine mesenteric lymphatics. *J. Physiol. (London)* **309**, 461–472

47. Allen, J.M., McHale, N.G. and Rooney, B.M. (1983) Effect of norepinephrine on contractility of isolated mesenteric lymphatics. *Am. J. Physiol.* **244**, H479–H486

48. Allen, J.M., McCarron, J.G., McHale, N.G. and Thornbury, K.D. (1988) Release of [³H]-noradrenaline from the sympathetic nerves to bovine mesenteric lymphatic vessels and its modification by α-agonists and antagonists. *Br. J. Pharmacol.* **94**, 823–833

49. Dobbins, D.E. (1992) Catecholamine-mediated lymphatic constriction: involvement of both alpha 1-adrenoreceptors and alpha 2-adrenoreceptors *Am. J. Physiol.* **263**, H473–H478

50. Ferguson, M.K., Shahinian, H.K. and Michelassi, F. (1988) Lymphatic smooth muscle responses to leukotrienes, histamine and platelet activating factor. *J. Surg. Res.* **44**, 172–177

51. Ferguson, M.K., Williams, U.E., Leff, A.R. and Mitchell, R.W. (1993) Heterogeneity of tracheobronchial lymphatic smooth muscle responses to histamine and 5-hydroxytryptamine. *Lymphology* **26**, 19–24

52. Dabney, J.M., Buehn, M.J. and Dobbins, D.E. (1991) Perfused prenodal lymphatics are constricted by prostaglandins. *Am. J. Physiol.* **260**, H1–H5

53. Azuma, T., Ohhashi, T. and Roddie, I.C. (1983) Bradykinin-induced contractors of bovine mesenteric lymphatics. *J. Physiol. (London)* **342**, 217–227

54. Zawieja, D.C., Greiner, S.T., Davis, K.L., Hinds, W.M. and Granger, H.J. (1991) Reactive oxygen metabolites inhibit spontaneous lymphatic contractions. *Am. J. Physiol.* **260**, H1935–H1943

55. Zawieja, D.C. and Davis, K.L. (1993) Inhibition of the active lymph pump in rat mesenteric lymphatics by hydrogen peroxide. *Lymphology* **26**, 135–142

56. Ohhashi, T., Watanabe, N. and Kawai, Y. (1990) Effects of atrial natriuretic peptide on isolated bovine mesenteric lymph vessels. *Am. J. Physiol.* **259**, H42–H47

57. Ohhashi, T., Olschowka, J.A. and Jacobowitz, D.M. (1983) Vasoactive intestinal peptide inhibitory innervation in bovine mesenteric lymphatics. *Circ. Res.* **53**, 535–538

13

Effects of reactive oxygen metabolites on lymphatic pumping function

Steven T. Greiner, Karen L. Davis and David C. Zawieja*

Department of Medical Physiology, Texas A&M University Health Science Center, College Station, TX 77843-1114, U.S.A.

Introduction

The importance of the lymphatic system in maintaining fluid homoeostasis has been evident since Starling's investigation of the basic forces responsible for producing fluid shifts between the cardiovascular system and the surrounding tissue compartments. The net result of the interaction of these forces normally favours a slow, incessant flow of fluid from the capillary to interstitium. It is clear that these forces must be balanced and carefully regulated to prevent gross oedema. However, what is often misunderstood is that the lymphatic system has an effect upon the balance of fluid movement through the interstitial space. Through the normal generation of lymph flow, the lymphatic system is responsible for returning plasma proteins which have traversed the capillary membrane as well as serving as one of the primary routes by which fluid is returned from the tissues to the vascular compartment.

The lymphatic system plays a dynamic role in fluid regulation and macromolecular exchange [1–4]. If such controls were lost or became abnormal, the end result would be oedema. Classically, oedema is thought to occur because of increased movement of fluid and/or protein to the interstitium from the blood. However, the interstitial space is supplied with both a blood and lymph vasculature. Thus, alterations in interstitial fluid volume can result from changes in either the inflow or the outflow of fluids from the blood and lymph vasculature respectively. The lymphatic system can work to buffer changes in interstitial volume by altering the lymphatic outflow. Thus the lymphatic system increases lymph flow in response to increases in interstitial volume or pressure [1,5]. Increases in lymph flow are accomplished by a number of different mechanisms. As fluid and protein collect in the interstitial space, the tissue pressure increases. This increased tissue pressure promotes flow of fluid and proteins from the tissue space into the lymphatic capillaries, increasing lymph formation. The precise means by which increases in lymph formation occur are not completely understood. However, it is well known that rises in lymph formation increase lymph flow by both passive and active mechanisms.

In many tissues, the active mechanisms rely on the spontaneous contractions of the lymph vessel. Most collecting and transport lymphatics are composed of smooth muscle surrounding an endothelial

---

*To whom correspondence should be addressed.

layer. Each segment of a lymphatic or lymphangion is terminated by a one-way valve [6]. The ability of the lymphangion to pump fluid relies on the co-ordinated contractions of the smooth muscle together with opening and closure of the appropriate valves [7–9]. This active lymph pump is found in many tissues and species. As the vessel contracts, the localized increase in pressure within the vessel will cause a small amount of retrograde movement of fluid which serves to close the downstream valves. Then as the contraction proceeds, the fluid 'bolus' is propelled into the next segment because of axial differences in lymph pressure. Propagation and co-ordination of these contractions along the vessel are important to efficient pump function [9]. As relaxation of the smooth muscle occurs, tissue attachments help re-establish lymphatic volume. Under normal conditions this spontaneous contractility has been shown to be of primary importance in the generation of lymph flow within many lymphatic vessels [10].

The function of the lymph pump can be regulated by neural, humoral and physical factors [1,7,11–16]. Numerous studies have described the impact of these different factors on lymphatic pumping. Of particular interest are the effects of the various humoral agents released during inflammation on lymphatic pumping. The importance of the lymphatic system during the inflammatory response is underscored by the findings that numerous inflammatory mediators alter the lymph pump [12,14,15]. Inhibition of the lymph pump will reduce the lymphatic outflow from the interstitial space, thus leading to the lymphatic generation of oedema. A number of inflammatory mediators or products of inflammation have been shown to stimulate the lymph pump, thus minimizing the formation of oedema. Others have been shown to inhibit the active lymph pump, thereby stimulating the formation of oedema. Reactive oxygen metabolites are produced during inflammation [17–19] and have been implicated in a number of pathologies [20–24]. These highly reactive species are produced and secreted during the respiratory burst seen in activated neutrophils and macrophages [18,19]. Reactive oxygen metabolites are also produced during the inflammatory oedema which occurs during ischaemia–reperfusion injury [22]. To our knowledge, the impact of reactive oxygen metabolites on lymphatic function is not known. Therefore, we conducted a series of studies which investigated the effects of reactive oxygen metabolites on the spontaneous contractile activity of collecting lymphatics in the rat mesentery [25,26]. We evaluated the hypothesis that reactive oxygen metabolites generated during inflammation alter the contractile activity of lymphatic vessels. Thus, these agents may alter lymphatic pumping function and impact on the formation of interstitial oedema.

Methods

Preparation
The rat is a suitable animal model for studies investigating the response of lymphatics to oxygen radical insult because it has mesenteric collecting lymphatics that contract spontaneously. Rats were housed in

an environmentally controlled AAALAC-approved vivarium. Animals weighing between 125–300 g were selected and fasted for 18–24 h before each experiment. Water was made available *ad libitum*. Each rat was anaesthetized with an intraperitoneal injection of pentobarbital sodium (50 mg/kg). Additional doses of anaesthetic were administered intra-venously to maintain anaesthesia. The trachea was cannulated to facilitate unassisted ventilation. A catheter was placed in the femoral vein to allow infusion of fluids to make up fluid losses and to provide drugs. An arterial femoral catheter was used to monitor systemic arterial pressure. During the entire experiment, mean arterial pressure was measured and recorded. If mean pressure dropped below 80 mmHg, the experiment was terminated and data discarded.

A mid-line abdominal incision (4 cm long) was made, through which a loop of small intestine (7–8 cm long) was exteriorized. Bleeding was controlled by heat cautery. The loop with attached mesentery was placed on a special viewing pedestal on a heated plexiglass preparation board. The loop was gently positioned so that lymphatics demonstrating spontaneous contractions were centred over an optical window. The exposed tissues were superfused with a modified Tyrode's solution. The solution was warmed to 37°C and bubbled with a 95% N/5% CO_2 solution to maintain pH at ~ 7.2. All experimental agents were dissolved in this modified Tyrode's solution. One series of experiments required the use of an enzyme–substrate scheme to generate superoxide. In this case the enzyme solutions and the substrate solutions were made up separately and pumped into a premixing chamber, mixed, heated and bubbled with gases, and then suffused on to tissues. The temperatures of the animal and exposed tissues were maintained between 36°C and 38°C.

Analysis of lymphatic contractions

To investigate the effects of oxy-radicals on the inherent pumping function of these vessels, we used intravital microscopy techniques [1,9]. The lymphatics were observed by placing the preparation on the stage of an intravital microscope. The selected actively contracting lymphatic was viewed at 100–200-fold magnification. The image was observed with a video camera, and recorded on to a video recorder for subsequent analysis. We evaluated the pumping function of the lymphatics by continuously monitoring the lymphatic diameter and calculating parameters which were analogous to those used to characterize cardiac pump function. Lymphatic diameters were measured from the videotape by either continuously tracking the diameter changes by hand using a video caliper [27] during slow motion playback of the experimental videotape or using digital image analysis hardware (Imaging Tech-nologies, Inc., Woburn, MA, U.S.A.) and software (Diamtrak, Vollum Inst., Portland, OR, U.S.A.) on a microcomputer [28].

Figure 1 depicts an example of the diameter tracing seen during a spontaneous contraction typically observed in these vessels. The lymphatic contraction cycle was separated into periods of lymphatic systole and lymphatic diastole [1]. These measures of lymphatic pumping activity were obtained directly from the lymphatic diameter trace: the end diastolic diameter (EDD, μm) of the lymphatic is the vessel diameter at the end of lymphatic diastole, just before the beginning of the lymphatic contraction; the end systolic diameter (ESD,

Figure 1

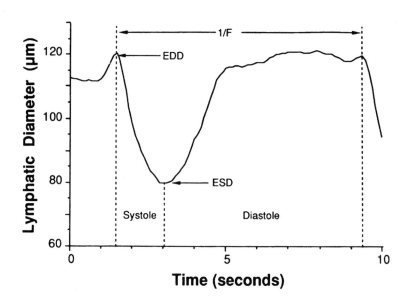

Measured Parameters

EDD (μm)
ESD (μm)
F (contr/min)

Calculated Parameters

$EDV = K*\Pi*EDD^2$
$ESV = K*\Pi*ESD^2$
$SV = EDV - ESV$
$EJF = SV/EDV$
$LPF = SV*F$

A representative lymphatic diameter tracing
Periods of lymphatic systole and diastole are separated by broken lines.
Examples of the end diastolic diameter (EDD), end systolic diameter (ESD), and
the lymphatic contraction frequency (F) are represented. The equations that
were used to calculate the following lymphatic contraction parameters are
shown: (1) end diastolic volume (EDV), where K is a constant that includes the
average lymphangion length; (2) end systolic volume (ESV); (3) lymphatic stroke
volume (SV); (4) lymphatic ejection fraction (EJF); (5) lymph pump flow,
generated by the lymphatic contraction (LPF). Reproduced from [25] with
permission.

μm) is the vessel diameter at the end of lymphatic systole; and the lymphatic contraction frequency (F, contractions/min) was evaluated from the time elapsed between consecutive contractions. Further characterization of lymphatic pumping was obtained by calculating the following lymphatic contractile indices: lymphatic stroke volume (SV); lymphatic ejection fraction (EJF); and lymph pump flow index (LPF). Figure 1 describes the calculations used to determine these parameters.

The propagation and co-ordination of the spontaneous lymphatic contractions along the vessels is important to overall lymph pumping function. We evaluated the propagation by monitoring lymphatic diameter at two separate sites along a vessel. An index of the lymphatic diameter at each site was simultaneously measured [9]. From the lymphatic diameter indices we determined the number of contractions that occurred at each lymphangion and the percentage of the contractions that were propagated (PC, %) along the vessel to the adjacent lymphangion.

Reactive oxygen metabolites exposure

During the conditions seen in inflammation and ischaemia–reperfusion a number of reactive oxygen metabolites can be produced; including superoxide anion, H_2O_2, hydroxyl radical, singlet oxygen and hypohalous acids among others [17]. Leucocytes, endothelium and other cell types are capable of generating reactive oxygen metabolites. Typically, the reactive oxygen species produced directly by these cells is superoxide anion $(O_2^{\cdot-})$. However, superoxide anion will be dismutated to form H_2O_2 in the presence or absence of the enzyme superoxide dismutase (SOD). H_2O_2 and $O_2^{\cdot-}$ can react to form hydroxyl radical. These radicals can lead to the formation of singlet oxygen and hypohalous acids. Thus, depending on conditions, a number of reactive oxygen metabolites can be produced during the inflammatory process.

Initially, reactive oxygen metabolites were generated in these studies using the enzyme xanthine oxidase, type III (Sigma, St. Louis, MO, U.S.A.). In the presence of oxygen and hypoxanthine, xanthine oxidase catalyses the oxidation of hypoxanthine to xanthine, generating superoxide anions in the process [29,30]. Xanthine can be further oxidized by this enzyme, yielding uric acid and another molecule of superoxide. Superoxide anions were generated at two different rates to evaluate a concentration dependence; a high rate, SH (hypoxanthine, 1 mM and xanthine oxidase, 0.05 unit/ml), of superoxide anion generation, and a low rate, SL (hypoxanthine, 1 mM and xanthine oxidase, 0.01 unit/ml). Since superoxide can yield a number of other reactive oxygen metabolites as breakdown products, we used special treatments to try to determine the role of superoxide itself as well as that of one of the breakdown products, H_2O_2. Superoxide anions undergo spontaneous dismutation to form H_2O_2. The enzyme SOD greatly accelerates the rate of the dismutation of superoxide anion, effectively lowering the concentration of superoxide anions but producing H_2O_2 in the process. We used SOD with hypoxanthine and xanthine oxidase to help determine the role of superoxide in the observed effects. We also evaluated the effects of H_2O_2 on lymphatic function by directly applying H_2O_2 'solutions': a low concentration of H_2O_2 (HPL; H_2O_2, 4 μM); and a high concentration of H_2O_2 (HPH; H_2O_2, 37 μM). Both of these concentrations of H_2O_2 fall within the range used in models of intestinal inflammation. However, both of these concentrations of H_2O_2 are higher than what would be seen at any point in time in either the SL, SH or SOD studies.

Experimental paradigm

The experimental protocol allowed selection of a suitable vessel which was followed by a stabilization period of 10–15 min. The tissues were continuously suffused with modified Tyrodes during this period. Three periods of data were collected: a 10 min control period; a 15–20 min experimental period; and a 15–20 min recovery period. The data were normally acquired and analysed for the last 5 min of each period. To determine the temporal pattern of the response, the data were acquired and analysed over the course of the whole experiment in 1 min sections in some experiments. During the experimental periods, the lymphatic was exposed to one of the test solutions described above in each experiment. In separate studies, suitable controls were run to account for effects of time, enzyme alone, substrate alone, etc.

Results

Controls

To verify that the observed results in the groups treated with reactive oxygen metabolites were not due to a time-dependent phenomenon, we evaluated lymphatic function for 45–60 min in a separate time control group. No significant alterations in any of the experimental parameters were observed in this time control group. To ensure that the results observed in the treated experiments were due to the reactive oxygen metabolites and not due to one of the substituents used to generate these metabolites, we evaluated the effects of hypoxanthine alone; xanthine oxidase alone; the ammonium sulphate buffer that is found in the commercial xanthine oxidase solution; and heat-inactivated xanthine oxidase in conjunction with the substrate. No significant changes in any of the experimental parameters were seen in these four control groups.

Superoxide anion and H₂O₂ treatment

Lymphatic pumping function was changed dramatically after the exposure to reactive oxygen metabolites. Figure 2(a) is a representative tracing of the lymphatic diameter during control conditions. Contraction frequency in this vessel was about 15 contractions per minute. Figure 2(b) shows the effects of H_2O_2 (HPH) on the same lymphatic diameter about 16 min after continuous exposure. Similar results were seen with HPH, SL and SH. Lymphatic diameter begins decreasing almost immediately after application of the H_2O_2. This can be seen in Figure 3. As seen in Figure 3, F, SV, EJF and LPF decreased dramatically in a time-dependent fashion during the HPH exposure. Similar results were observed for HPL, SL and SH treatments. In the superoxide-treated vessels, the effects tended to occur somewhat faster than those seen during treatment with H_2O_2. The contraction frequency and the lymph pump flow fell rapidly and precipitously after only 1 min of superoxide anion exposure. At the end of 5 min, F and LPF were effectively zero in these groups of vessels.

The effects of reactive oxygen metabolites on lymphatic function are summarized in Table 1. All reactive oxygen metabolite treatments tended to increase the diameter of the vessels although this effect was not significant. Reactive oxygen metabolites caused a dramatic, concentration-dependent decrease in the spontaneous contraction frequency. Exposure to superoxide caused a cessation of spontaneous lymphatic contractions during the last 5 min of exposure in the vast majority of experiments. The effects of H_2O_2 were similar, although not quite as dramatic. Reactive oxygen metabolites caused a concentration-dependent decrease in both the SV and EJF. Studies investigating lymphatic

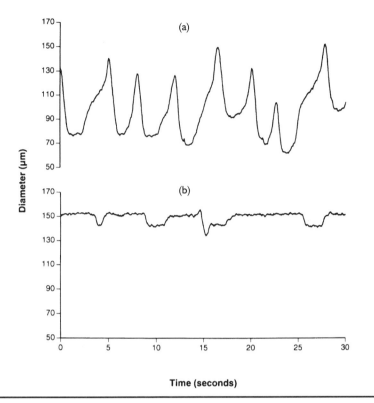

Diameter tracings depicting the effects of H₂O₂ (HPH, 37 μM) on spontaneous lymphatic contractions

(a) This panel depicts the lymphatic diameter during the control period. (b) This is the lymphatic diameter tracing of the same vessel about 16 min after the application of H₂O₂ to the preparation. Reproduced from [26] with permission.

contraction propagation were performed only in the experimental group that was exposed to the lower rate of generation of superoxides. During control experiments, $92 \pm 2\%$ of the contractions that were seen at either monitored segment propagated to the adjacent segment. After 5 min of superoxide anion exposure, the percentage of the lymphatic contractions that were propagated fell significantly to less than $56 \pm 8\%$. Thus, exposure of the lymphatics to the superoxide anion-generating solutions not only inhibited the mechanical pumping of the vessels, but it also profoundly inhibited the propagation and co-ordination of this contractile activity along the vessel. The overall result of these changes was a severe reduction in lymph pump flow in a concentration-dependent manner. This was true for both superoxide anion and H₂O₂ treatments. Lymph pump flow was reduced 87, 94, 55 and 98% in the HPL, HPH, SL and SH groups respectively. At the rates of damage produced by the concentrations of reactive oxygen metabolites we used, the damage was usually not reversible over the 10–20 min recovery period. In a few of the studies (both H₂O₂ and superoxide), some recovery was seen.

Figure 3

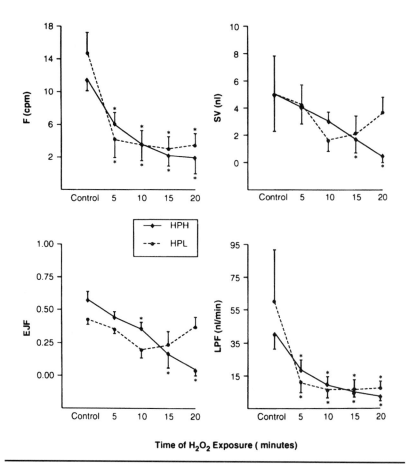

Temporal pattern of the effects of H₂O₂ (HPL, 4 μM and HPH, 37 μM) on lymphatic contraction characteristics

Each point represents the mean response from four different experiments. The upper left-hand panel depicts the lymphatic contraction frequency in contractions per minute (F) while the upper right-hand panel shows the lymphatic stroke volume (SV) in nanolitres. The lower left-hand panel represents the ejection fraction (EJF) and the lower right-hand panel depicts the lymph pump flow (LPF in nl/min). The x axis in each panel represents the 5 min period ending the control and 5, 10, 15 and 20 min after continuous exposure to H₂O₂. Reproduced from [26] with permission.

SOD treatments

In some experiments SOD was added to the superoxide-generating solution. Generally, SOD limited the effects of the superoxides on lymphatic contractile function. The decreases in ejection fraction, contraction frequency and lymph pump flow caused by the SH treatment were all significantly attenuated by the addition of SOD to the test solution (Figure 4). Indeed, LPF for the SOD-treated vessels was virtually identical to that of controls. In general, vessels that were treated with SOD appeared not to be significantly different from the corresponding time control vessels for all of the evaluated parameters.

Table I

	Control (H)	HPL	HPH	Control (S)	SL	SH
EDD	124±19	137±33	126.74±21	103±5	149.51±8	92±13
ESD	87±14	112±31	100±10	77±4	119.4±14	81±10
F	13.2±1.4	3.5±1.2*	1.9±1.9*	15.5±0.8	3.64±1.3*	0.8±0.7*
SV	5.04±1.39	3.69±1.15	0.47±0.47*	1.63±0.40		0.40±0.28*
EJF	0.499±0.046	0.373±0.074	0.047±0.047*	0.440±0.02	0.339±0.12	0.08±0.04*
LPF	50.5±15.9	7.7±4.1*	2.56±2.56*	41.0±5.2	18.6±7.4*	0.7±0.4*
PC				91.6±2.4	55.8±8.2*	

Lymph pump characteristics

Values are means ±S.E.M. Control (H), control period during H_2O_2 studies; HPL, low dose H_2O_2; HPH, high dose H_2O_2; Control (S), control period during superoxide studies; SL, low dose superoxide; SH, high dose superoxide; EDD, end diastolic diameter (μm); ESD, end systolic diameter (μm); F, contraction frequency (contractions/min); SV, stroke volume (nl); EJF, ejection fraction; LPF, lymph pump flow (nl/min); PC, propagated contractions (%). *Significantly different from the respective control at $P < 0.05$.

Figure 4

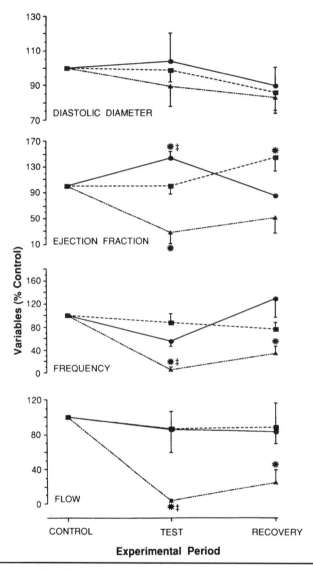

Inhibition of the effects of superoxides on lymphatic contraction parameters by SOD

*In all panels, each data point is the mean ±S.E.M. The data are expressed as percentages of the value obtained for that parameter during the control period. Each point represents the data obtained and analysed for the last 5 min of each period. TC, square symbols, shows the data from our time control studies (n=7). SH, triangular symbols, shows data from experiments using the higher rate (1 mM hypoxanthine and 0.05 unit/ml xanthine oxidase) of oxy-radical production (n=7). SOD, circular symbols, shows data from experiments in which SOD was added to the solution used to generate the higher rate (1 mM hypoxanthine, 0.05 unit/ml xanthine oxidase and 67 units/ml SOD) of superoxide production (n=4). *Significantly different from the initial control period of each experiment; P <0.05. ‡Significantly different from the corresponding period from the SOD studies; P <0.05. Reproduced from [25] with permission.*

Discussion

Fluid flow in the mesenteric lymphatics under normal conditions is thought to be primarily generated by the intrinsic contraction of these vessels. Total lymph flow due to pumping activity depends not only upon the strength of the individual lymphangion but also upon the co-ordination of the lymphangions. We evaluated the impact of reactive oxygen metabolites on the strength of the individual lymphangions, as well as the propagation of this pumping activity along the vessel. Some mediators of inflammation are known to alter the lymphatic pump [14,15]. The effects of reactive oxygen metabolites, a family of compounds that are released during inflammation and are thought to be responsible for oedema formation, on lymphatic pumping were determined in the mesenteric lymphatics of the rat small intestine [25,26].

Exposure of the lymphatics to reactive oxygen metabolites (both superoxides and H_2O_2) produced profound changes in the spontaneous contractile activity of these vessels. These changes were attenuated when SOD was added to the solutions generating superoxide anions. Thus, the effects observed in the superoxide studies were partially due to the action of the superoxide anions, although the exact contributions of the various reactive oxygen metabolites under these conditions remains to be determined. Exposure of the vessels to reactive oxygen metabolites produced rapid, profound reductions in contraction frequency. The decrease in lymphatic contraction frequency could be a result of either an alteration in the process that initiates a local spontaneous contraction or an inhibition of the ability of the contraction to propagate along the lymphatic. The cellular basis of the reduction in lymphatic contraction frequency caused by reactive oxygen metabolites is unknown.

Along with the decreases in contraction frequency were marked reductions in the strength of the lymphatic contraction during and after the exposure of the lymphatic to the reactive oxygen metabolites. This is shown by the decline in the ejection fraction and calculated stroke volume. Thus, even when the lymphatic vessel contracted, the strength of the contraction was markedly reduced. The exact mechanisms by which the reactive oxygen metabolites exert these effects and the active chemical species responsible for the altered function remain to be determined.

Taken together, reductions in the strength of the contraction and the lymphatic contraction frequency resulted in a tremendous decrease in the calculated lymph pump flow. If this degree of insult is representative of the situation that might exist during pathological states, these studies indicate that exposure of the lymphatics to reactive oxygen metabolites during the course of inflammation inhibits the pumping ability of these vessels. The inhibition of the pump occurs despite large increases in the transvascular flux of fluid and protein into the tissues caused by inflammation [21,23,31]. The role of the lymphatics as one of the 'safety factors against oedema' during inflammation may be compromised under these conditions. The inability of the lymphatics to remove the excess fluid and protein from tissues during inflammation could be a major factor contributing to the formation of interstitial oedema.

In summary, reactive oxygen metabolite exposure of the mesenteric collecting lymphatics in the rat intestine resulted in a marked inhibition of the spontaneous contractions of these vessels. This substantially reduced lymph pump flow, thus severely compromising one of the mechanisms thought to be responsible for the 'lymphatic oedema safety factor'. However, there are many mechanisms responsible for lymph flow and the relative importance of these different mechanisms to overall lymph flow varies dramatically depending upon the physiological or pathological conditions of the tissue. Their contribution to the 'lymphatic oedema safety factor' under different conditions remains to be determined.

Summary

The lymphatic system is a critical element in the regulation of fluid and macromolecular transport and is an important safety factor working against the formation of gross oedema. Many conditions which cause oedema also produce a number of different reactive oxygen metabolites. The effects of reactive oxygen metabolites on the contractile activity of the mesenteric collecting lymphatics were evaluated in the anaesthetized rat. Lymphatic contractions were monitored before, during and after the application of reactive oxygen metabolites. From the lymphatic diameter tracings, the following lymphatic contractile parameters were determined: contraction frequency (F), stroke volume (SV), ejection fraction (EJF), propagated contraction (PC) and lymph pump flow (LPF). The following reactive oxygen metabolite treatments were used: superoxide anion generation, low rate (SL: hypoxanthine, 1 mM and xanthine oxidase, 0.01 unit/ml); superoxide anion generation, high rate (SH: hypoxanthine, 1 mM and xanthine oxidase, 0.05 unit/ml); H_2O_2, low dose (HPL: H_2O_2, 4 μM); H_2O_2, high dose (HPH: H_2O_2, 37 μM). Exposure to reactive oxygen metabolites inhibited the lymphatic pumping mechanism in a time- and concentration-dependent fashion by decreasing F, SV, EJF, PC and LPF. We conclude that reactive oxygen metabolites significantly inhibit the lymph pump and that this inhibition could be an important factor contributing to the formation of interstitial oedema during inflammation.

We wish to thank Susan Gard, Linda LaFour, Harry Smalley and Mark Hinds for their assistance. This work was supported by Grants-in-Aid from the Texas Affiliate and the National Center of the American Heart Association, and grants from the National Heart, Lung and Blood Institute (HL21498, HL07688 and HL49601).

References

1. Benoit, J.N., Zawieja, D.C., Goodman, A.H. and Granger, H.J. (1989) Characterization of intact mesenteric lymphatic pump and its responsiveness to acute edemagenic stress. *Am. J. Physiol.* **257**, H2059–H2069
2. Casley-Smith, J.R. (1973) The lymphatic system in inflammation. In *The Inflammatory Process* (Zweifach, B.W., Grant, L. and McClusky, R.T., eds.), pp. 161–204, Academic Press, New York
3. Taylor, A.E. (1990) The lymphatic edema safety factor: the role of edema dependent lymphatic factors (EDLF). *Lymphology* **23**, 111–123
4. Taylor, A.E., Gibson, W.H., Granger, H.J. and Guyton, A.C. (1973) The interaction between intracapillary and tissue forces in the overall regulation of interstitial fluid volume. *Lymphology* **6**, 192–208

5. Granger, H.J., Laine, G.A., Barnes, G.E. and Lewis, R.E. (1984) Dynamics and control of transmicrovascular fluid exchange. In *Edema* (Staub, N.C. and Taylor, A.E., eds.), pp. 189–228, Raven Press, New York

6. Mislin, H. (1967) Structural and functional relations of the mesenteric lymph vessels. In *New Trends in Basic Lymphology* (Collette, M., Jantet, G. and Schoffeniels, E., eds.), pp. 87–96, Birkhaäser, Basel

7. Hargens, A.R. and Zweifach, B.W. (1979) Contractile stimuli in collecting lymph vessels. *Am. J. Physiol.* **233**, H57–H65

8. McHale, N.G. and Roddie, I.C. (1976) The effect of transmural pressure on pumping activity in isolated bovine lymphatic vessels. *J. Physiol. (London)* **261**, 255–269

9. Zawieja, D.C., Davis, K.L., Schuster, R., Hinds, W.M. and Granger, H.J. (1993) Distribution, propagation, and coordination of contractile activity in lymphatics. *Am. J. Physiol.* **264**, H1283–H1291

10. Benoit, J.N. (1991) Relationships between lymphatic pump flow and total lymph flow in the small intestine. *Am. J. Physiol.* **261**, H1970–H1978

11. Zweifach, B.W. and Schmid-Schönbein, G.W. (1985) Pressure and flow relations in the lymphatic system. In *Experimental Biology of the Lymphatic Circulation* (Johnston, M.G., ed.), pp. 45–79, Elsevier, Amsterdam

12. Johnston, M.G. (1985) Involvement of lymphatic collecting ducts in the physiology and pathophysiology of lymph flow. In *Experimental Biology of the Lymphatic Circulation* (Johnston, M.G., ed.), pp. 81–120, Elsevier, Amsterdam

13. McHale, N.G. (1985) Innervation of the lymphatic circulation. In *Experimental Biology of the Lymphatic Circulation* (Johnston, M.G., ed.), pp. 121–140, Elsevier, Amsterdam

14. Hanley, C.A., Elias, R.M., Movat, H.Z. and Johnston, M.G. (1989) Suppression of fluid pumping in isolated bovine mesenteric lymphatics by Interleukin-1: interaction with prostaglandin E2. *Microvasc. Res.* **37**, 218–229

15. Johnston, M.G., Kanalec, A. and Gordan, J.L. (1983) Effects of arachidonic acid and its cyclooxygenase and lipoxygenase products on lymph vessel contractility in vitro. *Prostaglandins* **25**, 85–98

16. Zweifach, B.W. and Prather, J.W. (1975) Micromanipulation of pressure in terminal lymphatics in the mesentery. *Am. J. Physiol.* **228**, 1326–1335

17. Halliwell, B. and Gutteridge, J.M. (1986) Oxygen free radicals and iron in relation to biology and medicine: some problems and concepts. *Arch. Biochem. Biophys.* **246**, 501–514

18. Babior, B.M., Curnette, J.T. and McMurrich, B.J. (1976) The particulate superoxide-forming system from human neutrophils. Properties of the system and further evidence supporting its participation in the respiratory burst. *J. Clin. Invest.* **58**, 989–996

19. Forman, H.J., Nelson, J. and Fisher, A.B. (1980) Rat alveolar macrophages require NADPH for superoxide production in the respiratory burst. Effect of NADPH depletion by paraquat. *J. Biol. Chem.* **255**, 9879–9883

20. Blaustein, A.S., Schine, L., Brooks, W.W., Fanburg, B.L. and Bing, O.H.L. (1986) Influence of exogenously generated oxidant species on myocardial function. *Am. J. Physiol.* **250**, H595–H599

21. Del Maestro, R.F., Bjork, J. and Arfors, K.-E. (1981) Increase in microvascular permeability induced by enzymatically generated free radicals. I. In vitro study. *Microvasc. Res.* **22**, 239–254

22. Granger, D.N., Rutili, G. and McCord, J. (1981) Superoxide radical in feline intestinal ischemia. *Gastroenterology* **81**, 22–29

23. Parks, D.A., Shah, A.K. and Granger, D.N. (1984) Oxygen radicals: effects on intestinal vascular permeability. *Am. J. Physiol.* **247**, G167–G170

24. Wei, E.P., Christman, C.W., Kontos, H.A. and Povlishock, J.T. (1985) Effects of oxygen radicals on cerebral arterioles. *Am. J. Physiol.* **248**, H157–H162

25. Zawieja, D.C., Greiner, S.T., Davis, K.L., Hinds, W.M. and Granger, H.J. (1991) Reactive oxygen metabolites inhibit spontaneous lymphatic contractions. *Am. J. Physiol.* **260**, H1935–H1943

26. Zawieja, D.C. and Davis, K.L. (1993) Inhibition of the active lymph pump in rat mesenteric lymphatics by hydrogen peroxide. *Lymphology* **26**, 135–142

27. Goodman, A.H. (1986) A simple television caliper for microvascular measurements (abstract). *Fed. Proc. Fed. Am. Soc. Exp. Biol.* **45**, 1147 (abstr.)

28. Neild, T.O. (1989) Measurement of arteriole diameter changes by analysis of television images. *Blood Vessels* **26**, 48–52

29. Fridovich, I.A. (1970) Quantitative aspects of the production of superoxide anion by milk xanthine oxidase. *J. Biol. Chem.* **245**, 4053–4057

30. McCord, J.M. and Fridovich, I.A. (1968) The reduction of cytochrome C by milk xanthine oxidase. *J. Biol. Chem.* **243**, 5753–5760

31. Del Maestro, R.F., Bjork, J. and Arfors, K.-E. (1981) Increase in microvascular permeability induced by enzymatically generated free radicals. II. Role of superoxide anion radical, hydrogen peroxide and hydroxyl radical. *Microvasc. Res.* **22**, 255–270

14

Nature of lymphatic innervation

Noel G. McHale

Department of Physiology, School of Biomedical Science,
The Queen's University of Belfast, 97 Lisburn Road,
Belfast BT9 7BL, Northern Ireland, U.K.

Introduction

There is wide agreement that extracellular fluid volume is controlled within very narrow limits [1,2] but there is less agreement on the exact nature of the mechanisms involved in this control. In Chapter 11 by Guyton, and Chapter 18 by Renkin and Tucker in this volume it is clear that the lymph pump is one of the 'operators' responsible for the regulation of interstitial fluid volume and it may be that it is also one of the sensors which detect changes in this compartment. An increase in interstitial fluid pressure increases the lymphatic filling pressure and this leads to increased pumping of the contractile collecting ducts. The sensitivity of this autoregulatory mechanism can by modulated by circulating vasoactive substances (as detailed in the chapter by Johnston in this book) and by nerves. The purpose of this chapter is to describe the evidence that lymph ducts are innervated and to examine the consequences of activation of these nerves.

Morphology

The fact that large lymph ducts are innervated has been known at least from the beginning of the 18th century [3], but most of this early work gives only a general anatomical picture of lymphatic innervation without precise detail of the types of nerves that make up the plexuses in the walls of lymph vessels and their relationship to smooth muscle cells. More detailed information has come from the application of the methods of histochemistry and electron microscopy to the study of lymphatic innervation. In 1973 Todd and Bernard [4] demonstrated dense plexuses of varicose fibres corresponding to the innervation of the vasa vasorum of the cervical lymph duct of the dog. From these branched a few fibres which ran separately from the blood vessels over the lymphatic's surface. These latter fibres, which were very sparse, were taken to be the true lymphatic innervation. They persisted following sympathectomy of the vagosympathetic trunk or section of the common carotid artery but disappeared following ligation of the entire carotid sheath. Under the electron microscope nerves were difficult to find, occurring only in the adventitia never closer than $1-2 \ \mu m$ to the outer smooth muscle of the media. All of the nerves identified were unmyelinated, some with only a partial Schwann cell covering and containing dense core vesicles characteristic of adrenergic nerves. Alessandrini *et al.* [5] also found the innervation of guinea-pig mesenteric lymphatics to be very sparse compared with that of veins and arteries. They found histochemical evidence of both cholinergic and adrenergic nerves. The latter disappeared after treatment of the animals with 6-hydroxydopamine. Under the electron microscope unmyelinated nerves of both types were seen in the adventitia, never closer than 200 nm to smooth muscle cells and frequently lying more than 400 nm away.

In vitro studies of bovine lymphatic vessels

It is possible to selectively stimulate the intramural nerves in isolated smooth muscle preparations by applying short-duration pulses via field electrodes immersed in the solution bathing the tissue [6]. When spontaneously contracting bovine mesenteric lymphatics were stimulated in this fashion at a frequency of 1 Hz the rate of spontaneous contraction was increased by about 60% while, during stimulation at 4 Hz, contraction frequency increased more than 3-fold (Figure 1, top

Figure 1

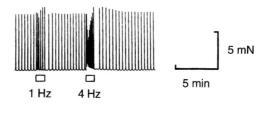

5 mN

5 min

1 Hz   4 Hz

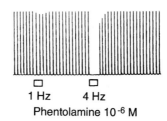

1 Hz   4 Hz
Phentolamine 10^{-6} M

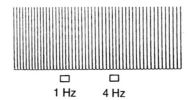

1 Hz   4 Hz
Phentolamine 10^{-6} M + Propranolol 10^{-6} M

The effects of field stimulation on the frequency of spontaneous isometric contractions in bovine mesenteric lymphatic rings
The excitatory effect of nerve stimulation was converted into an inhibitory one in the presence of the α-blocker phentolamine. This latter effect was in turn blocked by the β-blocker propranolol.

panel). The observed responses were due to nerve stimulation rather than direct activation of smooth muscle since they could be blocked by 3×10^{-6} M tetrodotoxin.

The α-adrenergic blocker phentolamine converted the normal excitatory effect of field stimulation into an inhibitory one (Figure 1, middle panel) and this could in turn be blocked by the β-blocker propranolol (Figure 1, bottom panel). This suggests that the transmitter being released is noradrenaline and that it can act on either α- or β-receptors in lymphatic smooth muscle. This is further supported by the observation that cocaine, which is known to block the uptake of noradrenaline into adrenergic nerve terminals, potentiated the effect of field stimulation [6]. No evidence was provided for the existence of a cholinergic innervation in these vessels since atropine failed to block the response to field stimulation.

The above results suggest that bovine mesenteric lymphatics have a noradrenergic innervation and this conclusion was supported when the vessels were incubated with ^{3}H-labelled noradrenaline and ^{3}H efflux in response to field stimulation was monitored [7]. Figure 2 shows the effect of four stimulus frequencies on ^{3}H efflux. At the points indicated by the double arrows (Figure 2a) the vessel was stimulated at frequencies of 0.25, 1, 4 and 8 Hz (0.3 ms pulses, 40 V nominal, 1 min train). With each train of pulses the spontaneous contraction rate and force were increased in proportion to stimulus frequency. Figure 2(b) shows corresponding ^{3}H flux in disintegrations/min. Stimulation at 0.25, 1, 4 and 8 Hz caused a progressively larger increase in ^{3}H overflow with increasing stimulus frequency. Figure 2(c) summarizes the average of six such experiments where ^{3}H efflux is plotted as a percentage of the total ^{3}H tissue content at the time of stimulation. ^{3}H efflux was potentiated by phentolamine and inhibited by noradrenaline and clonidine [7] but was little affected by either the $\alpha1$ agonist phenylephrine or the $\alpha1$ antagonist prazosin, suggesting that transmitter release was regulated via presynaptic $\alpha2$ receptors.

Electrical activity

Lymphatic electrical activity is discussed in detail in Chapter 15 by Van Helden *et al.* but an example of an experiment done on an isolated bovine mesenteric lymphatic using the single sucrose gap technique [8] is shown in Figure 3. This is a simultaneous recording of electrical activity (lower record) and isometric contractions (upper record) in a spontaneously active vessel. Each contraction was preceded by a single action potential and relaxation was usually complete before a second action potential was fired.

This is unlike most other types of smooth muscles such as portal vein, myometrium or taenia coli where contraction is initiated by a burst of action potentials. The contraction recorded from such tissues is in reality a fused tetanus. The effect of noradrenaline on these preparations is to increase the number of action potentials within a burst and thus increase tension generated. Lymphatic smooth muscle on the other hand behaves more like the heart with its well-defined one-to-one relationship

Figure 2

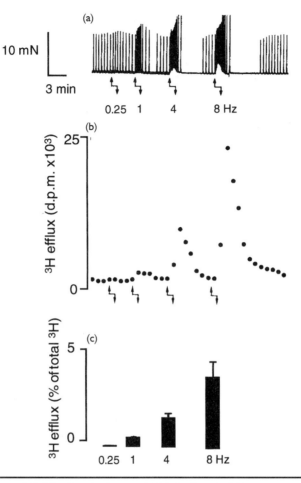

The effect of field stimulation at 0.25, 1, 4 and 8 Hz on spontaneous isometric contractions (a), the corresponding ³H efflux in d.p.m. (b) and the mean ³H efflux for six experiments of this type plotted as a percentage of total tissue ³H (c)
Reproduced from [7] with permission.

of single action potential and single contraction, and this probably reflects its function as a lymph pump.

The neuromuscular junction

When quiescent vessels were stimulated with single pulses in the double sucrose gap, electrical activity such as that shown in Figure 4 was recorded [9]. Each pulse elicited a small depolarization reminiscent of the excitatory junction potential (EJP) found in arterioles [10] but of slower time course (time to peak about 1 s). The amplitude of these

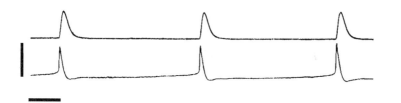

Figure 3

Simultaneous recording of mechanical (upper record) and electrical (lower record) activity in a spontaneously active segment of bovine mesenteric lymphatic

The vertical calibration represents 250 mg or 10 mV respectively. The horizontal calibration is 10 s (reproduced from [8] with permission).

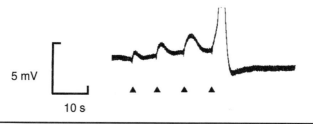

Figure 4

5 mV

10 s

Double sucrose gap recording of electrical activity in a bovine mesenteric lymphatic

Single pulses (0.3 ms duration) evoked depolarizations which showed facilitation on repeated stimulation. At the fourth stimulus threshold was reached and an action potential was fired. The gain of the recording is such that the peak of the action potential is lost (reproduced from [9] with permission).

increased with each successive pulse (facilitation) until the fourth one exceeded threshold and an action potential was fired.

Subthreshold depolarizations such as these are also capable of temporal summation when the interval between them is less than their duration, as Figure 5 illustrates. The depolarization in response to nerve stimulation in lymphatic vessels could be completely blocked by the α-antagonist phentolamine. In this respect lymphatics resemble the guinea-pig mesenteric vein and main pulmonary artery [11] but contrast with other vascular smooth muscle in which a slow depolarization and contraction following the EJP can be blocked with α-antagonists while the junction potential itself cannot [12,13]. Results such as these prompted Hirst and Neild to propose the existence of a novel type of receptor in the junctional region, later to be called the γ-receptor. No specific antagonist has ever been found to block such a receptor and the issue of its existence is still a matter of controversy. Nevertheless the concept of the smooth-muscle neuromuscular junction as a well-defined directed synapse similar to that found in skeletal muscle has recently been gaining ground. The argument that noradrenaline is released from varicosities up to 1 μm away from the nearest smooth-muscle cell and has its effect simply by diffusion across this relatively large distance

Figure 5

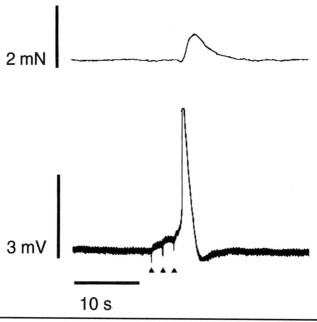

2 mN

3 mV

10 s

When the interval between pulses was less than the duration of the EJP these summed to reach threshold for action potential firing
The points of stimulation are indicated by the triangles below the record. The gain of the electrical record (lower trace) is such that the peak of the action potential is lost (reproduced from [9] with permission).

[14,15] is becoming harder to accept on both morphological and functional grounds. For example Hirst and Neild [16] showed that the response to nerve stimulation could only be mimicked by iontophoretic application of noradrenaline at a few restricted regions located within micrometres of varicose nerve bundles on the surface of the vessel. Although about 60 varicosities per 100 μm length of these arterioles can be counted in fluorescent micrographs, supramaximal stimulation released only one or two quanta of transmitter over the same length of vessel. We now know from the work of Cunnane and Stjarne [17] and Brock and Cunnane [18] that transmitter release from individual varicosities in sympathetic nerves occurs intermittently and that only a single quantum is released at a time.

Precise information about the innervation of lymphatic vessels is not available but there are several reasons to believe that similar neuromuscular specialization might exist. The very scant innervation when compared with that of arteries or veins [5] and the fact that such a small proportion of vesicles are known to be activated during sympathetic stimulation [17,18] makes it unlikely that such a diminutive amount of transmitter could remain effective after diffusing over the relatively large distances that are suggested by some morphological data. Bevan *et al.* [14], using the morphological data of Booz [19], have estimated that in portal vein (which has a much denser innervation than lymphatic vessels) the intrasynaptic equivalent noradrenaline concentration (at 10 Hz stimulation) rises as high as 10^{-5} M while perisynaptically it falls to 6×10^{-9} M. In lymphatics quite large doses of exogenously applied noradrenaline are required to mimic the effects of relatively low frequencies of nerve stimulation. This is particularly true *in vivo* where intravenous doses of 1 μg/kg per min [20] were required to produce the same increase in sheep hind-limb lymph flow as did 4 Hz stimulation of the sympathetic chain [21]. Similarly, *in vitro*, a dose of 1×10^{-6} M noradrenaline was required to mimic the effect of a 4 Hz field stimulation in spontaneously contracting bovine mesenteric lymphatics [22].

In vivo studies in sheep

To assess the role of nerves in the control of lymph flow in the living animal the sheep was chosen as a model. At first sight the innervation of sheep lymphatics appeared to be similar to that of the cow.

Figure 6 shows an example of an experiment [21] where the lumbar sympathetic chain was stimulated while recording arterial pressure (top record), tissue circumference (second from top) and lymph output and lymphatic outflow pressures (bottom two records). Lymph flow started to increase from its resting value of 30 μl/min within 15 s of the beginning of stimulation (1 Hz) and averaged

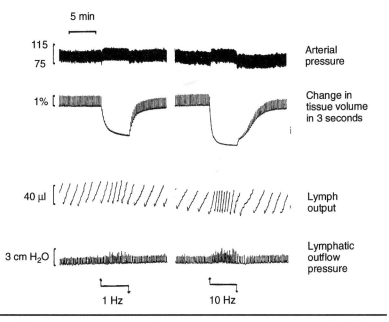

Figure 6

The effect of stimulating the left sympathetic chain at 1 and 10 Hz for 5 min periods (indicated by arrows)

The records are of arterial pressure (top), left hind-limb blood flow (second from top), left popliteal efferent lymph flow (second from bottom) and lymphatic contraction frequency (bottom) (reproduced from [21] with permission).

48 μl/min during the second half of the stimulus period. There was at the same time a marked decrease in hind-limb blood flow and limb circumference and this was accompanied by a slight rise in arterial pressure, suggesting that the decrease in blood flow was due to vasoconstriction. The effect on lymph flow of stimulation at 10 Hz was rather more dramatic (right panels). At this stimulus frequency it increased more than 3-fold. Thus, at a time when blood flow was depressed, lymph flow was increased and this almost certainly implies that the lymphatic vessels were working harder to expel their contents. It could be argued that this increase in lymph flow was somehow due to an increase in lymph formation rather than to any direct effect of sympathetic nerves on lymph ducts. To avoid this criticism Harty et al. [23] used the doubly cannulated preparation of sheep intestinal lymph duct developed by McHale and Thornbury [24] to examine direct effects of sympathetic stimulation on lymphatic pumping. This involved cannulating a length of the main intestinal duct at both ends, connecting the inflow to a constant pressure reservoir of either isotonic saline or artificial lymph (plasma 50%, isotonic saline 50%). The outflow was maintained at the same height as the inflow and all side branches were eliminated. Thus one had a length of lymph duct with its innervation and blood supply intact but which was isolated from the rest of the lymphatic system. Stimulation of the left greater splanchnic nerve caused an increase in both lymphatic contraction frequency and flow (Figure 7).

Under these conditions such increases can be due only to direct excitation of lymphatic smooth muscle in response to nerve stimulation. When an attempt was made to block this response by perfusing the inside of the lymphatic with phentolamine, or by injecting phentolamine intravenously, the response to splanchnic nerve stimulation was not blocked. This was a puzzling finding since Thornbury et al. [25] had demonstrated that the increase in mesenteric lymph flow in the sheep in response to splanchnic nerve stimulation was blocked by phentolamine. The increased pumping activity of the doubly cannulated sheep

Figure 7

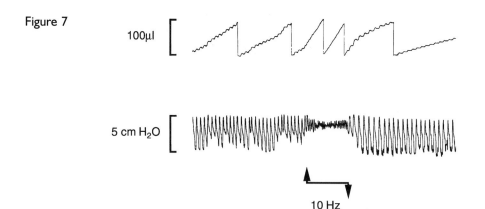

The effect of stimulating the left greater splanchnic nerve at 10 Hz on fluid pumping by a doubly cannulated intestinal lymph duct
Reproduced from [23] with permission.

mesenteric duct in response to intravenous injections of noradrenaline could also be blocked by phentolamine [26].

Innervation of sheep lymphatics

Having failed to block the increased pumping of the doubly cannulated sheep mesenteric lymphatic in response to splanchnic nerve stimulation we were forced to reassess our conclusions that sheep lymphatic ducts had a purely noradrenergic innervation similar to that of the cow. We decided to repeat the *in vitro* experiments described previously but using sheep rings instead of bovine rings [27]. Figure 8 shows an example of such an experiment. Field stimulation at 0.5 and 1 Hz increased frequency of spontaneous contraction as it did in bovine rings (upper panel). When phentolamine was added there was no blockade of the excitatory response to field stimulation nor was there any evidence of a β-inhibitory effect.

Other experiments in this study [27] made it clear that the excitatory response to field stimulation was not blocked by adrenergic or cholinergic blockers, nor by α,β-methylene-ATP and this led to the tentative conclusion that the innervation was not noradrenergic, cholinergic or purinergic. We therefore examined a range of possible transmitters including 5-hydroxytryptamine (5-HT) and neuropeptide Y (NPY). Although 5-HT has an excitatory effect similar to nerve stimulation in bovine vessels [28] its effect in sheep lymphatics was to cause a concentration-dependent inhibition of spontaneous rhythm [29], thus clearly ruling it out as a possible excitatory transmitter. NPY, on the other hand, did have an effect closely resembling field stimulation but the response to field stimulation could not be blocked by the NPY antagonist PYX-2 or by desensitizing with NPY [30].

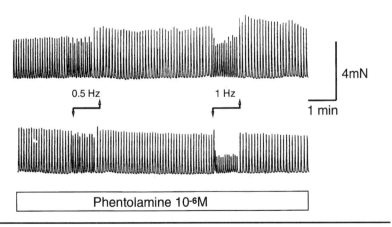

Figure 8

Two I min periods of field stimulation at 0.5 and 1 Hz before (upper record) and in the presence of 1×10^{-6} M phentolamine (lower record)

Reproduced from [27] with permission.

Guanethidine is known to block sympathetic nerves by a complex mechanism that is as yet incompletely understood. The action is probably a combination of a local anaesthetic effect (blocking action potential propagation), and depletion of neurotransmitter in nerve terminals [31]. When guanethidine was added to spontaneously contracting sheep mesenteric lymphatic rings it significantly reduced the effects of field stimulation. This suggests that these vessels have a sympathetic innervation but provides no indication of the nature of the transmitter, or transmitters, released by these nerves. Failure to implicate 5-HT or NPY led us to reappraise our previous conclusion that transmission was neither noradrenergic nor purinergic, since noradrenaline and ATP still appeared to be the most likely transmitters. The next obvious step was to load the vessels with ^{3}H-labelled noradrenaline to examine whether release of ^{3}H could be detected in response to field stimulation. Figure 9 shows such an experiment [32].

Figure 9 (upper panel) shows the effect on frequency of isometric contraction of field stimulation at a range of frequencies from 0.5 to 8 Hz, while the lower panel indicates the ^{3}H efflux from the tissue in disintegrations/min. At the beginning of the experiment the vessel was contracting spontaneously at a rate of 5 contractions/min. At the points indicated below the recording field stimulation was applied for 1 min

Figure 9

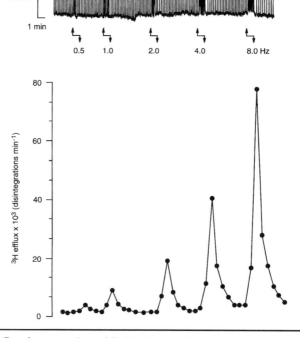

Effect of five frequencies of field stimulation on contraction frequency (upper panel) and ^{3}H efflux (lower panel) in the same lymphatic vessel
Reproduced from [32] with permission.

periods at the frequencies shown. Frequency of spontaneous contractions and ^{3}H efflux increased in parallel with increasing stimulus frequency. These results are very similar to those found in bovine lymphatic vessels [7] and suggest that noradrenaline was indeed a transmitter in sheep lymphatic vessels.

The demonstration by Chen *et al.* [33] that α,β-methylene-ATP did not block the ATP-induced contractile response in rabbit bladder alerted us to the possibility that ATP-induced increases in spontaneous rhythm in sheep lymphatics might be similarly resistant to the desensitizing effect of α,β-methylene-ATP. This was found to be the case, so it was clear that an antagonist that did block exogenous ATP would have to be found before we could assess the potential role of ATP as a neurotransmitter in these vessels. Suramin was chosen since it has been shown to block ATP and purinergic transmission in other tissues [34]. Having established that suramin blocked the effects of exogenously applied ATP and did not block those of noradrenaline it was of interest to examine its effects on field stimulation. Figure 10 shows an experiment where two 1 min periods of field stimulation were applied at 0.5 and 1 Hz in control conditions (top record) and in the presence of 1×10^{-4} M suramin. It is clear that suramin alone did not block the excitatory response at either frequency. However, when the α-blocker phentolamine $(3 \times 10^{-6}$ M) was also added, the excitatory effect of field stimulation was blocked.

Pretreatment of animals with reserpine is known to deplete adrenergic nerves of their noradrenaline stores. When rings were taken from such animals they still exhibited a vigorous excitatory response to field stimulation (top record, Figure 11). When 1×10^{-4} M suramin was added to the perfusate this excitatory response was completely blocked in the absence of adrenergic blocker. These results demonstrate that the excitatory innervation in sheep mesenteric lymphatics is mediated by the co-release of both ATP and noradrenaline in contrast to the single excitatory transmitter (noradrenaline) found in the closely related bovine species.

Physiological role of nerves in the lymphatic system

The foregoing evidence makes it clear that lymphatic vessels possess a sympathetic motor innervation. The question naturally arises as to what is the function of such an innervation in the living animal. The direct effect of nerve stimulation is to increase pumping activity of the ducts, at least at moderate levels of stimulation. At higher stimulating frequencies, or in the presence of large amounts of vasoactive agonists, the result may well be different. Lymphatic smooth muscle, while it bears a superficial resemblance to cardiac muscle, is nevertheless smooth muscle and thus has properties that are fundamentally different. Thus, while it is impossible to tetanize cardiac muscle by increasing its frequency of contraction, this is not true of lymphatic smooth muscle where driving it at high frequencies results in fusion of contractions into one sustained tetanus. This could have two consequences. If it were generalized throughout the lymphatic tree it could abolish lymph

Figure 10

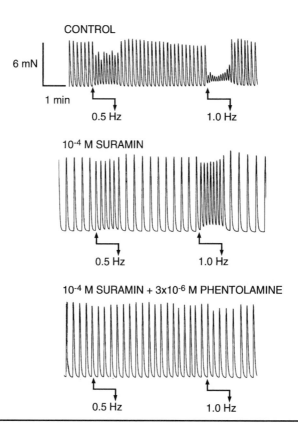

The effect of 1 min periods of field stimulation at 0.5 and 1 Hz under control conditions (top record), in the presence of suramin (middle record), and in the presence of both suramin and phentolamine (bottom record)
Reproduced from [32] with permission.

pumping, whereas if it were localized it could increase resistance to flow in the area affected making it harder for the lymphatics upstream of the constriction to pump fluid. It has been argued that, at least in some animals such as dogs and cats, lymphatics are not spontaneously active and act simply as passive conduits, and that lymph flows only because of external compression of the valved lymphatics. Under these conditions sympathetic stimulation and circulating catecholamines might act only to modulate the capacitance of lymphatic vessels or their resistance to flow.

A role for lymphatic nerves in the regulation of extracellular volume?

As detailed in Chapter 11 by Guyton, interstitial fluid volume is normally held constant due to the relationship between it and interstitial fluid pressure and the relationship between interstitial fluid pressure and lymph flow. Interstitial fluid pressure affects the degree of distension of

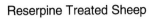

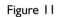

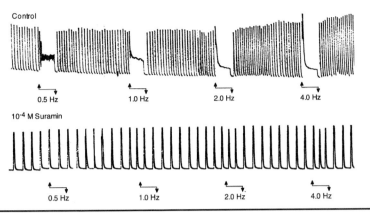

The effect of four frequencies of field stimulation on a spontaneously beating ring taken from a reserpinized sheep, under control conditions (upper panel) and in the presence of 1×10^{-4} M suramin (lower panel)
Reproduced from [32] with permission.

the collecting vessels, the rate and force of their contractions and thus lymph flow. If the lymph pump could be made more sensitive to distension this would result in the same lymph flow being achieved at a lower filling pressure and thus the interstitial fluid volume could be set to a lower value. In other words the tissues would be maintained in a relatively dehydrated condition. Conversely, if the lymph pump could be made less sensitive to distension interstitial fluid, volume could be maintained at a higher set point than normal (oedema).

There is evidence that the sensitivity of the lymph pump to distension can be modified in this manner. The curve relating distension to flow could be shifted to the left during stimulation of the intramural nerves in isolated cannulated bovine lymphatic vessels [35]. This might help to explain the apparently paradoxical result reported above that hind-limb lymph flow in the sheep was increased during sympathetic stimulation even though capillary filtration was almost certainly reduced [21]. This would be consistent with the body adjusting its set point for interstitial fluid volume to a lower value during a 'fight or flight' emergency in order to increase the available circulating fluid volume. The same mechanism might help explain the increased lymph flow observed in response to haemorrhage [36]. Equally there is evidence that the lymph pump can be made less sensitive to distension. Elias and Johnston [37] showed that the relationship between distension and flow in doubly cannulated sheep mesenteric lymphatic vessels could be shifted to the right when the vessels were perfused with lymph taken from sheep that had been treated with endotoxin. This topic is dealt with in detail in Chapter 12 by Johnston.

Conclusions

The evidence currently available suggests that the lymphatic vessels of most species have an autonomic innervation, although there is a surprising degree of variation in the precise nature of this even between such closely related species as cows and sheep. Stimulation of the excitatory sympathetic nerves can increase the frequency of lymphatic contractions and thus lymph flow. This has the effect of increasing the sensitivity of the pump to distension, causing increased flow at lower distending pressures. This may be important in fine tuning the relationship between interstitial fluid pressure and lymph flow such that lymph flow can be increased under conditions where capillary pressure is reduced, such as during haemorrhage or during the 'fight or flight' response.

My studies were supported by grants from the Medical Research Council, the DHSSNI, the Wellcome Trust, the British Heart Foundation and the European Commission.

References

1. Aukland, K. and Nicolaysen, G. (1981) Interstitial fluid volume: local regulatory mechanisms. *Physiol. Rev.* **61**, 556–643
2. Auckland, K. and Reed, R.K. (1993) Interstitial-lymphatic mechanisms in the control of extracellular fluid volume. *Physiol. Rev.* **73**, 1–78
3. McHale, N.G. (1985) Innervation of the lymphatic circulation. In *Experimental Biology of the Lymphatic Circulation* (Johnston, M.G., ed.), pp. 121–140, Elsevier, Amsterdam
4. Todd, G.L. and Bernard, G.R. (1973) The sympathetic innervation of the cervical lymph duct of the dog. *Anat. Rec.* **177**, 303–316
5. Alessandrini, C., Gerli, R., Sacchi, G., Pucci, A.M. and Fruschelli, C. (1981) Cholinergic and adrenergic innervation of mesenterial lymph vessels in guinea pig. *Lymphology* **14**, 1–6
6. McHale, N.G., Roddie, I.C. and Thornbury, K.D. (1980) Nervous modulation of spontaneous contractions in bovine mesenteric lymphatics *J. Physiol. (London)* **309**, 461–472
7. Allen, J.M., McCarron, J.G., McHale, N.G. and Thornbury, K.D. (1988) Release of noradrenaline from the sympathetic nerves to bovine mesenteric lymphatic vessels and its modification by α-agonists and antagonists. *Br. J. Pharmacol.* **94**, 823–833
8. Kirkpatrick, C.T. and McHale, N.G. (1977) Electrical and mechanical activity of isolated lymphatic vessels. *J. Physiol. (London)* **272**, 33–34P
9. Allen, J.M. and McHale, N.G. (1986) Neuromuscular transmission in bovine mesenteric lymphatics. *Microvasc. Res.* **31**, 77–83
10. Hirst, G.D.S. (1977) Neuromuscular transmission in arterioles of guinea-pig submucosa. *J. Physiol. (London)* **273**, 263–275
11. Suzuki, H. (1981) Effects of endogenous and exogenous noradrenaline on the smooth muscle of guinea-pig mesenteric vein. *J. Physiol. (London)* **321**, 495–512
12. Holman, M.E. and Surprenant, A.M. (1979) Some properties of the excitatory junction potentials recorded from saphenous arteries of rabbits. *J. Physiol. (London)* **287**, 337–351
13. Hirst, G.D.S. and Neild, T.O. (1980) Some properties of spontaneous excitatory junction potentials recorded from arterioles of guinea-pigs. *J. Physiol. (London)* **303**, 43–60
14. Bevan, J.A., Bevan, R.D. and Duckles, S.P. (1980) Adrenergic regulation of vascular smooth muscle. In *Handbook of Physiology. The cardiovascular system II*, American Physiological Society, Bethesda, MD
15. Vanhoutte, P.M., Verbeuren, T.J. and Webb, R.C. (1981) Local modulation of adrenergic neuroeffector interaction in the blood vessel wall. *Physiol. Rev.* **61**, 151–247
16. Hirst, G.D.S. and Neild, T.O. (1981) Localization of specialized noradrenaline receptors at neuromuscular junctions on arterioles of the guinea-pig. *J. Physiol. (London)* **313**, 343–350
17. Cunnane, T.C. and Stjarne, L. (1984) Transmitter release from individual varicosities of guinea-pig and mouse vas deferens: highly intermittent and monoquantal. *Neuroscience* **13**, 1–20
18. Brock, J.A. and Cunnane, T.C. (1987) Characteristic features of transmitter release from sympathetic nerve terminals. *Blood Vessels* **24**, 253–260
19. Booz, K.H. (1978) Zur innervation der autonom pulsierendon Vena portae der weissen Ratte. Eine histochemische und electronmicroscopische Untersuchung. *Z. Zellforsch. Microskop. Anat.* **117**, 394–418
20. McHale, N.G. and Roddie, I.C. (1983) The effect of intravenous adrenaline and noradrenaline infusion on peripheral lymph flow in the sheep. *J. Physiol. (London)* **341**, 517–526

21. McGeown, J.G., McHale, N.G. and Thornbury, K.D. (1987) The effect of electrical stimulation of the sympathetic chain on popliteal efferent lymph flow in the anaesthetised sheep. *J. Physiol. (London)* **393**, 123–133

22. McHale, N.G., Allen, J.M. and McCarron, J.G. (1988) Transient excitatory responses to sustained stimulation of intramural nerves in isolated bovine lymphatic vessels. *Q. J. Exp. Physiol.* **73**, 175–182

23. Harty, H., McGeown, J.G., McHale, N.G. and Thornbury, K.D. (1988) Modulation of pumping activity in mesenteric lymphatics following splanchnic nerve stimulation in the anaesthetized sheep. *J. Physiol. (London)* **403**, 87P

24. McHale, N.G. and Thornbury, K.D. (1986) A method for studying lymphatic pumping activity in conscious and anaesthetised sheep. *J. Physiol. (London)* **378**, 109–118

25. Thornbury, K.D., Harty, H.R., McGeown, J.G. and McHale, N.G. (1993) Mesenteric lymph flow responses to splanchnic nerve stimulation in the sheep. *Am. J. Physiol.* **264**, H604–H610

26. McHale, N.G. and Adair, T.H. (1989) Reflex modulation of lymphatic pumping in sheep. *Circ. Res.* **64**, 1165–1171

27. Harty, H.R., Thornbury, K.D. and McHale, N.G. (1993) Neurotransmission in isolated sheep mesenteric lymphatics. *Microvasc. Res.* **46**, 310–319

28. Hutchinson, S.P., Hollywood, M.A., Burke, E.P., Allen, J.M. and McHale, N.G. (1992) Effects of 5-HT on spontaneous contractility in isolated bovine mesenteric lymphatics. *Br. J. Pharmacol.* **107**, 37P

29. Hollywood, M.A. and McHale, N.G. (1993) Serotonin has both inhibitory and excitatory effects on spontaneous contractility in isolated sheep mesenteric lymphatics. *J. Physiol. (London)* **467**, 305P

30. Hollywood, M.A. (1994) Innervation of sheep mesenteric lymphatics. Ph.D. Thesis, The Queen's University of Belfast, Belfast

31. Brock, J.A. and Cunnane, T.C. (1988) Studies of the mode of action of bretylium and guanethidine in post-ganglionic sympathetic nerve fibres. *Naunyn-Schmiedeberg's Arch. Pharmacol.* **338**, 504–509

32. Hollywood, M.A. and McHale, N.G. (1994) Mediation of excitatory neurotransmission by the release of ATP and noradrenaline in sheep mesenteric lymphatic vessels. *J. Physiol. (London)* **481**, 415–423

33. Chen, H.I., Fan, P.L., Hu, P. and Brading, A.F. (1992) Effects of ATP on the lower urinary tract smooth muscles from rabbit and cat. In *Urology 1992* (Giulani, L. and Pippo, P., eds.), pp. 179–183, Monduzzi, Milano

34. Dunn, P.M. and Blakeley, A.G.H. (1988) Suramin: a reversible P2-purinoceptor antagonist in the mouse vas deferens. *Br. J. Pharmacol.* **93**, 243–245

35. McCullough, J.S. and McHale, N.G. (1988) Pressure flow relationships in isolated bovine mesenteric lymphatics during field stimulation. *J. Physiol. (London)* **396**, 177P

36. Hayashi, A., Johnston, M.G., Nelson, W., Hamilton, S. and McHale, N.G. (1987) Increased intrinsic pumping of intestinal lymphatics following haemorrhage in anaesthetised sheep. *Circ. Res.* **60**, 265–272

37. Elias, R.M. and Johnston, M.G. (1990) Modulation of lymphatic pumping by lymph-borne factors after endotoxin administration in sheep. *J. Appl. Physiol.* **68**, 199–208

15

Electrophysiology of lymphatic smooth muscle

D.F. Van Helden*, P.-Y. von der Weid and M.J. Crowe
The Neuroscience Group, Discipline of Human Physiology,
Faculty of Medicine and Health Sciences, University of Newcastle, Callaghan,
NSW 2308, Australia

Introduction

Lymphatic vessels are profusely present throughout the body to an extent similar to blood vessels. They provide the pathway for removal of extracellular debris and thus serve a key role in tissue fluid homoeostasis. They are also integral to the immune system in interconnecting lymphoid tissue and providing the return path for immune cells to the bloodstream.

Mammalian lymphatic vessels are divided into many small tubular chambers (Figure 1) through frequently occurring unidirectional valves. These chambers provide the means for propelling lymph which occurs when any chamber is compressed. Compression results when one or a number of chambers are externally compressed by structures such as skeletal muscle. Alternatively, and most importantly, compression can occur intrinsically.

Intrinsic lymphatic pumping is a property of many of the collecting lymphatics which generally have a wall structure containing smooth muscle, the constriction of which actively pumps lymph [1–4]. Vessels can be activated either by stretching of the vessel wall by filling [5,6] or by endogenous or exogenous stimulation through substances such as the sympathetic neurotransmitter noradrenaline [7–11]. It is known that an action potential precedes each transient constriction of lymphatic smooth muscle [12–14]. Yet, little is known about the mechanisms underlying generation of these action potentials. Resolution of this problem is crucial to understanding the physiological basis for lymphatic pumping.

The lymphangion

The observation that many individual chambers in guinea-pig mesenteric lymphatics constrict independently (as illustrated in Figure 2) led Mislin [5] to consider each chamber as a primitive heart, which he referred to as a lymphangion. This definition was based on both his work and that of Horstmann [15] who had morphologically shown that there was discontinuity in the smooth muscle in the region of valves (see Figure 3). Mislin described the lymphangion as "a segment with a central muscle band or 'sleeve', with a muscle-free valve formed by folds of the

*To whom correspondence should be addressed.

Figure I

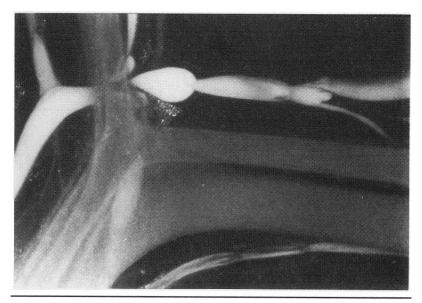

A lymphatic vessel (lacteal) in the guinea-pig mesentery (upper vessel)
The variable size and shape of the individual chambers is to be noted. An artery (the smaller vessel) and a vein lie underneath the lymphatic vessel. The small vessel at the bottom of the photograph, while initially of similar size to the upper vessel, became highly constricted consequent to damage. The largest diameter of the lymphatic vessel is about 280 μm (central chamber).

tunica intima (formed by a single layer of endothelial cells) at either end" (see [2]). However, some lymphatic vessels have smooth muscle which is continuous in the region of the valves [16,17]. Therefore, the lymphangion *per se* cannot be considered universally as the elementary contractile unit. Regardless of this, constriction in the smooth muscle, be it in a single chamber or a number of electrically coupled chambers, causes forward propulsion of lymph. Each constriction is phasic and brief (less than 10 s) compared with other smooth muscle (see [18]). Taken together, contractile lymphatic vessels can be considered as pumping lymph through a vast network of lymphangions, acting both in series and in parallel.

The action potential

A number of different procedures have been used to study the action potential in lymphatic smooth muscle.

Extracellular recording of the action potential
Extracellular electrical recording was first used to record the electrical activity of lymphatic smooth muscle (see [2,19]). Mislin referred to these recordings as electrolymphangiograms (ELGs). The ELG, which he

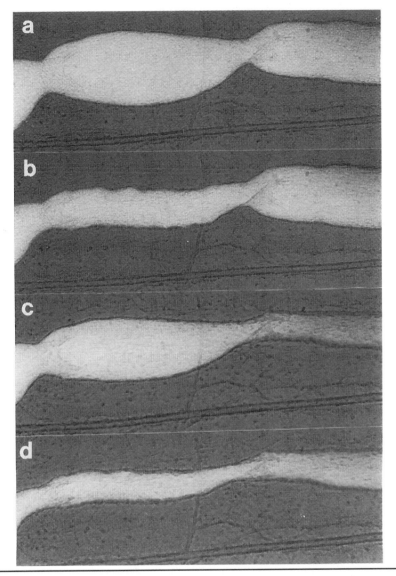

Spontaneous constrictions in a lymphatic vessel perfused with physiological saline containing 1 μM fluorescein and viewed with a fluorescence microscope (Nikon diaphot, fluorescein filter set)
The vessel is shown (a) in its relaxed state, (b) with the middle chamber constricted, (c) with the right-hand chamber constricted and (d) with all three chambers constricted. The maximum diameter of the vessel was 228 μm (a, middle chamber). Reproduced from [23] with permission.

considered to reflect the action potential, consisted of a series of peaks of short duration followed by a slower 'after-potential'. The initial peak of the ELG preceded constriction by some 0.22 s. He also noted that single peaks could even be recorded from relaxed vessels.

Figure 3

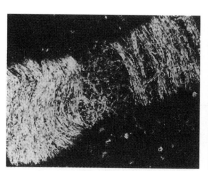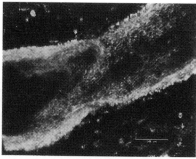

A confocal microscopic image of a guinea-pig mesenteric lymphatic vessel in the region of a valve

The image was taken with a Bio-Rad MRC 600 confocal microscope attached to a Zeiss axiovert 10 microscope with oil immersion × 40 objective (numerical aperture 1.3). The vessel was exposed to 1 μM 3,3'-diethyloxadicarbocyanine (DiOC₂ [5]). The left-hand image shows a discontinuity in the circularly oriented smooth muscle. The right-hand sectional image through the vessel shows the position of the valve and confirms that the discontinuity in smooth muscle occurred at this region. It is to be noted that this example represents a morphological subset, as the majority of lymphatic chambers in the guinea-pig mesentery exhibit a partial continuity in the region of valves with a few exhibiting almost continuous smooth muscle in this region (see [17]). The scale bar represents 50 μm.

Sucrose gap recording of the action potential

Measurements of intracellular voltage changes have primarily been made using the sucrose gap technique. This procedure, while not producing reliable measurements of absolute membrane potential, does provide an approximate dynamic description (although somewhat filtered; see [20]) of intracellular voltage changes when applied to tissues such as lymphatic vessels. The sucrose gap technique was first used to study lymphatic vessels by Orlov *et al.* [21]. The procedure was subsequently used to confirm a correlation between action potentials and constrictions [12–14]. These studies made on bovine mesenteric lymphatics recorded the action potential as a single spike followed by a gradually declining plateau with a mean duration at half amplitude of about 1 s.

Intracellular microelectrode recording of the action potential

Intracellular microelectrode recordings have provided measurements of membrane potential and the characteristics of the action potential in lymphatic smooth muscle. Ohhashi and Azuma [22] reported a mean membrane potential of −48 mV from bovine mesenteric lymphatic smooth muscle, while Ward *et al.* [20] measured a mean resting potential of −61 mV in the same tissue. This latter value compares with a mean value of −66 mV for the smooth muscle of guinea-pig mesenteric lymphatics [23]. The small difference between values may relate to differences in the method of tissue pinning (see below), or to the observation that bovine vessels showed consistent spontaneous action potentials and most guinea-pig vessels were quiescent.

Ward *et al.* [20] reported action potentials of average amplitude 58 mV, which only rarely exhibited an overshoot (1 to 2 mV). The mean duration and half amplitude was 1 s. The main difference between their observations and those previously made using the sucrose gap technique (see above) was that the bovine action potential had an initial transient followed by several spikes superimposed on the plateau phase. Guinea-pig mesenteric lymphatic action potentials also showed an initial transient followed by a plateau phase (Figure 4). The principal difference is that the guinea-pig smooth muscle generally did not show a short burst of 'spikes' during the plateau phase. It is not known whether this difference from the bovine recordings is a species-, size- or method-related difference. One obvious difference is that the bovine study was undertaken with vessels cut open and tightly pinned, with impalements made by a luminal approach. By comparison, the guinea-pig recordings were made on relaxed, non-perfused, intact vessels.

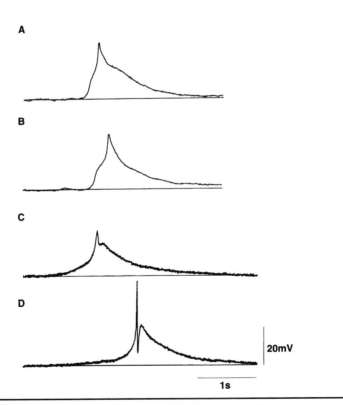

Figure 4

Intracellularly recorded action potentials from a small and a large lymphatic vessel

A and B, sample action potentials recorded from a single impalement in the smooth muscle of a small (diameter 200 μm) lymphatic vessel (intervalve spacing 1400 μm; resting membrane potential −55 mV). C and D, sample action potentials from a single impalement from a large (diameter 500 μm) lymphatic vessel (intervalve spacing not measured; membrane potential −65 mV).

Shape characteristics of the action potential

The records in Figure 4 demonstrate some important characteristics of lymphatic action potentials. First, the initial rise (generator phase) of the action potential differed between vessels. For example, records A and B, obtained from a small vessel (non-perfused diameter 200 μm), showed a rapid onset compared with the more uniform initial depolarization which occurred in a large vessel (non-perfused diameter 500 μm; records C and D). Secondly, the action potential displayed variations in shape even for sequential recordings at the same location (compare C and D). The action potentials occurred at various intervals (between 15 and 40 s), generally alternating in shape between the two waveforms shown (Figures 4C and 4D). Both types of action potential caused phasic constrictions; however, whether one was more forceful than the other was not assessed. The fact that the slow phase of each action potential was very similar indicates that this action potential is composed of at least two separate components.

Ionic dependence of the action potential

Like most smooth muscles [18], lymphatic action potentials are primarily carried by the entry of Ca^{2+} ions. Azuma *et al.* [12] showed that spontaneous action potentials, while unaffected by tetrodotoxin (1×10^{-6} g/ml), were inhibited when Mn^{2+} ions (1×10^{-6} g/ml) were added to the bathing 'Ringer' solution. They also demonstrated that spontaneous constrictions were abolished when Ca^{2+} ions were omitted from this solution. McHale *et al.* [24] showed that removal of Ca^{2+} had a direct effect on the action potential (and not the underlying pacemaker mechanisms) as evoked action potentials were abolished in Ca^{2+}-free (plus 1 mM EGTA) Ringer solution. This same study also showed that replacement of NaCl in the Ringer solution with LiCl shortened the action potentials, but did not alter their amplitude. A detailed pharmacological characterization of the type(s) of Ca^{2+} channels underlying the action potential has yet to be made.

K$^+$ channels also play a role in the action potential, as indicated by the effects of tetraethylammonium ions (TEA, 10 mM), a known blocker of most types of K$^+$ channels. TEA increased the amplitude of the rapid component (the 'initial spike') and caused marked prolongation of the slow phase (the 'gradually declining plateau') of the action potential [24,25]. Generally, a series of oscillations resembling 'spontaneous spikes' occurred during the prolonged plateau. It is not known whether these effects were due to blockage of K$^+$ channels involved in the resting membrane conductance and/or direct inhibition of K$^+$ channels opened during the action potential. However, lymphatic smooth muscle exhibits at least two types of K$^+$ channels, an inward rectifying channel [25] and a Ca^{2+}-activated K$^+$ channel [26]. Interestingly, 4-aminopyridine (10 mM) blocked inward rectification but had little effect on the action potential [25]. Ba^{2+} ions, which are known to block K$^+$ channels, caused a decrease in membrane conductance, a depolarization and greatly increased action potential duration [25].

Pharmacological modulation of the action potential

There have been a number of studies showing that various pharmacological agents have either a positive or negative effect on the strength of constrictions (e.g. see [2]). Noradrenaline is known to increase the force of lymphatic phasic constrictions. The basis for this was shown to be primarily an increase in the duration of the slow phase of the action potential [24].

Lymphatic pacemaking

One of the primary determinants of intrinsic lymph propulsion is the lymphatic pumping rate, which is dependent on the underlying pace-making mechanisms. This section considers present understanding of these mechanisms.

Mechanical modulation of pacemaking

At present it is known that many stimuli modulate pumping rate. A key modulator is vessel filling [5–8,27]. An example of such modulation is presented in Figure 5 where the contractile behaviour of a perfused segment of vessel cut from a small lymphangion is shown. The contractions have been recorded videoscopically *in vitro* using an edge-tracking program [28].

The behaviour of the segment was typical of single lymphangions in guinea-pig mesenteric lymphatics. The interval between constrictions showed considerable variability. Interestingly, constrictions in larger vessels such as bovine mesenteric lymphatics appear to occur more regularly (e.g. see [13]). While the segment of Figure 5 showed no

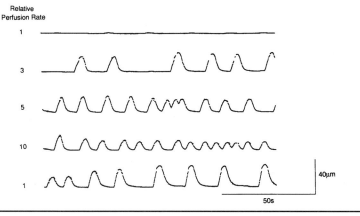

Figure 5

Relative
Perfusion Rate

Spontaneous constrictions in a perfused lymphatic segment
This segment (length approx. 450 µm; diameter approx. 200 µm) was cut from a small lymphangion in the region of the valves. The vessel was perfused by abutting a perfusion electrode against the inflow site and perfused with an oxygenated tissue saline solution. The vessel responded to increased flow, showing the maximum constriction frequency at relative perfusion rate 10 (the highest rate examined). The stroke volume was decreased at this higher perfusion rate. It is to be noted that the spontaneous constrictions persisted upon return to the original low perfusion rate.

contractile activity at a low perfusion rate (relative rate 1), the frequency of constrictions increased with faster perfusion rates. Characteristic of a 'heart', the stroke volume decreased when the frequency of constriction was high. Importantly, the vessel segment continued to constrict upon return to the starting perfusion rate (although this activity stopped after about 5 min; results not shown). Electrophysiological investigation of pressure/flow modulation of pacemaking has been examined by extra-cellular recording. Mislin [19] noted that the extracellularly recorded action potential (composed of a series of peaks followed by a slower 'after-potential') which preceded each constriction occurred at higher frequency with increased pressure. It was noted that there were both large- and small-amplitude peaks. Increasing the pressure caused more large-amplitude peaks. Interpretation of such observations is difficult. Mislin speculated that the findings were consistent with stretch causing depolarization of the smooth muscle, this then leading to increased electrical activity.

Pharmacological modulation of pacemaking

Many studies on the lymphatics have examined the effects of a wide range of substances on the pumping activity of lymphatic vessels, with many causing either an increase or decrease in spontaneous lymphatic constrictions [2–4,25,29]. The effect of the sympathetic nerve trans-mitter noradrenaline has been studied in detail. As well as its effect on the action potential, noradrenaline also causes an increase in the frequency of spontaneous contractions [7–9,11]. The study by McHale and Roddie [11] indicated that noradrenaline had a dual action and indeed high concentrations of noradrenaline were found to inhibit spontaneous constrictions through stimulation of β-adrenoceptors [9–11,30,31]. The mechanism underlying this inhibition relates to a β-adrenoceptor-mediated hyperpolarization and an increase in membrane potassium conductance [31].

The effects of adrenergic excitation through α-adrenoceptors were studied in detail using the sucrose gap technique [11,24,32]. It was shown that the slope of the slow-depolarizing pacemaker potential which preceded each action potential was increased by noradrenaline, consistent with the increased rate of action potential firing [14,32,33]. McHale *et al.* [24] demonstrated that noradrenaline caused a depolarization and a decrease in membrane potassium conductance.

Spontaneous transient depolarizations (STDs): the pacemaker potential in small lymphangions

Our laboratory has investigated the electrophysiological basis for pace-making using guinea-pig mesenteric lymphatics. Most of our experi-ments have been undertaken on short segments of lymphatic vessel. These have electrically simplified properties approximating the electrical circuit of a spherical cell. This means that electrical events such as pacemaker activity can be recorded without decrement by impaling any of the smooth muscle cells present in the short segment [23,34]. It was found that short segments (length $<300\ \mu m$, diameter 70–200 μm) were effectively isopotential, as injection of a current pulse produced an exponential voltage response (i.e. they had the simplified circuit of a resistor and capacitor in parallel; see Figure 10). These segments had measurable input resistance and time constants with mean values of about 36 MΩ and 180 ms respectively [23]. Some 20% of short, non-perfused segments constricted spontaneously in a manner similar to that demonstrated in Figure 5 (for intermediate perfusion rates), with segments normally relaxing before undergoing further constriction.

Electrophysiological recording from such segments demonstrated normal resting membrane potentials (usually between −55 and −75 mV [35]). The membrane potential record often demonstrated brief spontaneous transient depolarizations (STDs). Of note is the finding that action potentials, when they occurred, were preceded by such activity. An example is presented in Figure 6. An initial STD occurred followed by two action potentials. Figure 6(B) shows the STD and the action potentials on an expanded time scale. The activity at the foot of the action potential generally appeared as though it was composed of either one or more STDs. The biphasic nature of the action potentials is also apparent with a rapid onset and a brief inflection followed by a slower

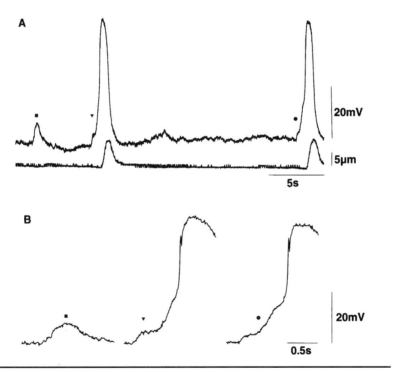

Figure 6

Recordings of membrane potential and associated constriction of a short segment of lymphatic vessel (length 220 μm, diameter 130 μm) undergoing spontaneous constrictions

A, the smooth muscle exhibited spontaneous, transient depolarizing potentials and action potentials. STDs (■) were monophasic and did not cause constriction whereas action potentials (▼,●) were biphasic and caused constriction. B, the STD and the action potentials marked in A are shown on an expanded time scale. The smooth muscle of the segment had a membrane potential of −61 mV and an input resistance of 44 MΩ. Reproduced from [23] with permission.

depolarizing component. STDs did not cause constriction, whereas action potentials always did, with constriction commencing 250–400 ms from the beginning of the rapid rising component of the action potential. Slow-depolarizing pacemaker potentials were never observed in these segments.

The possibility that cut segments behaved differently to intact vessels was examined by recording intracellularly from small lymphangions which constricted independently of adjacent lymphangions. These behaved similarly to cut segments, exhibiting a depolarizing potential rising from an apparently stable resting potential which then initiated the action potential. An example is presented in Figure 7. Figure 7(B) demonstrates that this lymphangion also exhibited STDs of variable amplitude (arrowheads). Again, the action potential caused constriction, whereas the STDs did not. Small lymphangions such as this one exhibited the electrical characteristics of a short cable. They responded to injection of a constant current with an exponential voltage response (Figure 7D). Therefore, the initial depolarizing phase leading

Figure 7

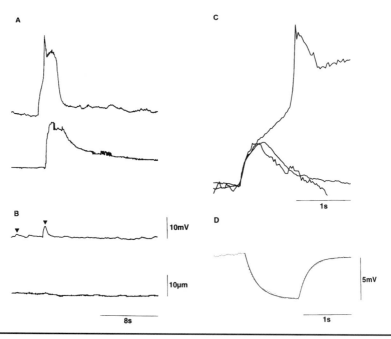

Records of membrane potential and constriction in a non-perfused lymphangion

The resting potential of a lymphangion (length 390 μm, diameter 150 μm) was −60 mV. A, the action potential was biphasic and caused constriction. B, STDs were of variable size and were monophasic. They did not cause constriction directly. Two STDs have been marked (arrowheads). C, the action potential and STDs (of A and B). The STDs have been amplitude-scaled to that of the foot of the action potential. D, the voltage response to injection of a current pulse (amplitude −0.2 nA). The solid curve represents the exponential of best fit to the 'on' and 'off' transients of the voltage response. A and B are represented on the same scale. Reproduced from [23] with permission.

16

Microcirculation of lymph through lymph nodes

T.J. Heath*, C.S. Lowden and G.T. Belz
Department of Anatomical Sciences, University of Queensland, Brisbane,
Queensland 4072, Australia

Introduction

Many illustrations of lymph nodes show all afferent lymphatic vessels joining the subcapsular sinus almost at right angles and the subcapsular sinus being continuous, through the trabecular sinuses, with a network of medullary sinuses which converge on a few efferent lymphatics emerging at a well-defined hilus [1–5]. We have an interest in the lymphatic system of domestic animals, and it soon became clear that this was, at best, an oversimplification of the situation, at least in sheep, pigs and horses.

We used a variety of methods to study the lymph pathways through lymph nodes in sheep and horses. The main methods involved filling the lymph spaces with either the latex casting material Microfil (Stecca Associates, San Francisco, CA, U.S.A.) and viewing with light microscopy after clearing the tissue with methyl salicylate, or using the hard casting material Batsons #17 (Paul Valley Industrial Park, Warrington, PA, U.S.A.), then digesting away the tissue and viewing with the scanning electron microscope. We also used traditional light microscopy, scanning electron microscopy and transmission electron microscopy.

The microcirculation of lymph flow through lymph nodes in sheep and horses is described under the following four headings: (1) pathways of lymph flow into the node; (2) pathways of lymph flow through the cortex of the node; (3) pathways of lymph flow through the medulla of the node; and (4) pathways of lymph flow from the node.

Under each heading, a comparison will be made with the patterns of lymph flow in nodes of other species studied, with the exception of those in pigs, which have a very different structure and will therefore be considered separately.

Pathways of lymph flow into the node

As the afferent lymphatics approach the node they divide sequentially, forming a radiating pattern of primary, secondary and terminal vessels on the surface of the node [6–9]. In sheep, each afferent lymphatic may give rise to up to 30–40 terminal vessels [8,9] which enter over the entire surface of the node apart from the hilar depression [10] (Figure 1). These terminal vessels follow either one of two courses. First, some

---

*To whom correspondence should be addressed.

Figure 1

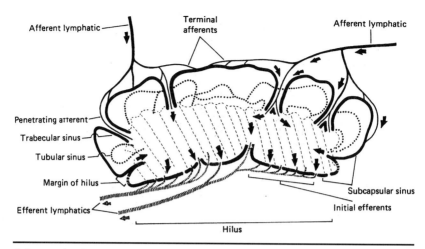

Afferent lymphatic

Terminal afferents

Afferent lymphatic

Penetrating afferent

Trabecular sinus

Tubular sinus

Margin of hilus

Efferent lymphatics

Subcapsular sinus

Initial efferents

Hilus

Schematic diagram of the lymph pathways within an iliofemoral lymph node of a sheep

Afferent lymphatics approach the dorsal surface of the node and divide into terminal afferents which either enter the subcapsular sinus (full line), or penetrate within trabeculae. Lymph reaches the sinuses of the medulla (broken line) from these penetrating afferents, or through invaginations of the subcapsular sinus around the trabeculae. Tubular sinuses (dotted line) within the cortex also join medullary sinuses. Initial efferent lymphatics arise over a large area of hilus. Most have their origin in the hilar subcapsular sinus or adjacent medullary sinuses. The initial efferents join together as they pass across the hilar surface, forming two efferent vessels which carry lymph towards the lumbar trunks. Reproduced from [14] with permission.

vessels enter the subcapsular sinus, and the lymph flows through the subcapsular sinus to the trabecular sinuses as shown in traditional illustrations. The second pathway is quite different: it involves a lymphatic vessel penetrating the node within a trabeculum [9,11], and delivering the lymph through holes in its wall deep into the cortex of the node [11] (Figure 1). Therefore, although some lymph enters the node through the subcapsular and trabecular sinuses, some — and it is not known what proportion — enters the sinuses deep within the cortex.

Like those in sheep and horses, the afferent lymphatics of rabbit mesenteric nodes [3] branch to form a radiating pattern on the surface of the node, and lymph is distributed over a large area of nodal tissue. In rats, however, a single afferent lymphatic delivers lymph preferentially to a discrete cortical unit [1,12,13], suggesting that the nodes are comprised of separate physiological compartments. This concept of physiological compartmentalization does not seem to apply in sheep or horse lymph nodes. The reasons for this conclusion include: (1) the large area of nodal tissue covered by a single afferent via the radiating pattern; and (2) the entry of terminal afferent lymphatics into trabecular sinuses continuous with parts of the subcapsular sinus supplied by an adjacent vessel [6–9].

Pathways of lymph flow through the cortex

Some lymph flows through the cortex in sinuses which surround the trabeculae. However, there are other types of sinuses within the cortex of sheep and horse nodes. Some of these have a meshwork of reticular cell processes supporting macrophages and other cells as do most sinuses in the node, but there are many, especially in sheep, which lack such processes. These sinuses are tubular in outline and measure 20–100 μm across in sheep and 10–30 μm across in horses [6,7,14]. They may have holes in their walls and they extend through the cortical parenchyma, often close to blood vessels. These sinuses have been termed as cortical tubular sinuses [6–8,14,15], and they occur throughout the cortical tissue, with the exception of the nodules, and are confluent with subcapsular, trabecular or medullary sinuses (Figure 1). Cortical tubular sinuses appear comparable with the 'lymph labyrinths' [16] and 'mudstreams' [17] described in rodents, and the 'tubular sinuses' [3] described in rabbits. However, they appear to differ from the 'paracortical sinuses' of rabbits [18], and the 'paracortical lymphatics' of sheep [4] for which few connections to surrounding sinuses could be demonstrated. Many of the sinuses in the cortex lie close to lymph nodules [15] and may be important in the wide distribution of lymph constituents within the cortex. In sheep, this is supported by observations on the distribution of Microfil [8,14] and carbon particles [6] over a wide area of the node after they had been introduced into a single afferent lymphatic. An important point, however, is that each of the nodules is surrounded by a meshwork of sinuses, and these must play a role in the transport of cells and cell products [15]. It has been shown that stimulation of the node by dextran causes changes to the sinuses, and a reduction in the filtering capacity of the node [19]. There is no evidence, however, as to whether any comparable morphological changes occur during antigenic stimulation under normal conditions.

Pathways of lymph flow through the medulla

Most lymph flows through the medullary sinuses that surround medullary cords [14,15] (Figure 1). These medullary sinuses are crossed by numerous reticular processes which are continuous with the cells lining the sinuses. Studies in sheep have shown that the lining cells, in turn, form a continuous layer throughout the sinuses except where cells are migrating between medullary cords and sinuses, or between the deep cortical parenchyma and medullary sinuses at the cortex/medulla interface [14]. There is no indication that the medullary sinuses in sheep [14] converge towards efferent lymphatics as described by Kurokawa and Ogata [3] in rabbits.

In addition, there are sinuses within many of the medullary cords: small vessels less than 30 μm across, but which differ from the medullary sinuses by lacking the complex network of processes [7,8]. What is the role of medullary cord sinuses? Perhaps it is to increase the surface area for exchange, although no evidence is currently available.

The complex arrangement of the lymph pathways through the node may provide an increased contact area for fluid exchange between the lymph and blood compartments of the node. It has been suggested that post-nodal lymph is not representative of interstitial fluid because the lymph protein concentration may be modified during lymph node transit [20–22]. This indicates that lymph nodes may act as a fluid-exchange chamber, with the composition of lymph determined by transport dynamics across a surface described as the nodal blood–lymph barrier [20,21].

A question which has exercised workers for many years is whether lymph can flow along the subcapsular sinus around the periphery of the node to the efferent lymphatics, without entering the substance of the node [23]. This still does not seem to have been answered clearly. Perusal of illustrations in standard textbooks could lead one to the conclusion that no impediment exists to such lymph flow [24,25]. In the rabbit, however, the subcapsular sinus apparently does not extend into the hilus [3].

In sheep, Microfil preparations revealed some continuity between the subcapsular sinus over the cortex and that within the hilus [14]. However, the margin of the hilus did contain a high concentration of trabecular and reticular processes, and it is considered that these may decrease the volume of the sinus and thus increase the resistance to lymph flow in this region. Furthermore, the trabeculae at the hilar margin may divert some lymph from the cortical subcapsular sinus along the trabecular sinus and into the depths of the node.

Pathways of lymph flow from the node

Lymph leaves the medulla through initial efferent lymphatic vessels. Some of these initial efferent vessels begin immediately under the capsule and their lumens communicate through holes in their wall with the medullary sinuses [7,8,14], while others have their origins deep within the medulla; they begin, by the coalescing of cell processes, to form a progressively more complete wall [7,8].

It is difficult to estimate the total number of initial efferent lymphatics within a node, although 60–100 were counted in some sheep popliteal nodes [14]. These lymphatics, which were 30–70 μm across in sheep nodes and 40–100 μm across in horse nodes [8,11,14], then drain into slightly larger vessels within the medullary trabeculae — some of which have valves — and they emerge on to the surface of the node (Figure 1). Initial efferent lymphatics arising within the node have not been reported in rats. In this species, as Sainte-Marie and Sin [26] reported, the medullary sinuses join together with the end-portion of the subcapsular sinus at the hilus to form the efferent lymphatics.

Some of the small vessels that emerge into the hilar depression might not be evident on first examination, as many are embedded in a tight pad of fat [8,14]. This fat provides protection and support to the tiny, fragile vessels before they coalesce to form the major efferent lymphatics that emerge from the vicinity of the node.

The situation in horse and sheep nodes, where lymph leaves the node through many efferent vessels over a significant portion of the

node surface, over the whole medulla [7,10,14] (Figure 1), differs substantially from the situation represented in most publications on lymph
nodes; namely 1–3 lymph vessels emerging from a single depression
which resembles a renal hilus [1,23,24,26,27].

In summary then, lymph approaching a lymph node, at least in
the sheep and horse, might take one of a number of pathways through
the node. It may enter at the surface or more deeply; it may then enter
sinuses that are crossed by numerous processes that support macrophages and other cells, or sinuses that are tubular and essentially free
from processes. The lymph pathways are closely associated with the
lymph nodules in the cortex, and with the cords in the medulla. Finally,
the lymph enters initial efferent lymphatics deep within the medulla or
at its surface, and emerges over an appreciable area of the surface, then
flows into one or more major efferent vessels which transport it either
to the next node in the chain, or to the bloodstream in the neck.

Microcirculation of lymph nodes in pigs

The lymph nodes of the pig differ significantly from those of most other
mammals in having a somewhat inverted structure [28–34]. Dense
nodular tissue, which corresponds to the cortical tissue in other species,
is located mainly towards the centre of the node, while diffuse tissue,
which contains relatively few lymphocytes and is the counterpart of
medullary tissue, is located mainly at the periphery [32,33] (Figure 2).
Larger lymph nodes appear to be formed by the fusion of several node
anlages [29,35].

The flow of lymph through the lymph node in the pig has been
described as being comparable with that in other species [29]. That is,
lymph flows first through the 'cortical' tissue, albeit in a central position,
and then proceeds through the 'medullary' tissue [29,30]. Although this
general flow pattern was evident in our experiments [32,33], the flow
pattern appears to be rather more complex.

The afferent lymphatics enter the node either together, or at
separate sites over the node surface where the capsule is invaginated to
form trabeculae. These trabeculae, containing the afferent lymphatics,
ramify through the dense nodular tissue located centrally in the node
(Figure 2). The nodular tissue which is located superficially is covered by
a subcapsular sinus, and this is continuous with the trabecular sinuses.
The afferent lymphatics give rise to numerous branches which open into
sinuses surrounding the trabeculae. Usually lymph enters the subcapsular
sinus from the trabecular sinuses; however, direct communications may
occur between branches of afferent lymphatics and the subcapsular sinus
over dense nodular tissue. Valves are present in virtually all afferent
lymphatics, both outside the nodes and within them [32,33].

After flowing through the nodular tissue, lymph enters the
diffuse tissue. The diffuse tissue generally surrounds the dense nodular
tissue except where an afferent lymphatic enters the node (Figure 2).
The sinuses in the diffuse tissue consist of those bordered partially
y trabeculae and the capsule, as well as those bordered only by
parenchyma. The sinus walls consist of reticular lining cells and a few

Figure 2

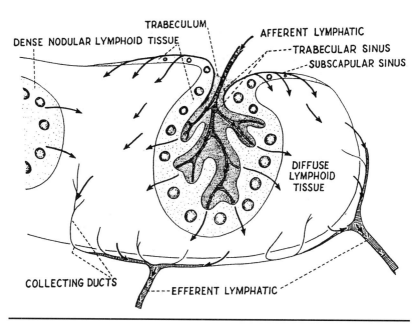

DENSE NODULAR LYMPHOID TISSUE

TRABECULUM

AFFERENT LYMPHATIC

----TRABECULAR SINUS

---SUBSCAPULAR SINUS

DIFFUSE
LYMPHOID
TISSUE

COLLECTING DUCTS

----EFFERENT LYMPHATIC

Schematic diagram of the lymph pathways within a superficial inguinal lymph node of a pig

An afferent lymphatic enters and penetrates within a trabeculum into the dense nodular ('cortical') tissue of the node. Some dense nodular tissue extends over the periphery of the node from the point of entry of the afferent lymphatic. This tissue is overlain by a subcapsular sinus, and this is continuous with the trabecular sinus. To avoid cluttering the diagram, we did not show the small trabeculae, each surrounded by a trabecular sinus, which penetrate the dense nodular tissue in two locations: as branches of the central trabeculum, and extending inward from the capsule over the superficial part of the dense nodular tissue. The diffuse lymphoid ('medullary') tissue extends to the periphery over most of the node, and collecting ducts emerge from the sinuses of this tissue and join efferent lymphatics. The portion of dense nodular tissue shown on the left is thought to be derived from a different node anlage, and at the lower left, collecting ducts emerge from deep within the node along what is believed to be the line of fusion of the two node anlages. Major pathways for the flow of lymph are represented by arrows. Reproduced from [14] with permission.

collagen fibres, but contain many gaps up to 10 μm across. The sinus lumen is continuous with the interstices of the diffuse tissue through some of these gaps. The trabeculae and capsule adjacent to the sinuses are lined by a single continuous layer of lining cells [32,33].

Lymph flows from the sinuses of the diffuse tissue into efferent lymphatics (Figure 2); these are usually in the capsule or along the plane of fusion of adjacent node anlagen. Some sinuses of the diffuse tissue connect more or less directly with the efferent lymphatics. More commonly they join collecting ducts which, unlike the efferent lymphatics, do not possess valves. The collecting ducts are very similar in appearance to some of the initial efferents found in sheep and horse nodes [7,8,11,34]. Collecting ducts are extensively distributed at the node surface where the diffuse tissue is peripherally located (Figure 2), and generally lie within the substance of the capsule and communicate with it through holes (up to 80 μm across) in their walls. Some also occur within the diffuse tissue, and others are present in trabeculae [32,33].

The collecting ducts join the efferent lymphatics either after a very short course, or after passing over the node surface and joining with other collecting ducts (Figure 2). In studies of the superficial inguinal lymph centre in the pig [32], the efferent lymphatics from different nodes converged and interconnected, forming up to five or sometimes more draining lymphatic trunks.

Therefore, the lymph nodes of pigs have a distinctively different structure, particularly in the central location of the dense nodular tissue. However, the significance of this positioning is not clear. Lymph still reaches the sinuses adjacent to the dense nodular tissue directly from the afferent lymphatics, as in other species, and the orientation of the nodules towards the incoming lymph is the same [36].

Further similarities between the lymph flow in pig lymph nodes and conventional lymph nodes can be found. In pigs, afferent lymphatics can communicate directly with the subcapsular sinus, as is usually the case in other species, and afferent lymphatics often penetrate the node within trabeculae. The collecting ducts are also very similar to some initial efferent vessels in sheep and horse nodes. These similarities, and the increasing awareness that cortical and medullary tissue in other species are not always classically arranged in a peripheral and central postion in the node [30,37], suggest that the unusual distribution of the dense nodular tissue and diffuse tissues in the pig may have little functional significance. It certainly seems unlikely that the distribution of these tissues is fundamental to the unusual pattern of lymphocyte recirculation in the pig as suggested by Bennell and Husband [38].

References

1. Sainte-Marie, G., Peng, F.-S. and Belisle, C. (1982) *Am. J. Anat.* **164**, 275–309
2. Steinmann, G., Foldi, E., Foldi, M., Racz, P. and Lennert, K. (1982) *Lab. Invest.* **47**, 43–50
3. Kurokawa, T. and Ogata, T. (1980) *Acta Anat.* **107**, 439–466
4. Nicander, L., Nafstad, P., Landsverk, T. and Engebretsen, R.H. (1991) *J. Anat.* **178**, 203–212
5. Schummer, A., Wilkens, H., Vollmerhaus, B. and Habermehl, K.-H. (1981) *The Circulatory System, the Skin, and the Cutaneous Organs of the Domestic Mammals*, 1st edn., vol. 3, Verlag Paul Parey, Berlin and Hamburg
6. Heath, T.J., Kerlin, R.L. and Spalding, H.J. (1986) *J. Anat.* **149**, 65–75
7. Nikles, S.A. and Heath, T.J. (1992) *Anat. Rec.* **232**, 126–132
8. Lowden, S. and Heath, T. (1993) *J. Anat.* **183**, 13–20
9. Heath, T.J. and Kerlin, R.L. (1986) *J. Anat.* **144**, 61–70
10. Heath, T. and Brandon, R. (1983) *Anat. Rec.* **207**, 461–472
11. Heath, T.J. and Perkins, N.R. (1989) *Anat. Rec.* **223**, 420–424
12. Sainte-Marie, G. and Peng, F.-S. (1986) *Cell Tissue Res.* **245**, 481–486
13. Sainte-Marie, G. and Peng, F.-S. (1985) *Cell Tissue Res.* **239**, 31–35
14. Heath, T.J. and Spalding, H.J. (1987) *J. Anat.* **155**, 177–188
15. Heath, T.J. and Nikles, S.A. (1991) *J. Anat.* **178**, 39–43
16. He, Y. (1985) *Arch. Histol.* **48**, 1–15
17. Soderstrom, N. and Stenstrom, A. (1969) *Scand. J. Haematol.* **6**, 186–196
18. Kelly, R.H. (1975) *Int. Arch. Allergy Appl. Immunol.* **48**, 836–849
19. Spalding, H.J. and Heath, T.J. (1991) *Res. Vet. Sci.* **51**, 100–106
20. Adair, T.H., Moffatt, D.S., Paulsen, A.W. and Guyton, A.C. (1982) *Am. J. Physiol.* **243**, H351–H359
21. Adair, T.H. and Guyton, A.C. (1983) *Am. J. Physiol.* **245**, H616–H622
22. Adair, T.H. and Guyton, A.C. (1985) *Am. J. Physiol.* **249**, H777–H782

23. Drinker, C.K., Field, M.E. and Ward, H.K. (1934) *J. Exp. Med.* **59**, 393–405

24. Weiss, L. (1984) *The Blood Cells and Haematopoietic Tissues*, 2nd edn., Elsevier, New York

25. Raviola, E. (1975) in *A Textbook of Histology* (Bloom, W. and Fawcett, D.W., eds.), 10th edn., pp. 471–486, W.B. Saunders, Philadelphia

26. Sainte-Marie, G. and Sin, Y.M. (1968) *Rev. Can. Biol.* **27**, 191–207

27. Banks, W.J. (1993) *Applied Veterinary Histology*, 3rd edn., Mosby-Year Book, Inc., St. Louis

28. Hoshi, N., Hashimoto, Y., Kitigawa, H. and Kon, Y. (1986) *Jpn. J. Vet. Sci.* **48**, 1097–1107

29. Bouwman, F.L. (1959) Ph.D. Thesis, Michigan State University, East Lansing

30. Binns, R.M. (1982) *Vet. Immunol. Immunopathol.* **3**, 95–146

31. Binns, R.M. and Pabst, R. (1988) in *Migration and Homing of Lymphoid Cells* (Husband, A., ed.), vol. 2, pp. 137–174, CRC Press, Boca Raton

32. Spalding, H. and Heath, T. (1987) *Anat. Rec.* **217**, 188–195

33. Spalding, H.J. and Heath, T.J. (1989) *J. Anat.* **166**, 43–54

34. Spalding, H.J. (1990) Ph.D. Thesis, University of Queensland, Brisbane

35. Kampmeier, O.F. (ed.)(1969) *Evolution and Comparative Morphology of the Lymphatic System*, 1st edn., Charles C. Thomas, Springfield

36. Hunt, A.C. (1968) *Br. J. Exp. Pathol.* **49**, 338–339

37. Kowala, M.C. and Schoefl, G.I. (1986) *J. Anat.* **148**, 25–46

38. Bennell, M.A. and Husband, A.J. (1981) *Immunology* **42**, 469–474

17

Lymphocyte circulation

John B. Hay* and Alan J. Young
Department of Immunology and Pathology, University of Toronto, Toronto, Canada

Introduction

The circulation of lymphocytes is a complex, continuous physiological process which only occurs in the whole animal. It is absolutely dependent upon an intact blood vascular and lymphatic system. Parts of the process can and have been dissected and analysed in simpler systems using a variety of techniques. These types of study have led to our current knowledge regarding some of the mediators and molecules which might modulate the migration of lymphocytes, and to the concept that molecules on the surface of the lymphocyte interact with complementary molecules on the surface of endothelial cells, particularly in post-capillary venules. One challenge is to now test whether the conclusions drawn from these simpler models adequately represent the physiological process.

We welcome this opportunity to describe some experiments which we feel attempt to preserve the physiological integrity to analyse lymphocyte recirculation, but still permit a quantitative approach and the advancement of experimentally testable ideas relevant to the mechanisms. Too often our audience is composed of immunologists who are more oriented towards molecules and less adept than physiologists at dealing with more complex integrated tissue, organ and whole animal responses to immunological challenges.

We have dealt with the following topics in much the same way as they were presented at the Symposium in Glasgow and the intent has been to illustrate some experimental approaches that we and others have used to investigate this fundamental problem and to outline the deficiencies in our knowledge. Detailed and much more comprehensive reviews can be found which concentrate on the individual components of lymphocyte traffic and we have attempted to identify these to the reader.

Numbers of lymphocytes

Before one can comprehend the magnitude, kinetics and relevance of lymphocyte circulation, it is pertinent to be reminded of a few background facts regarding the numbers of these cells and their origin and distribution in the body.

Since our experiments involve sheep, the numbers are based upon this species, but most likely apply, for the most part, to other mammalian species (including humans) of comparable size and age.

*To whom correspondence should be addressed at: Trauma Research Program, Sunnybrook Health Science Centre, 2075 Bayview Avenue, North York, Ontario M4N 3M5, Canada.

There are approximately 10^{12} lymphocytes in a 30 kg, 6-month-old (near the age of sexual maturity) sheep. This includes cells found in the thymus (which is approximately 25 g but is already starting to involute), the spleen (approx. 100 g but half non-lymphoid), the lymph nodes (estimated to total 70 g), the bone marrow and various areas of diffuse lymphoid cell accumulation underlying mucosal tissues. It is interesting that the blood contains only about 1% of the total found in the fixed lymphoid tissues. The recirculating lymphocyte pool has been estimated to be about 10 times the blood pool or 10% of the total. This estimate is based upon draining lymph from the thoracic duct and other major lymphatics, and observing that nearly 80% of the normal lymphocyte output can be removed (usually within a few days) [1,2]. However, several questions and problems with this balance sheet immediately come to mind. For example, most of the lymphocytes in the thymus (thymocytes) do not yet recirculate or participate in immunological responses to foreign antigens. Is the spleen really a static representation of the blood? The phenotypic pattern of lymphocyte subsets in the spleen is very similar to that in blood and quite different from the pattern in lymph nodes, afferent lymph and efferent lymph. If the recirculating lymphocyte pool can be drained off with chronic lymph collection, does this mean that the residual lymphocytes seen in lymph cannot recirculate between blood and lymph? It is our observation and that of others that the residual lymphocytes seen after such lymph drainage reach a stable plateau at this lower output [1,2]. Does this mean that rapidly proliferating (i.e. short-lived) cells make up this steady-state population? The question of lymphocyte turnover and lifespan is dealt with later. Qualitative analyses show that chronic lymph drainage depletes lymphocytes from the fixed lymphoid tissues, as judged by the histological appearance, but the degree of depletion has not been adequately quantified. Although fixed versus recirculating lymphocytes have been referred to for many years, we really do not know the relationship between the two. Given that recirculating lymphocytes are responsible for immune surveillance in nearly all tissues, and that recirculating lymphocytes are responsible for the dissemination of immune responses and for the systemic distribution of immunological memory, what could be the function of fixed lymphocytes? Are they lymphocytes which are either immature or near the end of their life? Lymphocytes which become antibody-forming cells seem to have a more sessile existence and do not recirculate [3] but memory lymphocytes are clearly recirculating cells [4–6]. If the recirculating lymphocyte pool is 10 times greater than the blood pool, and this pool can be drained in 2 days, then assuming a steady state the blood lymphocytes must be replaced every 48 h/10 (i.e. 4.8 h). This assumes that all of the lymphocytes in the blood are part of the recirculating pool. However, this does not match data obtained by tracking labelled cells, as discussed later. If one assumes that the spleen is really an extension of the blood pool of lymphocytes and is in equilibrium with the blood, then together they represent about 6×10^{10} lymphocytes. This means that the blood pool is about 60% of the recirculating pool and that the blood pool is replaced about every 29 h. To compound the problem, maybe a significant proportion of blood lymphocytes do not recirculate. We simply do not know, although some recent data lead to this conclusion (A.J. Young, unpublished work).

Some of the questions posed can be tested experimentally but adequate experimental systems are crucial. In most small animals it is not even feasible to sequentially sample blood lymphocytes over long periods of time. In addition, although thoracic duct lymph can be continuously collected for a few days in rats and even mice, the physiological integrity of the animal is quickly compromised due to the loss of fluid, protein and cells [7,8]. Other lymphatics are too small and nearly impossible to cannulate and keep flowing, and the collection of afferent lymph poses an even larger problem. We think it justifiable to state that more is known about the physiology of lymphocyte circulation in sheep than in any other species [9,10] and the following synopsis of some of the relevant literature attempts to validate our claim. The chronic collection of lymph from conscious animals [11] is the single most important development which permitted these experiments.

The single lymph node

What are the dynamics of the input and output of lymphocytes through a single lymph node? A great deal of our knowlege comes from experimental studies by the late Bede Morris and a series of his research trainees [9–11]. More recent experiments have documented the distribution of a variety of phenotypically different lymphocytes entering a single lymph node via the afferent lymph and via the blood [12–14]. In summary, a 1 g popliteal lymph node (containing at least 10^9 lymphocytes) has a cell output in efferent lymph of 3×10^7 lymphocytes/h. This relationship of lymphocyte output per g holds for all lymph nodes which have been studied and the list includes prefemoral, lumbar, renal, hepatic, mesenteric, prescapular, cervical, testicular, uterine, ovarian and others [15]. A much smaller number of lymphocytes enter via the afferent lymph, although there is some indication that this may not apply to mesenteric nodes. Typically, single afferent lymphatic vessels flow at about 1 ml/h and have a cell output of 1×10^6 cells/h. Although not usual, we have continuously collected normal afferent lymph for periods up to 3 months. In the resting state, over 90% of the cells leaving a lymph node in efferent lymph come from the post-capillary blood venules within the lymph node. These values have been recorded in relation to the blood flow (and therefore lymphocyte delivery) to lymph nodes, and it was found that one out of every four lymphocytes which enter a resting lymph node in the blood, crosses from the blood, migrates through the node and is collected in efferent lymph [16]. Collectively, this means that about 10^9 lymphocytes/h are returned to the blood via the thoracic duct (flowing at an average of 80 ml/h [17]) and another 6×10^8 lymphocytes are returned to the blood from the two prescapular and cervical vessels which drain the head, neck and shoulder regions. With a blood pool of 10^{10} lymphocytes this means that, again assuming a steady state, the turnover in the blood is 6–7 h. If some of the blood lymphocytes are not part of the recirculating pool, as more recent data suggest (A.J. Young, unpublished work), the turnover is shorter, maybe every 2–3 h! Less than 5% of the lymphocytes recovered in efferent lymph will incorporate [³H]thymidine following a short pulse *in vitro*, indicating that the overwhelming majority of lymphocytes returned to the blood via the lymphatic system are quiescent lymphocytes.

The cells found in afferent lymph are quite different from those found in efferent lymph. Although lymphocytes are unique among leucocytes in that they continuously recirculate between blood and lymph, monocytes and their derivatives have an aborted circulatory pattern through the interstitium of most tissues. Although their numbers are low, for the most part they do not pass through lymph nodes to enter efferent lymph. Recently, we have begun to use the techniques previously applied to tracking lymphocytes to monitor the movement of monocytes between blood and afferent lymph (W. Andrade, M.G. Johnston and J.B. Hay, unpublished work). It is interesting to note that a subpopulation of cells in afferent lymph is derived from Langerhans cells in the skin and other tissues, and that these cells are extremely potent antigen-presenting cells [18]. They appear to be identified within lymph nodes as dendritic cells. The percentage of B cells is much lower in afferent compared with efferent lymph [19]. Using a battery of monoclonal antibodies produced against lymphocyte surface constituents, Brandon, Mackay and colleagues from the University of Melbourne, Cahill, Kimpton and associates, and also Hein, Mackay and colleagues from Basel, have carried out exhaustive phenotypic analyses on the lymphocytes in lymph, blood and other lymphoid tissues [20–23]. As discussed in a later section, the application of these markers to studies involving the tracking of labelled cells in a variety of lymphatic vessels makes data obtained from sheep unique and so far unobtainable from any other species.

Although afferent lymph can and has been continuously and quantitatively collected from sheep, the vessels are still small. Several laboratories have capitalized on an earlier observation by Morris that, a month or so after surgical extirpation of lymph nodes, the afferent vessels re-anastomose with the remaining efferent duct. Subsequently afferent lymph (sometimes referred to as pseudoafferent) [24] can be collected by cannulating the larger and more muscular efferent duct [25]. This in itself poses interesting questions regarding the similarities and differences between the lymphatic and blood vascular systems. Because of this re-anastomosis of lymphatic vessels one might suppose that lymphatic capillaries are quite different from blood vascular capillaries. Are lymphatic endothelial cells different from blood vascular endothelial cells? A number of laboratories have grown lymphatic endothelial cells and, so far, they are indistinguishable from blood vascular endothelial cells [26–28]. They both have Factor VIII antigens, take up labelled acetylated low-density protein, bind lymphocytes *in vitro*, can be induced to bind lymphocytes more efficiently following exposure to cytokines like tumour necrosis factor α (TNF-α) and interferon γ (IFNγ) [27] and express genes responsible for the production of plasminogen activator and plasminogen activator inhibitor [28]. Some feel that endothelial cells which have been grown to confluence and passaged *in vitro* revert to a common phenotype and lose the properties associated with small vessels, or perhaps lymphatic vessels, as they exist *in situ*.

There are many studies on the immune response of single lymph nodes, the kinetics of antibody production and the role of the lymphatic system in the dissemination of immunity. These studies are beyond the scope of this paper but several reviews have been published [15,29–31]. It seems clear to us that the data support the notion that lymphocytes which have crossed into lymph nodes from the blood can only return to the blood via an intact lymphatic system. Experiments by Smith et al. [5] and Chin and Cahill [32] demonstrate this most convincingly. It is interesting that the importance of lymph nodes continues to be debated in the clinical literature. As often as not, lymph nodes are removed to stage cancer or to debulk metastatic cells found within the nodes. Removal of a few lymph nodes seems to have little consequence and does not obviously compromise the immune status. A new mutant strain of mice has recently been reported which lacks lymph nodes altogether and these animals are clearly immunodeficient [33].

Tracking labelled lymphocytes

As with any tracer-labelling procedure there are certain assumptions made about the nature of the labelled versus unlabelled constituents of an overall population. Perhaps the most important assumption is that both labelled and unlabelled populations behave the same. This situation is equally important with lymphocyte labels which have been used to track lymphocytes *in vivo*. One very important observation is that lymphocytes must be viable to recirculate. Dead or dying cells which are injected intravenously do not reach the lymph but are removed in the lungs, liver and spleen. Over the years our laboratory has standardized the recovery of labelled cells in lymph by choosing the manageable but arbitrary time of 40 h after the intravenous injection to calculate the recovery. To normalize the data for small and large lymph nodes we have divided the recovery by 1×10^9 lymphocytes collected, and expressed this as the percentage of the total injected. Obviously, if one collects lymph from a large intestinal lymphatic or the thoracic duct this recovery of labelled cells can be a large proportion of the lymphocytes injected. One must optimize the dose and conditions of labelling and take care to not use lymph collections which are greater than about 16 h old. By comparing data obtained over many years using the radiolabels ^{51}Cr and ^{111}In, and the fluorescent labels fluorescein isothiocyanate, substituted rhodamine (or lymphocytes labelled simultaneously with both of the latter dyes) [34], and more recently the PKH (Zynaxis Cell Science) membrane dyes, the combined average recovery is near 0.5% of the intravenously injected dose/10^9 cells collected per 40 h [35]. Using our earlier estimate of 70 g of lymph nodes (with a total lymphatic lymphocyte output of 2×10^9 lymphocytes/h) this means that about $2 \times 40 \times 0.5$ or 40% of the total is recoverable in lymph within 40 h. The remainder of the cells are in the spleen or other tissues, particularly the lymphoid tissue of the small intestine. The use of the PKH dyes has opened new possibilities in physiological experiments and these are discussed in a subsequent section.

When labelled lymphocytes are injected as a bolus into the venous (or arterial) blood about half of them initially disappear from the blood in approx. 2–3 h [36]. Thereafter the rate of disappearance more closely resembles an exponential decay curve. Labelled lymphocytes can be detected thereafter in the efferent lymph within the first hour. However, they typically reach their highest concentration in lymph after about 21 h [29]. What then is the average transit time for the migration from blood to lymph? Is it less than an hour, since some cells negotiated the lymph node this fast? Or is this 21 h peak a physiological entity? It is interesting that the kinetics of reappearance of labelled cells in afferent lymph are not noticeably different from the kinetics of appearance in efferent lymph [29]. The kinetics through the liver may be an exception to this [37]. The kinetic curves that have been reported for the thoracic duct of rats and mice are also similar to those of the sheep [38]. If the transit time is short (as the turnover rate in the blood would suggest) then one would expect to recover large numbers of the intravenously injected cells in the lymph nodes soon (say 3–5 h) after the injection. However, this is not observed. A few hours after injection most of the labelled cells are in the lung, liver and spleen. Does this mean that all labelled lymphocyte experiments, with a variety of labels, generate a substantial artifact simply as a consequence of handling the cells *in vitro* during the labelling procedure? Several *in vitro* tests for viability, proliferative capacity and even the capacity to incite graft-versus-host reactions *in vivo* (a property of living lymphocytes only) demonstrate that the labelled lymphocytes are functional and indistinguishable from the unlabelled population. The labelling time for PKH dyes is 2 min and the handling minimal. It is therefore with a certain degree of embarrassment that our interpretation of these seemingly simple experiments remains somewhat of an enigma. Are normal lymphocytes which are continually re-entering the venous blood via the lymphatics in the major veins in the neck physiologically detained in the large microcirculatory beds of the lung, liver and spleen, even though they do not cross out of the blood vascular space? Experiments by Pabst *et al.* [39] suggest this. In order to reach the lymph nodes via the arterial blood the probability is low as only about 1–2% of the cardiac output is delivered to lymph nodes [16].

One may ask the question whether all lymph nodes are the same? Very early studies by Yoffey showed that some lymph nodes have higher proliferation rates than others and that the proportion of lymphoblasts is therefore higher in the efferent lymph from these nodes. These tended to be mesenteric and cervical lymph nodes, presumably because they drain mucosal surfaces which are under continuous antigen bombardment. It seems very clear that lymphocytes with a rapid cell cycle (lymphoblasts) preferentially localize in the gut-associated lymphoid tissues following labelling and intravenous injection [40]. Lymphoblasts do not recirculate. When Cahill *et al.* [41] first demonstrated the non-random migration of lymphocytes to the intestinal lymph the conclusion was criticized because it was felt that the phenomenon was due to lymphoblasts [42]. However, comparable experiments were not technically feasible in mice. It was shown that this homing to intestinal lymph was a property of small T-lymphocytes and not lymphoblasts [43]. Furthermore, the preferential homing to the intestinal lymph was not seen in fetal lambs [44]. Lymphocytes recovered from older sheep, however, would home to the intestinal lymph in the fetal environment, indicating that this capacity was a property of the lymphocytes more than the lymph node [45]. It was shown by Reynolds *et al.* [46] that cells harvested from lymph nodes of sheep did not show this migratory bias.

There is little question that lymphocytes recirculate in a non-random fashion. The unequal proportions of various lymphocytes [e.g. memory versus naive; TCR1 (T-cell receptor 1) versus TCR2 (T-cell receptor 2) lymphocytes; T- versus B-lymphocytes] in various lymph and blood compartments suggests this (recognizing that these are recirculating cells and assuming that the phenotypic profile is stable). However, our recent data suggest that the intestinal homing population may be fairly small and that the non-random pattern may only be evident for about 10 days [47]. This observation could be explained by differences in lifespan of subpopulations of lymphocytes or by changes in their phenotypic profile with time.

The battery of newly defined molecules called vascular addressins and different selectins (demonstrable on the surface of lymphocytes and/or vascular endothelial cells) may eventually explain these patterns but the picture is not clear at present [48–51]. For example, the peripheral lymph node homing receptor (L-selectin or MEL 14) is quite prominent on cells recovered from intestinal lymph as well as from peripheral lymph [47]. In fact it is also expressed on neutrophils [50]. The hypothesis that B1 integrin-positive lymphocytes preferentially home to the skin while B7 integrin-positive lymphocytes home to the intestine is also not absolute [47]. These controversies underlie the need to study the relevance of the newly defined molecules in a physiological context rather than only in binding reactions *in vitro*. Nevertheless, it seems that we are closer than ever before to selectively regulating the recirculation of lymphocytes both experimentally and clinically [52].

Traffic through non-lymphoid tissues

This topic is possibly more relevant to pathology than to physiology but some of the observations enhance our knowledge regarding the recirculatory capacity of lymphocytes. The very fact that lymphocytes are continuously migrating through nearly all tissues and can be recovered in afferent lymph illustrates that lymphocyte migration is not just facilitated by lymph nodes. The second fundamental feature is that lymphocyte traffic sites can be induced virtually anywhere and that the local traffic can equal that through lymph nodes. A few examples illustrate this. The blood to afferent lymph migration of lymphocytes through a rejecting renal allograft in sheep is spectacular. During the 8 or so days to rejection as much as 50 g wet weight of cells can be recovered in this lymph. This is approximately 100 times that which can be collected from normal afferent renal lymph. Although some of these cells are the result of replication within the kidney, a high proportion are migrating as has been shown by tracking labelled cells [53]. Another example is a delayed hypersensitivity lesion in the skin, bowel or joint synovium [36]. Chronic granulomatous lesions induced by the injection of Freund's adjuvant also induce local lymphocyte traffic sites [54]. What then is the mechanism of creation of a lymphocyte traffic site? We approached this problem by screening a variety of potential mediator molecules. These included: C5a desarg of the complement system, prostaglandins, interleukin (IL)-1, IL-2, IL-6, IL-8 and bacterial peptides like formylmethionyl-leucyl-phenylalanine. To assay for the induction of a lymphocyte traffic site, we used a well-characterized, quantitative lymphocyte localization assay consisting of a 3 h intravenous pulse of ^{111}In-labelled lymphocytes [55]. All of the potential mediators listed above were negative at all times and doses tested. It was not until TNF-α and IFNγ were tested that significant numbers of lymphocytes extravasated into the injection site. The maximal accumulation occurred about 12 h after injection. Since these are both molecules which are produced in delayed hypersensitivity reactions, they must be considered potentially relevant mediators. Secondly, both of these molecules can enhance the binding of lymphocytes to blood vascular endothelial cells grown *in vitro* and can upregulate the appearance of adhesion molecules on the surface of these endothelial cells [56]. In our search to identify potential mediators in the lymph-draining delayed hypersensitivity reactions, we were unable to find TNF-α and, at present, we postulate that IFNγ may be more relevant (A.J. Young, B. Au, L.S. O'Hara, W. Phillipson, A. Kalaaji, L. Tam and J.B. Hay, unpublished work).

Tracking lymphocytes long-term and the determination of cellular turnover and lifespan

Some experiments involving the tracking of lymphocytes have been carried out using nuclear labels [57]. In some cases quantitative autoradiography was used to monitor the labelled cells [58]. The more commonly used labels have been those which bind to proteins within the lymphocytes or on the cell surface. Since proteins are continually turning over, it takes only a few days *in vivo* until the labelled cells are not easily detectable. Nearly all of the lymphocyte tracking experiments described so far have involved protocols which, in general, do not exceed 4–5 days.

Two relatively recent developments now make possible a range of experiments which were impossible a few years ago. The first is the introduction of lipophilic membrane linker compounds to which fluorescent or other labels can be attached. The turnover of plasma membranes is less rapid than the turnover of most proteins. This now allows the experimentalist to track lymphocytes for weeks and even months [35,47,59]. The second technology greatly improves the data analysis and removes the labour intensive assays such as quantitative autoradiography. Flow cytometry, with contemporary multi-parameter data aquisition and storage combined with computer-assisted analysis, enables the processing of large numbers of samples and the rapid and reproducible assessment of the proportion of labelled cells, even when the proportion of labelled cells is low. When these two techniques are combined and optimized by using two-or-more-colour fluorescence and cell sampling numbers of 10^4–10^6 per sample, combined with the capacity to simultaneously monitor several blood, lymph and tissue compartments in the same sheep, the 'art of the possible' reaches new heights. Recent experiments performed by Young have involved the analysis of several hundred such samples taken continuously over 2–3 months following the bolus injection of 2×10^9 PKH 26-labelled lymphocytes into an individual sheep. The sheep hosted a variety of lymphatic and blood sampling catheters and many of the compartments were analysed with samples collected simultaneously. The single most important experiment, to our minds, that is now possible involves the measurement of lymphocyte turnover and lifespan.

The lifespan of any cell type *in vivo* is a highly relevant parameter, and absolutely fundamental to an understanding of biology. The area, however, is fraught with misunderstandings in terminology and methodology. For example, some use the term 'lifespan' to be a measure of the life of a cell between cell divisions. This, of course, is a perfectly valid definition. The turnover rate of cells *in vivo* is sometimes related, but the meaning is different in different biological systems. We have begun by asking, "How long does it take for the recirculating lymphocytes to be completely replaced?" We have used erythrocytes as a standard to which we compare our data. The question of lymphocyte lifespan has been with immunology for many years. There has been discussion of short-lived versus long-lived lymphocytes. Immunological memory is a hallmark of the acquired immune response and since memory is clearly carried by recirculating lymphocytes, and as immunological memory is long-lasting, perhaps the recirculating lymphocytes are long-lasting as well, although more recent experiments claim that memory is related to long-term retention of antigen instead [60].

The experimental data on lifespan are presently being prepared for publication elsewhere (A.J. Young and J.B. Hay, unpublished work). We have found that erythrocytes turn over completely every 150 days and that one-half of the recirculating lymphocytes turnover completely every 15 days. Furthermore, using the PKH dyes and by monitoring the time taken for the fluorescence intensity to halve (by flow cytometry) we found that the intensity of erythrocytes does not diminish over periods of several weeks. The lymphocyte intensity does diminish and this could be the direct consequence of cell division. Therefore, we hope to be in a position to comment on the 'lifespan' of lymphocytes as well. Of course it is well established that lymphocytes are composed of many subpopulations and that they are stimulated to proliferate in immune reactions. Comparisons of turnover and lifespan are now feasible in this array of cells as well as in many other cellular systems. Basic, physiological questions pertaining to lymphocyte migration can continue to be asked and tested with quantitative methods in the intact animal.

References

1. Gowans, J.L. (1957) *Br. J. Exp. Pathol.* **38**, 67–78
2. Borgs, P. (1993) Ph.D. Thesis, Australian National University, Canberra
3. Hay, J.B., Murphy, M.J., Morris, B. and Bessis, M.C. (1972) *Am J. Pathol.* **66**, 1–25
4. Gowans, J.L. (1959) *J. Physiol. (London)* **146**, 54–69
5. Smith, J.B., Cunningham, A.J., Lafferty, K.J. and Morris, B. (1970) *Aust. J. Biol. Med. Sci.* **48**, 57–70
6. Mackay, C.R., Marston, W.L. and Dudler, L. (1990) *J. Exp. Med.* **171**, 801–817

7. Bollman, J.L., Cain, J.C. and Grindlay, J.H. (1948) *J. Lab. Clin. Med.* **38**, 1349–1352
8. Sprent, J. (1973) *Cell. Immunol.* **7**, 10–39
9. Hall, J.G. and Morris, B. (1963) *Q. J. Exp. Physiol.* **48**, 235–247
10. Hall, J.G. and Morris, B. (1965) *J. Exp. Med.* **121**, 901–910
11. Hall, J.G. and Morris, B. (1962) *Q. J. Exp. Physiol.* **47**, 360–369
12. Mackay, C.R., Kimpton, W.G., Brandon, M.R. and Cahill, R.N.P. (1988) *J. Exp. Med.* **167**, 1755–1765
13. Washington, E.A., Kimpton, W.G. and Cahill, R.N.P. (1988) *Eur. J. Immunol.* **18**, 2093–2096
14. Kimpton, W.G., Washington, E.A. and Cahill, R.N.P. (1988) *Immunology* **66**, 69–75
15. Trnka, Z. and Morris, B. (1985) in *Immunology of the Sheep* (Morris, B. and Miyasaka, M., eds.), pp. 1–18, Editiones Roche, Basle
16. Hay, J.B. and Hobbs, B.B. (1977) *J. Exp. Med.* **145**, 31–44
17. Abernethy, N.J., Chin, W., Hay, J.B., Rodela, H., Oreopoulos, D. and Johnston, M.G. (1991) *Am. J. Physiol.* **260**, 353–358
18. Kelly, R.H., Balfour, B.M., Armstrong, J.A. and Griffiths, S. (1978) *Anat. Rec.* **190**, 5–22
19. Miller, H.R.P. and Adams, E.A. (1977) *Am. J. Pathol.* **87**, 59–80
20. Maddox, J.F., Mackay, C.R. and Brandon, M.R. (1985) *Immunology* **55**, 739–748
21. Mackay, C.R., Maddox, J.F. and Brandon, M.R. (1986) *Eur. J. Immunol.* **16**, 19–25
22. Ezaki, T., Miyasaka, M., Beya, M.-F., Dudler, L. and Trnka, Z. (1987) *Int. Arch. Allergy Appl. Immunol.* **82**, 168–177
23. Hein, W.R. and Mackay, C.R. (1991) *Immunol. Today* **12**, 30–34
24. Hopkins, J., Dutia, B.M., Bujdoso, R. and McConnell, I. (1989) *J. Exp. Med.* **170**, 1303–1318
25. Dandie, G.W., Watkins, F.Y., Ragg, S.J., Holloway, P.E. and Muller, H.K. (1994) *Immunol. Cell Biol.* **72**, 79–86
26. Johnston, M.G. and Walker, M.A. (1984) *In Vitro* **20**, 566–571
27. Borron, P. and Hay, J.B. (1994) *Lymphology* **27**, 6–13
28. Pepper, M.S., Wasi, S., Ferrara, N., Orci, L. and Montesano, R. (1994) *Exp. Cell Res.* **210**, 298–305
29. Chin, G.W., Pearson, L.D. and Hay, J.B. (1985) *Experimental Biology of the Lymphatic Circulation* (Johnston, M.G., ed.), Elsevier, Amsterdam
30. Miyasaka, M. and Trnka, Z. (1986) *Immunol. Rev.* **91**, 87–114
31. Abernethy, N.J. and Hay, J.B. (1992) *Lymphology* **25**, 1–30
32. Chin, G.W. and Cahill, R.N.P. (1984) *Immunology* **52**, 341–347
33. Miyawaki, S., Nakamura, Y., Suzuka, H., Koba, M., Yasumizu, R., Ikehara, S. and Shibata, Y. (1994) *Eur. J. Immunol.* **24**, 429–434
34. Abernethy, N.J., Chin, G.W., Lyons, H. and Hay, J.B. (1985) *Cytometry* **6**, 407–413
35. Teare, G.F., Horan, P.K., Slezak, S.E., Smith, C. and Hay, J.B. (1991) *Cell. Immunol.* **134**, 157–170
36. Teare, G.F. (1990) M.Sc. Thesis, Department of Immunology, University of Toronto, Toronto
37. Young, A.J., Hare, G.T. and Hay, J.B. (1994) *Hepatology* **19**, 758–763
38. Hay, J.B. and Cahill, R.N.P. (1982) *Animal Models of Immunological Processes* (Hay, J.B., ed.), p. 97, Academic Press, London
39. Pabst, R., Binns, R.M., Licence, S.T. and Peter, M. (1987) *Am. Rev. Respir. Dis.* **136**, 1213–1218
40. Guy-Grand, D., Griscelli, C. and Vassalli, P. (1974) *Eur. J. Immunol.* **4**, 435–443
41. Cahill, R.N.P., Poskitt, D.C., Frost, H. and Trnka, Z. (1977) *J. Exp. Med.* **145**, 420–428
42. Freitas, A.A., Rose, M.L. and Parrott, D.V.M. (1977) *Nature (London)* **270**, 731–733
43. Chin, W. and Hay, J.B. (1980) *Gastroenterology* **79**, 1231–1242
44. Cahill, R.N.P., Poskitt, D.C., Hay, J.B., Heron, I. and Trnka, Z. (1979) *Eur. J. Immunol.* **9**, 251
45. Kimpton, W.G. and Cahill, R.N.P. (1985) in *Immunology of the Sheep* (Morris, B. and Miyasaka, M., eds.), pp. 306–326, Editiones Roche, Basle
46. Reynolds, J.D., Heron, I., Dudler, L. and Trnka, Z. (1982) *Immunology* **47**, 415–421
47. Young, A.J. (1994) Ph.D. Thesis, Department of Immunology, University of Toronto, Toronto
48. Duijvestijn, A. and Hamann, A. (1989) *Immunol. Today* **10**, 23–28
49. Stoolman, L.M. (1989) *Cell* **56**, 907–910
50. Berg, E.L., Goldstein, I.A., Jutila, M.A., Nakache, M., Picker, L.J., Streeter, P.R., Wu, N.W., Zhou, D. and Butcher, E.C. (1989) *Immunol. Rev.* **18**, 5–18
51. Hynes, R.O. (1987) *Cell* **48**, 549–554
52. Issekutz, T.B. and Stoltz, J.M. (1989) *Cell. Immunol.* **120**, 165–173
53. Pedersen, N.C. and Morris, B. (1974) *Transplantation* **17**, 48–56
54. Issekutz, T.B., Chin, W. and Hay, J.B. (1980) *Cell. Immunol.* **54**, 79–86
55. Borgs, P. and Hay, J.B. (1986) *J. Leukocyte Biol.* **39**, 333–342
56. Abernethy, N.J. and Hay, J.B. (1989) *Int. Immunol.* **1**, 414–423
57. Freitas, A.A. and Rocha, B.B. (1993) *Immunol. Today* **14**, 25–29
58. Michie, C.A., Mclean, A., Alcock, C. and Beverley, P.C.C. (1992) *Nature (London)* **360**, 264–265
59. Horan, P.K. and Slezak, S.E. (1990) *Nature (London)* **340**, 167–169
60. Gray, D. and Matszinger, P. (1991) *J. Exp. Med.* **174**, 969–974

18

Integration of capillary, interstitial and lymphatic function

E.M. Renkin* and V.L. Tucker

Department of Human Physiology, University of California, Davis, CA 95616, U.S.A.

Introduction

As an introduction to the chapters that follow, we present an overview of the contributions of capillaries, interstitium and lymphatics to extracellular fluid homoeostasis. Figure 1 illustrates the daily circulation of extracellular fluid in the human body. Fluid (plasma ultrafiltrate) and plasma protein flow from the vascular system through the interstitial compartments of the body's organs and tissues to the lymphatic system and back again to the bloodstream. Each compartment and flow path in the diagram represents the contributions of many organs and tissues, and 'plasma protein' represents a multiplicity of components.

A large amount of 'plasma' protein resides outside the vascular compartment, more than half by even the most conservative estimate. The fluid volume turnover (including the volume reabsorbed in the lymph nodes) normally approaches two-thirds of the entire interstitial fluid volume every 24 h. Plasma protein turnover in the same time is roughly equal to the entire amount of protein in the plasma. In the steady state, extravasation of fluid and protein is balanced by lymph drainage and return to the vascular system. Thus plasma and interstitial fluid volumes and protein contents are maintained in constant proportion. Because of the magnitude of these exchanges, even brief departures from steady-state conditions can lead to large displacements of fluid and protein. Normal homoeostasis is maintained by action of both passive forces ('Starling forces') and active processes (local and extrinsic mechanisms involving cellular signal transduction, conduction and implementation).

Regional extracellular fluid distribution

Figure 2 is a bar graph showing the proportions of plasma (P), interstitial fluid (ISF), intracellular water (ICW) and dry solids in several rat tissues. Each ISF pool is divided into two compartments, one of which is accessible to plasma albumin ('free' ISF) and one which excludes albumin but allows entry of water and small ions and molecules, such as those used to measure extracellular fluid (ECF) volume. The data shown in the Figure were obtained by Helge Wiig in our laboratory using ^{131}I-albumin to measure plasma volume, ^{51}Cr-EDTA to measure ECF volume, ^{125}I-albumin equilibrated for more than 3 days to measure albumin distribution volume and desiccation to measure total tissue

*To whom correspondence should be addressed.

Figure I

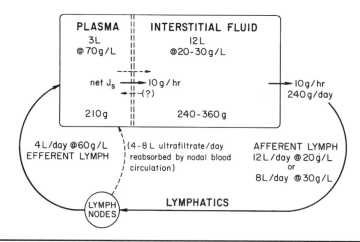

Diagram illustrating the recirculation of fluid and plasma protein from plasma to interstitium to lymph and back to plasma via the lymphatics

The figures are estimates for a 65 kg human, based largely on previous summaries by Courtice [1], Landis and Pappenheimer [2] and Mayerson [3] and modified by the recent demonstration by Adair et al. [4] of substantial reabsorption of protein-free fluid from lymph in the lymph nodes. Reproduced from [5] with permission.

water [6]. Extravascular albumin distribution volume (VA) was calculated at steady-state ISF albumin concentration ([ISF]/[P]=0.6–0.8). In all tissues shown, VA was significantly less than the distribution volume of ^{51}Cr-EDTA ([ISF]/[P]=1).

The Figure shows that there are large differences in relative volumes of ISF (ISFV) in the different tissues. ISFV is smaller in skeletal muscle than in skin and tendon, which have a much lower cell content. The proportion of ISFV which excludes albumin and other plasma proteins is less variable: in these tissues it depends largely on the collagen content of the interstitial matrix, and to a lesser extent on its content of glycosaminoglycans [7,8]. On a comparative basis, lymph flow and total protein turnover appear to be proportional to ISFV in these tissues, rather than to total tissue mass or water content. Lymph flow and protein flux in skin are 4–5 times lymph flow and protein flux in skeletal muscle [9,10].

Partition of ECF volume (ECFV) between plasma and ISF volumes depends on factors acting in each organ or tissue: (1) at the microvascular level to control fluid and protein exchange across the walls of capillaries and non-muscular venules; (2) on components of interstitial compartment matrices which determine interstitial compliance, exclusion and possibly also resistance to fluid and protein transit; and (3) on the lymphatic system to control the rate of lymphatic return to the vascular system [11]. Our presentation is concerned with the homoeostatic, physiological controls acting through passive and active mechanisms.

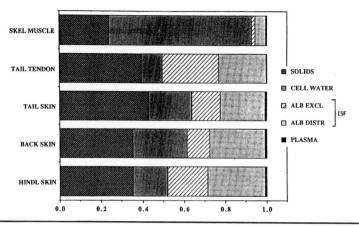

Figure 2

Solids and fluid volumes in selected tissues of rats
Interstitial fluid is partitioned into albumin-accessible and albumin-excluding fractions. Data from [6].

Control of transcapillary fluid and protein exchange

Passive controls ('safety factors')
The basic principle governing fluid movement across exchange vessel walls is Starling's Hypothesis, which delineates the balance of hydrostatic forces (Δp) against colloid osmotic forces ($\Delta \Pi$). A modern mathematical expression of this balance is as follows [12]:

$$J_v = L_p S \left[(p_c - p_i) - \sigma (\Pi_c - \Pi_i) \right] \tag{1}$$

where J_v represents the net rate of fluid (volume) flow out of a microvessel or microvascular network into its interstitial pool, L_p the hydraulic conductivity of the microvessel wall and S its surface area. p_c is the hydrostatic pressure within the vessel, or the average pressure in a network of vessels, p_i the ISF pressure outside. The Greek letters Π_c and Π_i represent plasma and ISF colloid osmotic pressures and σ (sigma) is a solute reflection coefficient, which is a function of the permeability of microvascular walls to the macromolecular solutes responsible for the Πs ($\sigma = 1$ means completely impermeable; $\sigma = 0$ means freely permeable).

Microvascular hydrostatic pressure (p_c) depends on the relative values of upstream and downstream resistances. Arteriolar vasodilation tends to increase p_c, arteriolar vasoconstriction to lower it. There is substantial evidence that exchange-vessel pressures are regulated by local, intrinsic microcirculatory ('stretch') responses to intraluminal pressure changes. This stabilized pressure is subject to further modulation by extrinsic control mechanisms. ISF pressure (p_i) is a non-linear function of ISFV, subatmospheric at low to normal volumes, rising to values slightly above atmospheric with expansion. Π_c depends on plasma concentrations of the various plasma proteins; the relatively small plasma proteins like albumin (68 kDa) make greater contributions than the larger molecules. The relationship between Π and protein concentration is non-linear (self-augmenting) and is usually described by a power series in which the coefficients depend on the ratio of low-molecular-mass components to high-molecular-mass ones [13].

Steady-state Π_i depends on the relative rates of fluid and protein extravasation, i.e. on the ratio J_s/J_v, where J_s is the net outward plasma protein flux, since this ratio determines the protein concentration of the net filtrate. Transiently, ISF protein concentrations and Π_i can deviate from steady-state values, as more concentrated or more dilute filtrate mixes with and displaces previously formed ISF into the lymphatics. In peripheral tissues (skin and muscle, which make up the bulk of body mass) such transients may be of very long duration, i.e. half-time 12–24 h [8].

As a consequence of this relationship, the rate of extravasation of plasma proteins, particularly of albumin, is an important determinant of the partition of ECF between plasma and interstitial compartments. J_s for a macromolecular solute is dependent on J_v and on the product of exchange-vessel permeability to that solute (P) and surface area (S). The simplified formula below illustrates the contributions of convection (bulk flow), diffusion and dissipative transport by vesicular exchange to the total solute transport:

$$J_s = J_v(1-\sigma)C_p + PS(C_p' - C_i) + \alpha Q_v(C_p - C_i) \qquad (2)$$

C_p is the plasma concentration of the protein and C_i its ISF concentration. C_p' is a function of C_p, equal to C_p at low J_v, but decreasing as J_v becomes larger, and approaching C_i as J_v increases without limit. The first term on the right of the equals sign represents convective transport, proportional to fluid flow; the factor $(1-\sigma)$ is often called the solvent drag coefficient. The second term is diffusive transport, which according to Fick's law is proportional to the mean concentration difference across the membrane. The third term represents vesicular exchange, which also depends on concentration differences. Its form is similar to the second: P is replaced by the vesicular volume turnover rate per unit surface area (Q_v), multiplied by a partition coefficient (α) between vesicular contents and free fluid. Eqn. (2) shows the three potential transport mechanisms and identifies their driving forces, but it does not express the interaction of convection and diffusion which is responsible for the variation of C_p' with J_v. The more complex formulation below incorporates this relation:

$$J_s = J_v(1-\sigma)[(C_p - C_i e^{-Pe})/(1 - e^{-Pe})] + \alpha Q_v(C_p - C_i) \qquad (3)$$

Pe is a modified Peclet number expressing the ratio of convective to diffusive velocities; $Pe = J_v(1-\sigma)/PS$ [14,15]. Eqn. (3) is valid for membranes in which diffusion and convection take place through channels which all have the same width (radius) and reflection coefficient. Microvascular endothelium behaves as if it has channels of at least two distinct sizes with markedly different σ values: the so-called small-pores and large-pores pathways. For such membranes, it is necessary to apply the first two terms of the equation separately to both pathways independently, and to combine their contributions to J_s and J_v. An important consequence for heteroporous membranes is that basal (steady state; no volume change) convective leakage of protein becomes proportional to $(\Pi_c - \Pi_i)$, and may be mistaken for a purely diffusive flux [16].

Eqns. (2) and (3) predict that for constant σ, PS and αQ_v, the ratio of J_s to J_v, and thus the ratios C_i/C_p and Π_i/Π_p, will decrease as J_v increases. Consequently the difference between Π_p and Π_i will increase, and through eqn. (1) will act as a restoring force ('safety factor') tending to reduce J_v. Another passive safety factor is the rise in ISF pressure as ISFV is increased. This decreases the transcapillary hydrostatic pressure difference and increases the driving force for lymph flow out of the interstitium [11,17]. The passive homoeostatic mechanisms are effective against small disturbances of microvascular fluid balance, particularly against declining J_v [12]. However, the restoring forces are non-linearly related to J_v, and become less effective as increases in J_v become large [11,18]. To prevent large, uncontrolled deviations of fluid flows and plasma and interstitial volumes, active responsive regulatory mechanisms are required.

Active (reflex) control mechanisms

The actions of the passive mechanisms sketched out above on transcapillary fluxes of fluid and macromolecular solutes and on plasma and ISF volumes have been developed extensively in the past few years, and we shall not expound them further here (see the recent review of Aukland and Reed [11], and Chapter 11 by Guyton in this volume). What we are interested in now are the actions of physiological regulatory mechanisms (local and extrinsic; cellular, nervous and hormonal) which contribute responsively to control of ECF partition and distribution. Since these mechanisms must necessarily operate by way of these passive principles, we must keep them in mind at all times.

(i) Active mechanisms controlling microvascular pressures

There is abundant evidence that hydrostatic pressures in exchange vessels (capillaries and post-capillary venules) in many tissues and organs are kept within narrow limits as arterial pressure is varied over a wide range. Stabilization of exchange-vessel pressures against changes in arterial pressure appears to be one of the functions of myogenic autoregulation [19–23]. Figure 3 shows one example of autoregulatory control in isolated perfused skeletal muscle. Capillary pressures in both resting and contracting muscle are stabilized against experimentally induced changes in arterial perfusion pressure by locally induced changes in arteriolar and venular smooth muscle. Intrinsic control of pre- and post-capillary resistance (R_A and R_V respectively) diminishes the rise of capillary pressure with metabolic vasodilation and the fall with nervous vasoconstriction. However, following blood loss, increased sympathetic vasoconstrictor nerve activity decreases exchange-vessel pressures and promotes reabsorption of fluid [25,26]. Autoregulation of capillary pressure appears to be suppressed by the action of circulating adrenaline (epinephrine) on β-2 receptors in arteriolar smooth muscle [27]. The full extent of such control mechanisms has not been fully explored, particularly with respect to plasma volume regulation, and deserves further study.

Figure 3

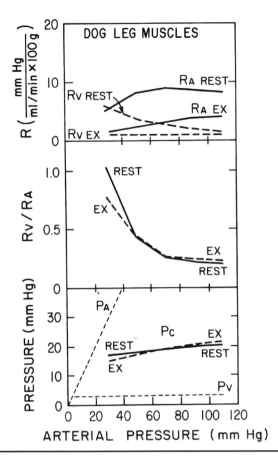

Autoregulatory stabilization of capillary pressure (P_C) against experimentally induced changes in arterial perfusion pressure (PA) by changes in precapillary (R_A) and post-capillary (R_V) resistances in resting and contracting (EX) skeletal muscle

P_C calculated from the data of Thulesius and Johnson [24]. Reproduced from [19] with permission.

(ii) Active mechanisms controlling microvascular permeability and surface area

Permeability and surface area are considered together here, first because it is not always feasible to separate them on the basis of available information, and secondly because these two parameters appear as products (PS or L_pS) in transport equations, and are thus functionally connected. In the example of microvascular pressure control described above (haemorrhagic hypotension), β-adrenergic vasodilation is believed also to increase functional exchange-vessel surface area and thus to augment fluid reabsorption [28]; however, the experimental evidence for this is a measured increase in the capillary filtration coefficient, L_pS, per unit tissue mass, and might just as well be ascribed to an increase in L_p (hydraulic conductivity — permeability to filtrate) as to an increase in surface area (S).

Blood volume expansion with whole blood, plasma or colloid volume expanders is known to increase protein extravasation into many tissues [29,30] more than can be accounted for by passive safety factors [31]. On the other hand, volume contraction (dehydration, haemorrhage) has been reported to decrease protein leakage [32]. Reduction of plasma protein content by plasmapheresis has also been reported to reduce permeability to plasma proteins [33]. These responses tend to restore plasma volume by altering the partition of ECF protein between plasma and ISF [eqns. (2) and (3)], and thus the difference between Π_c and Π_i [eqn. (1)].

Figure 4 shows some of our own measurements of tracer-albumin uptake (expressed as plasma clearance of albumin $J_{s,alb}/C_{p,alb}$) of several tissues in control and in colloid volume-expanded rats [31]. Blood volume was increased by 50%, causing central venous pressure to rise initially by 5 mmHg, falling back to control levels as fluid was redistributed. The increases in V_A were larger in the visceral organs than in skin or skeletal muscles, and were not correlated with any gains in water content. Passive elevation of peripheral exchange-vessel pressures by venous congestion [34], or diminution of plasma colloid osmotic pressure by infusion of saline [35], does not increase albumin clearances to this extent, and the small increases observed under these conditions are closely coupled to transcapillary fluid movement. On the basis of these observations, we concluded that the increase in albumin transport is dissipative, due to increased diffusion (increased PS) and/or increased vesicular transport (increased αQ_v), rather than convective transport.

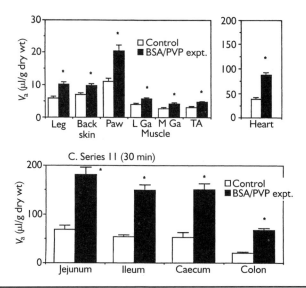

Figure 4

Influence of plasma volume expansion with colloids [iso-oncotic BSA or polyvinylpyrrolidone (PVP)] on tracer-albumin uptake (V_a)

V_a = 30 min extravascular distribution volume of albumin at plasma concentration. *P < 0.05, significantly different from control. Abbreviations used: LGa, lateral gastrocnemius; MGa, medial gastrocnemius; TA, tibialis anterior. Reproduced from [31] with permission.

The increases in albumin extravasation are brought about by a systemic, homoeostatic response to the volume expansion, and appear to be due largely to increased endothelial permeability to large molecules, with possibly some increase in exchange-vessel surface area. There is abundant evidence that atrial natriuretic peptide (ANP), a hormone of cardiac origin, is the controlling factor.

Atrial stretch produced by volume expansion or after impairment of cardiac function is a potent stimulus for ANP release [36]. Furthermore, elevated plasma ANP levels following plasma volume loading have been repeatedly documented (e.g. [37,38]). When we infused graded doses of synthetic ANP intravenously in anaesthetized rats that were given lactate–Ringer containing 2% albumin to keep plasma volume and plasma protein concentration from decreasing, albumin clearances into small and large intestine, fat, kidney and skeletal muscle were increased 1.5–4.6-fold. At plasma levels of ANP within the range reported for plasma volume expansion or congestive heart failure, observed increases in albumin clearance were similar in tissue distribution and magnitude to those observed during colloid volume expansion (Figure 5) [39].

As further proof of the ability of ANP to increase albumin clearance independently of the rise in central venous pressure or any other consequence of volume expansion, we tested the effects of interfering with the release of ANP by atrial appendectomy [40]. Figure 6 shows the results of this procedure. The initial increase in central

Figure 5

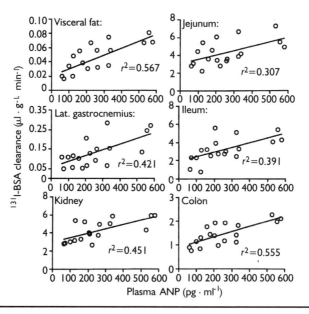

Infusion of exogenous ANP in anaesthetized rats

Tracer-albumin clearances in selected tissues and organs are plotted in relation to plasma ANP concentrations. Each point represents one animal; controls and low- and high-infusion-rate experiments are plotted together. Least-squares slopes (solid lines) are significantly different from zero for all tissues shown. For skin and lungs, no significant correlation was observed. Reproduced from [39] with permission.

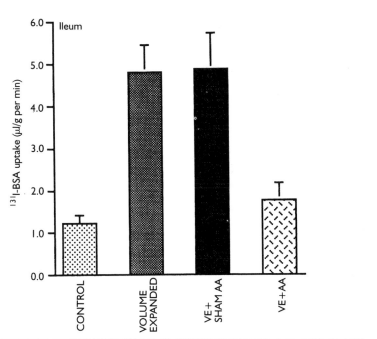

Figure 6

Influence of atrial appendectomy on the response of albumin transport in the rat ileum to colloid volume expansion
Abbreviations: VE, volume expansion (3% body wt. iso-oncotic BSA); AA, atrial appendectomy (V.L. Tucker, unpublished work).

venous pressure (CVP) was the same (5 mmHg) for volume-expanded controls, sham-operated controls and atrial-appendectomized (AA) animals, but in the AA rats, the fall in CVP after expansion was greatly retarded. Plasma ANP concentration rose only slightly in the AA rats, and albumin clearances did not rise significantly above control values.

Whether the atrial stretch–ANP reflex is responsible for the decreases in albumin clearance which have been reported in plasma volume contraction and after reduction of plasma protein concentration is not clear. Compared with the plasma levels reached after expansion, baseline ANP concentrations are relatively small, and, if the relationship of clearances to concentration are linear, they do not appear to allow much scope for albumin transport reduction. Plasma ANP levels are decreased after haemorrhage [41,42], but plasma vasopressin (known to contribute to the regulation of extracellular volume by the kidney) is elevated [43] and may contribute to the control of ECF partition between plasma and ISF. Angiotensin II and adrenaline are also candidate transport-regulating hormones [44]. Further investigation of plasma volume contraction and of the actions of these substances on transcapillary exchange is called for. A technical problem is that baseline plasma protein clearances are low, and thus reductions may be harder to demonstrate than increases.

Control of interstitial fluid volume and protein content

Passive mechanisms

(i) The increase of ISF pressure with increasing ISFV provides for passive feedback control of local ISFVs. Under normal conditions (baseline V_i) in most tissues and organs, P_i is slightly subatmospheric, and is close to the 'turning point' of the P_i/V_i curve [11,45]. When V_i decreases, P_i falls steeply, producing a strong opposing force to further reduction of V_i. However, when V_i increases more than a few percent above baseline, and P_i has reached atmospheric pressure, the slope of the P_i/V_i curve is greatly reduced, and further increase of P_i is limited.

(ii) The inverse relationship of capillary filtrate protein concentration (and thus Π_i) with filtration rate described by eqns. (2) and (3) above provides a more substantial degree of protection against increases in ISFV. The ratio of filtrate to plasma protein concentration decreases with increasing filtration rate, thereby increasing the difference between Π_c and Π_i, and increasing the colloid osmotic force opposing movement of fluid from plasma to interstitium and lymph [46]. The opposing force depends on both PS and σ and on the rate of fluid shift rather than on the increase in V_i itself. As filtration rate increases and the filtrate/plasma protein concentration ratio approaches its limit of $1 - \sigma$, the colloid osmotic restraining force reaches a maximum (normally approx. 20–25 mmHg) and can provide no further protection against greater increases in hydrostatic driving force. Decreasing PS, particularly at low to moderate rates of filtration, and increasing σ can increase the feedback to some extent, but cannot increase the maximum opposing force above Π_p.

(iii) It has been suggested that changes in the fraction of interstitial volume which excludes plasma proteins, and only allows entry and passage of water and small solutes, may contribute to regulation of ISFVs [11,47]. Variation of exclusion volume does not change steady-state ISF protein concentrations or colloid osmotic pressures, which depend on rates of trans-endothelial fluid flow and solute fluxes determined according to eqns. (2) and (3) above. However, increased exclusion promotes washout of plasma proteins from tissue interstitia, and return of proteins to the blood circulation.

Another effect of macromolecular exclusion is the creation of an osmotic barrier between protein-accessible and protein-excluding regions. This barrier causes the volume of the protein-excluding region to decrease as the protein concentration (and colloid osmotic pressure) of the 'free' ISF increases. The flowpaths for proteins through the interstitial compartment from plasma to lymph are limited to the free ISF, and do not include the bundles of collagen fibres, which may nevertheless serve as pathways for transit of water and small ions and molecules [48] (see also Chapter 8 by Bert and Martinez, and Chapter 9 by Taylor in this volume). Changes in the extent of the free fluid pathways may result in a kind of autoregulation of interstitial resistance to fluid flow: as the protein concentration of ISF rises, the volume available to protein distribution and transit increases, due to osmotic shrinkage of the protein-excluding regions (Figure 7).

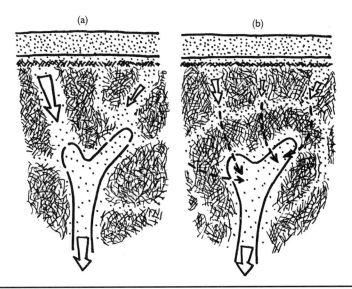

Figure 7

Model diagrams showing alternative interstitial flow-paths for fluid and proteins to illustrate the influence of exclusion and restriction in the interstitial fibre matrix on interstitial transport and distribution of plasma protein and protein-free fluid

(a) Free-fluid pathways from exchange vessel to lymphatic. (b) Restrictive pathways through the matrix. The cross-hatched areas represent fibre matrix or gel phase, the stippled areas free fluid. The stippled band at the top of each diagram represents a capillary, the Y-shaped object below a lymphatic. The density of stippling is supposed to represent protein concentration. In (a), contraction of gel-phase volume by increased colloid osmotic pressure of the free fluid would increase the width of free-fluid channels and decrease resistance to lymph flow. In (b), contraction of the gel phase would increase resistance to fluid and protein transit. Reproduced from [56] with permission.

Active mechanisms

The extent to which hormonal or other cell-mediated control mechanisms actively contribute to interstitial volume control by modulating interstitial compliance or molecular exclusion is not known. Clearly, there are great possibilities for homoeostatic control of these characteristics in the formation, destruction and replacement of interstitial matrix components by the cellular elements of the interstitium. However, although much has been learned about pathological alterations of interstitial matrices [49–52] (see also Chapter 7 by Reed in this volume), little has been done to elucidate normal homoeostatic controls. The recent studies of hyaluronan distribution and its removal by lymph conducted by Laurent, Reed and others hold promise of future development of our knowledge of such controls [11,53,54] (see also Chapter 1 by Laurent and Chapter 7 by Reed in this volume).

Lymph flow and the return of ISF and protein to plasma

The final process which operates to control ISF and plasma volumes is the transport of fluid and plasma proteins from the interstitial compartment to the plasma. Figure 7 illustrates alternative configurations of fluid and protein flowpaths within the interstitial compartment. Both passive and active mechanisms contribute to the return of lymph [3,55].

Passive mechanisms
These include elastic recoil of matrix fibres and surrounding structures, movement of structures within the interstitium (e.g. muscular contractions, arterial pulsations) and along the course of the valved conducting lymphatics (respiratory movements, limb movements) [57,58]. Expansion of the interstitial compartment may also facilitate entry of fluid into terminal lymphatics by widening the intercellular junctions [59,60]. Lymph drainage from skin and skeletal muscles is more consistently related to ISFV than to ISF pressure [11]. Thus lymph flow is a strong volume-regulating mechanism at high filtration rates and high ISFVs, when other passive safety factors have reached their limits. Not only is excess fluid removed from the interstitium, but the interstitial content of protein is washed out. On the other hand, reduction of lymph flow below baseline values is not an effective plasma-volume conserving mechanism, because continued accumulation of plasma proteins in the interstitial compartment raises Π_i [12]. All of the protein removed in the lymph is returned to the circulation via lymphatic-to-vein junctions, mainly the right and left thoracic ducts [3]. However, as noted above and in Figure 1, a variable proportion of protein-free fluid is reabsorbed into the plasma in the lymph nodes [4,56].

Active mechanisms
Aspects of lymph propulsion in conducting lymphatics are described more fully in the chapters by Johnston (Chapter 12) and McHale (Chapter 14) in this volume. Lymphatic smooth muscle contractions appear to be stimulated by increased delivery of fluid to the conducting lymphatics [61,62], presumably due to the direct stimulating action of mechanical stretch [63,64]. Rhythmic contractions of lymphatic smooth muscle are not dependent on innervation or hormonal control, but can be modulated by these extrinsic agencies. Conducting lymphatics are innervated by both adrenergic and cholinergic nerves [65–67]. α-Adrenergic receptors increase spontaneous contraction frequency and volume transport; this is the dominant effect of sympathetic nerve activity. β-Adrenergic inhibition is revealed after α blockade [65]. Cholinergic and peptidergic receptors may also inhibit lymphatic contractions [68,69]. *In vivo*, the rate at which fluid is supplied by the terminal lymphatics seems to be the dominant factor controlling lymphatic pumping [63,70]. The extent to which nervous and hormonal controls of lymphatic smooth muscle are involved in regulation of plasma and interstitial volumes is not known, and deserves further study. It is interesting in this connection that ANP has been reported to increase contraction amplitude and frequency of isolated, perfused conducting lymphatics [71].

Conclusion

Division of ECF volume between circulating plasma and ISF compartments of the diverse tissues and organs of our bodies is a complex process involving several physiological systems: (1) the heart and large blood vessels, which provide the flow of blood; (2) the arterioles and muscular venules, which control flow distribution and exchange-vessel pressures and functional surface areas; (3) the exchange vessels themselves, capillaries and non-muscular venules, the endothelial walls of which determine hydraulic conductivity and solute permeabilities; (4) the interstitial matrices of individual tissues and organs, whose compliances and exclusion properties determine the relation of ISFV to ISF pressure and protein concentration; and finally (5) the lymphatic system which returns extravasated fluid and protein to the circulating plasma.

In health, whole body plasma volume and regional ISFVs are maintained within relatively narrow limits, partly through the action of passive forces acting on exchange-vessel walls ('Starling forces'), interstitial matrix components and lymphatics, but also by reflex hormonal (and possibly nervous) mechanisms that may act on one or more of these systems.

Our own experimental studies described in this presentation were supported by National Institutes of Health grant HL-18010 and NIH-NRSA Fellowship HL-07957 to V.L.T.

References

1. Courtice, F.C. (1971) Lymph and plasma proteins: barriers to their movement throughout the extracellular fluid. *Lymphology* **4**, 9–17
2. Landis, E.M. and Pappenheimer, J.R. (1963) Exchange of substances through the capillary walls. In *Handbook of Physiology, 1st edn. Sect. 2: Circulation, Vol. II* (Hamilton, W.F., vol. ed.; Dow, P., series ed.), pp. 961–1034, Am. Physiol. Soc., Washington, D.C.
3. Mayerson, H.S. (1963) The physiologic importance of lymph. In *Handbook of Physiology, 1st edn., Sect. 2: Circulation, Vol. II* (Hamilton, W.F., vol. ed.; Dow, P., series ed.), pp. 1035–1073, Am. Physiol. Soc., Washington, D.C.
4. Adair, T.H., Moffatt, D.S., Paulsen, A.W. and Guyton, A.C. (1982) Quantitation of changes in lymph protein concentration during lymph node transit. *Am. J. Physiol.* **243**, H351–H359
5. Renkin, E.M. (1986) Some consequences of capillary permeability to macromolecules: Starling's hypothesis reconsidered. *Am. J. Physiol.* **250**, H706–H710
6. Wiig, H., DeCarlo, M., Sibley, L. and Renkin, E.M. (1992) Interstitial exclusion of albumin in rat tissues measured by a continuous infusion method. *Am. J. Physiol.* **263**, H1222–H1233
7. Wiederhielm, C.A. and Black, L.L. (1976) Osmotic interaction of plasma proteins with interstitial molecules. *Am. J. Physiol.* **231**, 638–641
8. Bert, J.L. and Pearce, R.H. (1984) The interstitium and microvascular exchange. In *Handbook of Physiology, 2nd edn., Sect. 2: The Cardiovascular System, Vol. IV, Microcirculation* (Renkin, E.M. and Michel, C.C., vol. eds.; Geiger, S.R., series ed.), pp. 521–547, Am. Physiol. Soc., Bethesda, MD
9. Bach, C. and Lewis, G.P. (1973) Lymph flow and lymph protein concentration in the skin and muscle of the rabbit hind limb. *J. Physiol. (London)* **235**, 477–492
10. Mullins, R.J. and Bell, D.R. (1982) Changes in interstitial volume and masses of albumin and IgG in rabbit skin and skeletal muscles after saline volume loading. *Circ. Res.* **51**, 305–313
11. Aukland, K. and Reed, R.K. (1993) Interstitial-lymphatic mechanisms in the control of extracellular fluid volume. *Physiol. Rev.* **73**, 1–78
12. Michel, C.C. (1984) Fluid movements through capillary walls. In *Handbook of Physiology, 2nd edn., Sect. 2: The Cardiovascular System, Vol. IV, Microcirculation* (Renkin, E.M. and Michel, C.C., vol. eds.; Geiger, S.M., series ed.), pp. 375–409, Am. Physiol. Soc., Bethesda, MD
13. Nitta, S., Ohnuki, T., Ohkuda, K., Nakada, T. and Staub, N.C. (1981) The corrected protein equation to estimate plasma colloid osmotic pressure and its development on a nomogram. *Tohoku J. Exp. Med.* **135**, 43–49
14. Patlak, C.S., Goldstein, D.A. and Hoffman, J.F. (1963) The flow of solute and solvent across a two-membrane system. *J. Theor. Biol.* **5**, 426–442

15. Curry, F.E. (1984) Mechanics and thermodynamics of transcapillary exchange. In *Handbook of Physiology, 2nd edn., Sect. 2: The Cardiovascular System, Vol. IV, Microcirculation* (Renkin, E.M. and Michel, C.C., vol. eds., Geiger, S.R., series ed.), pp. 309–374, Am. Physiol. Soc., Bethesda, MD

16. Haraldsson, B. (1988) Diffusional transport of albumin from interstitium to blood across small pores in the capillary walls of rat skeletal muscle. *Acta Physiol. Scand.* **133**, 63–71

17. Taylor, A.E., Gibson, W.H., Granger, H.J. and Guyton, A.C. (1973) The interaction between intracapillary and tissue forces in the overall regulation of interstitial fluid volume. *Lymphology* **6**, 192–208

18. Wiig, H. and Reed, R.K. (1985) Interstitial compliance and transcapillary Starling pressures in cat skin and skeletal muscle. *Am. J. Physiol.* **248**, H666–H673

19. Renkin, E.M. (1984) Control of microcirculation and blood-tissue exchange. In *Handbook of Physiology, 2nd edn., Sect. 2: The Cardiovascular System, Vol. IV, Microcirculation* (Renkin, E.M. and Michel, C.C., vol. eds., Geiger, S.R., series ed.), pp. 627–687, Am. Physiol. Soc., Bethesda, MD

20. Johnson, P.C. (1986) Autoregulation of blood flow. *Circ. Res.* **59**, 483–495

21. Björnberg, J., Gründe, P.-O., Maspers, M. and Mellander, S. (1988) Site of autoregulatory reactions in the vascular bed of cat skeletal muscle as determined with a new technique for segmental vascular resistance recordings. *Acta Physiol. Scand.* **133**, 199–210

22. Davis, M.J. (1988) Control of bat wing capillary pressure and blood flow during reduced perfusion pressure. *Am. J. Physiol.* **255**, H1114–H1129

23. Shore, A.C., Sandeman, O.D. and Tooke, J.E. (1993) Effect of an increase in systemic blood pressure on nailfold capillary pressure in humans. *Am. J. Physiol.* **265**, H820–H823

24. Thulesius, O. and Johnson, P.C. (1966) Pre- and postcapillary resistance in skeletal muscle. *Am. J. Physiol.* **210**, 869–872

25. Lewis, D.H. and Mellander, S. (1962) Competetive effects of sympathetic control and tissue metabolites on resistance and capacitance vessels and capillary filtration in skeletal muscle. *Acta Physiol. Scand.* **56**, 162–188

26. Mellander, S., Maspers, M., Björnberg, J. and Anderson, L.-O. (1987) Autoregulation of capillary pressure and filtration in cat skeletal muscle in states of normal and reduced vascular tone. *Acta Physiol. Scand.* **129**, 337–351

27. Gründe, P.-O. and Mellander, S. (1979) Beta adrenergic inhibitory interference with myogenic vascular reactivity during experimental intervention. *Acta Physiol. Scand.* **106**, 87–89

28. Lundvall, J. and Hillman, J. (1978) Fluid transfer from skeletal muscle to blood during hemorrhage. Importance of beta adrenergic vascular mechanisms. *Acta Physiol. Scand.* **102**, 450–458

29. Smith, E.L., Huggins, R.A. and Deavers, S. (1965) Effect of blood volume on movement of protein and volume distribution of albumin in the dog. *Am. J. Vet. Res.* **26**, 829–836

30. Manning, R.D. and Guyton, A.C. (1982) Control of blood volume. *Rev. Physiol. Biochem. Pharmacol.* **93**, 69–114

31. Renkin, E.M., Tucker, V., Rew, K., O'Loughlin, D., Wong, M. and Sibley, L. (1992) Plasma volume expansion with colloids increases blood-tissue albumin transport. *Am. J. Physiol.* **262**, H1054–H1067

32. Wraight, E.P. (1974) Capillary permeability to protein as a factor in the control of plasma volume. *J. Physiol. (London)* **237**, 39–47

33. Kramer, G.C., Harms, B.A., Bodai, B.I., Demling, R.H. and Renkin, E.M. (1982) Mechanisms for redistribution of plasma protein following acute protein depletion. *Am. J. Physiol.* **243**, H803–H809

34. Renkin, E.M., Gustafson-Sgro, M. and Sibley, L. (1988) Coupling of albumin flux to volume flow in skin and muscles of anesthetized rats. *Am. J. Physiol.* **255**, H458–H466

35. Renkin, E.M., Rew, K.T., Wong, M.S., O'Loughlin, D. and Sibley, L. (1989) Influence of saline infusion on blood-tissue albumin transport. *Am. J. Physiol.* **257**, H525–H533

36. Edwards, B.S., Zimmerman, R.S., Schwab, T.R., Heublin, D.M. and Burnett, J.J.C. (1988) Atrial stretch, not pressure, is the principal determinant controlling the acute release of atrial natriuretic factor. *Circ. Res.* **62**, 191–195

37. Lang, R.E., Thölken, H., Ganten, D., Luft, F.C., Ruskoaho, H. and Unger, T. (1985) Atrial natriuretic factor — a circulating hormone stimulated by volume loading. *Nature (London)* **314**, 264–266

38. Anderson, J., Christofides, N. and Bloom, S. (1986) Plasma release of atrial natriuretic peptide in response to blood volume expansion. *J. Endocrinol.* **109**, 9–13

39. Tucker, V.L., Simanonok, K.E. and Renkin, E.M. (1992) Tissue-specific effects of physiological ANP infusion on blood-tissue albumin transport. *Am. J. Physiol.* **263**, R945–R953

40. Villarreal, D., Freeman, R.H., Davis, J.O., Verburg, K.M. and Vari, R.C. (1986) Effects of atrial appendectomy on circulating atrial natriuretic factor during volume expansion in the rat (42385). *Proc. Soc. Exp. Biol. Med.* **183**, 54–58

41. Verburg, K.M., Freeman, R.H., Davis, J.O., Villarreal, D. and Vari, R.C. (1986) Control of atrial natriuretic factor release in conscious dogs. *Am. J. Physiol.* **251**, R947–R956

42. Windle, R.J., Forsling M.L., Smith, C.P. and Balment , R.J. (1993) Patterns of neurohypophysial hormone release during dehydration in the rat. *J. Endocrinol.* **137**, 311–319

43. Share, L. (1988) Role of vasopressin in cardiovascular regulation. *Physiol. Rev.* **68**, 1248–1284

44. Bealer, S.L., Haddy, F.J., Diana, J.N., Grega, G.J., Manning, R.D.J., Rose, J.C. and Gann, D.S.

(1986) Neuroendocrine mechanisms of plasma volume regulation. *Fed. Proc. Fed. Assoc. Soc. Exp. Biol.* **45**, 2455–2463

45. Aukland, K. and Nicolaysen, G. (1981) Interstitial fluid volume: local regulatory mechanisms. *Physiol. Rev.* **61**, 556–643

46. Brace, R.A. and Guyton, A.C. (1977) Interaction of transcapillary Starling forces in the isolated dog forelimb. *Am. J. Physiol.* **223**, H136–H140

47. Reed, R.K., Bowen, B.D. and Bert, J.L. (1989) Microvascular exchange and interstitial volume regulation in the rat: implications of the model. *Am. J. Physiol.* **257**, H2081–H2091

48. Bert, J.L. and Pinder, K.L. (1983) From which compartment in the interstitium does lymph originate? *Microvasc. Res.* **26**, 116–121

49. Witte, C.L., Witte, M.H. and Dumont, A.E. (1984) Pathophysiology of chronic edema, lymphedema and fibrosis. In *Edema* (Staub, N.C. and Taylor, A.E., eds.), pp. 521–542, Raven Press, New York

50. Lund, T., Onarheim, H., Wiig, H. and Reed, R.K. (1989) Mechanisms behind increased dermal imbibition in acute burn edema. *Am. J. Physiol.* **256**, H940–H948

51. Reed, R.K. and Rodt, S.Å. (1991) Increased negativity of interstitial fluid pressure during the onset stage of inflammatory edema in rat skin. *Am. J. Physiol.* **260**, H1985–H1991

52. Reed, R.K., Rubin, K., Wiig, H. and Rodt, S.Å. (1992) Blockade of b1-integrins in skin causes edema through lowering of interstitial fluid pressure. *Circ. Res.* **71**, 978–983

53. Reed, R.C., Laurent, T.C. and Taylor, A.E. (1990) Hyaluronan in prenodal lymph from skin: changes with lymph flow. *Am. J. Physiol.* **259**, H1097–H1100

54. Reed, R.K., Laurent, U.B.G., Fraser, J.R.E. and Laurent, T.C. (1990) Removal rate of [³H]-hyaluronan injected subcutaneously in rabbits. *Am. J. Physiol.* **259**, H532–H535

55. Schmid-Schönbein, G.W. (1990) Microlymphatics and lymph flow. *Physiol. Rev.* **70**, 987–1028

56. Renkin, E.M. (1979) Lymph as a measure of the composition of interstitial fluid. In *Pulmonary Edema* (Fishman, A.P. and Renkin, E.M., eds.), pp. 145–159, Am. Physiol. Soc., Bethesda, MD

57. McGeown, J.G., McHale, N.G. and Thornbury, K.D. (1987) The role of external compression and movement in lymph propulsion in the sheep hind limb. *J. Physiol. (London)* **387**, 83–93

58. Schmid-Schönbein, G.W. (1990) Mechanisms causing initial lymphatics to expand and compress to promote lymph flow. *Arch. Histol. Cytol.* **53** (Suppl.), 107–114

59. Leak, L.V. (1987) Lymphatic endothelial interstitial interface. *Lymphology* **20**, 196–204

60. O'Morchoe, P.J., Yang, V.V. and O'Morchoe, C.C.C. (1980) Lymphatic transport pathways during volume expansion. *Microvasc. Res.* **20**, 275–294

61. Hogan, R.D. and Unthank, J.L. (1986) The initial lymphatics as sensors of interstitial fluid volume. *Microvasc. Res.* **31**, 317–324

62. Benoit, J.N., Zawieja, D.C., Goodman, A.H. and Granger, H.J. (1989) Characterization of intact mesenteric lymphatic pump and its responsiveness to acute edemagenic stress. *Am. J. Physiol.* **257**, H2059–H2069

63. McHale, N.G. and Roddie, I.C. (1976) The effect of transmural pressure on pumping activity in isolated bovine lymphatic vessels. *J. Physiol. (London)* **261**, 255–269

64. Ohhashi, T., Azuma, T. and Sakaguchi, M. (1980) Active and passive mechanical characteristics of bovine mesenteric lymphatics. *Am. J. Physiol.* **239**, H88–H95

65. McHale, N.G., Roddie, I.C. and Thornbury, K.D. (1980) Nervous modulation of spontaneous contractions in bovine mesenteric lymphatics. *J. Physiol. (London)* **309**, 461–472

66. Alessandrini, C., Gerli, R., Sacchi, R., Ibba, L., Pucci, A.M. and Fruschelli, C. (1981) Cholinergic and adrenergic innervation of mesenterial lymph vessels in guinea pig. *Lymphology* **14**, 1–6

67. Ohhashi, T., Kobayashi, S., Tsukahara, S. and Azuma, T. (1982) Innervation of bovine mesenteric lymphatics: from the histochemical point of view. *Microvasc. Res.* **24**, 377–385

68. Ohhashi, T., Kawai, Y. and Azuma, T. (1978) The response of lymphatic smooth muscle to vasoactive substances. *Pflüger's Arch.* **375**, 183–188

69. Ohhashi, T., Olschowka, J.A. and Jacobowitz, D.M. (1983) Vasoactive intestinal peptide inhibitory innervation in bovine mesenteric lymphatics. A histological and pharmacological study. *Circ. Res.* **53**, 535–538

70. Benoit, J.N. (1991) Relation between lymphatic pump flow and total lymph flow in the small intestine. *Am. J. Physiol.* **261**, H1970–H1978

71. Ohhashi, T., Watanabe, N. and Kawai, Y. (1990) Effects of atrial natriuretic peptide on isolated bovine mesenteric lymphatics. *Am. J. Physiol.* **259**, H42–H47

19

Myocardial interstitium and lymphatics: pathophysiology and effects on cardiac function

Glen A. Laine*, Uwe Mehlhorn, Karen L. Davis and Steven J. Allen
Center for Microvascular and Lymphatic Studies, Department of Anesthesiology, University of Texas Medical School, Houston, TX, U.S.A. and Microcirculation Research Institute, Department of Veterinary Physiology and Pharmacology, College of Veterinary Medicine, Texas A&M University, College Station, TX, U.S.A.

Introduction

In this chapter we will evaluate the current level of understanding about the myocardial interstitium and myocardial lymphatic system. Two factors contribute significantly to disturbances of the interstitium; they are (1) the accumulation of interstitial fluid or oedema and (2) the accumulation of excess or altered interstitial matrix material or fibrosis. Oedema fluid may accumulate in response to increased myocardial microvascular pressures, changes in myocardial microvascular permeability or reductions in myocardial lymph flow rate. Although interstitial fibrosis may develop secondarily to various pathologies we shall focus on interstitial changes resulting from the presence of interstitial oedema. Figure 1 depicts schematically factors that can induce myocardial oedema, interstitial fibrosis and compromised cardiac function. We shall begin our discussion by outlining the clinical importance of interstitial and lymphatic pathologies of the heart.

Clinical importance of the myocardial interstitium and lymphatics

Various pathologies of the myocardial interstitium and lymphatic system can lead to myocardial dysfunction. These pathologies may be acute or chronic in nature and are collectively referred to as interstitial heart disease. Cardiopulmonary bypass [1–4], cardiac transplantation [5,6], sepsis [7], myocarditis [8,9], myocardial infarction [10,11], as well as acute and chronic arterial and pulmonary hypertension, have all been shown to produce myocardial oedema and manifestations of interstitial heart disease. We have demonstrated compromised contractility [1,4], as well as diastolic cardiac function, both active (relaxation) and passive (compliance), following accumulation of myocardial oedema [1,4]. These changes may enhance the development of ischaemia, not only by increasing the diffusion distance for oxygen, but also by increasing

*To whom correspondence should be addressed.

Figure 1

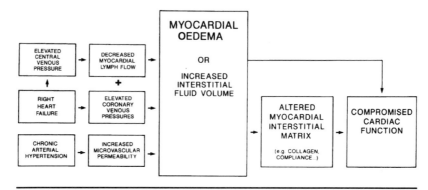

Schematic representation of factors which may lead to myocardial oedema and interstitial fibrosis
Reproduced from [16] with permission.

myocardial oxygen demand for a given amount of cardiac work [12,13]. Clinical management of myocardial oedema is dissimilar from the management of pulmonary oedema since we do not have a bedside technique for monitoring myocardial water content. Several techniques ranging from direct endomyocardial biopsy to various imaging techniques demonstrate promise for the quantification of clinically relevant myocardial oedema. Quantifying myocardial oedema presents an added problem since very small fluid volume changes, of the order of 10%, may compromise cardiac function, in contrast with pulmonary oedema which may double lung weight before significant pathology is observed. Significant new research is needed in the areas of myocardial oedema and fibrosis resolution, as well as interventions that either decrease myocardial microvascular filtration rate or enhance myocardial lymph flow rate. We have demonstrated that decompressing the lymphatic system by thoracic duct cannulation and drainage significantly decreases pulmonary oedema in an animal model [14]. Efforts are under way to determine whether similar benefit may be realized in the treatment of cardiac oedema.

Myocardial interstitium

Physicochemical properties
Although staining techniques for some elements of the interstitial matrix exist, direct microscopic visualization of the functional properties of the interstitium remains problematic. Approaches which are proving useful include evaluating various physicochemical properties, biochemistry and molecular biology of the myocardial interstitium. Physicochemical properties are those fundamental factors such as compliance and permeability which are determined by the structural elements of the interstitium. Biochemistry and molecular biology can be used to evaluate the concentration, turnover and gene regulation of interstitial constituents.

The relationship between myocardial interstitial pressure (P_{INT}) and interstitial fluid volume is referred to as compliance. When we speak of myocardial interstitial compliance, we refer to compliance of the myocardial wall and not chamber compliance. The myocardial interstitium is a relatively stiff or non-compliant structure in which pressure increases significantly for a given increase in interstitial volume [15]. As P_{INT} increases and the heart wall becomes stiff, cardiac function is adversely affected [16]. As pointed out earlier, various pathologies can alter myocardial interstitial compliance, thus directly impacting on cardiac function.

P_{INT} can be measured using acute and chronic techniques such as porous polyethylene capsules, wicks or needles [17]. The baseline value for P_{INT} is approximately 15 mmHg during diastole [17]. P_{INT} varies throughout the cardiac cycle and is recorded during diastole as this is the phase during which microvascular fluid exchange takes place.

Fluid and proteins enter the myocardial interstitium from the myocardial microvascular exchange vessels and must exit via the myocardial lymphatics or as pericardial effusions. Interstitial fluid volume is normally expressed as the (wet − dry)/dry weight ratio corrected for residual blood volume within the tissues [16]. Newer techniques utilizing radioactive tracers differentiate myocardial fluid volume into vascular, cellular and interstitial compartments [18]. The introduction of linear density-gradient columns allows the accurate determination of water content in small endomyocardial biopsies [19].

As fluid and protein leave the microvasculature, they must travel across multiple barriers including the microvascular exchange-vessel wall and interstitium before exiting via the lymphatics. Permeability of these barriers is an important physiological factor since increases in microvascular permeability can lead to myocardial oedema, even at normal microvascular pressures. An index of microvascular permeability to plasma proteins may be obtained by determining the osmotic reflection coefficient (σ or sigma) using a variety of techniques [17]. Although the usefulness of absolute numerical values for σ may be debatable, variations in σ provide a useful index of changes in microvascular permeability. Control values for σ in the heart are about 0.42 for albumin and 0.95 for β-lipoprotein, with a lymph to plasma total protein concentration ratio of approx. 0.82. Although experimentally more difficult to obtain, determinations of the filtration coefficient or hydraulic conductivity will provide more useful information as to the permeability of the exchange barrier to water. Permeability may be either increased or decreased depending upon pathological insult. For example, chronic arterial hypertension increases microvascular permeability in the heart while chronic venous pressure elevation decreases permeability [20].

Two other factors which help to characterize the myocardial interstitium further are 'protein-excluded volume' and 'free fluid channels'. The concept of exclusion originates since the interstitium is a tight matrix of various macromolecules which can either physically or sterically exclude plasma proteins from a portion of the interstitial matrix. Albumin, for example, is excluded from over 50% of the myocardial interstitium [18]. This process is responsible for protein concentration and thus osmotic pressure amplification of interstitial fluid not bound within the matrix. The excluded volume for plasma proteins decreases significantly as the interstitium is hydrated or becomes oedematous, thus reducing osmotic amplification. The existence of free fluid channels leading through the interstitium from the microvascular exchange barrier to the lymphatics has long been postulated. The existence of such channels could explain the rapid appearance in lymph of substances placed within the circulation. By introducing equimolar concentrations of two molecules of similar charge and geometry but differing size into the coronary circulation and recording their rate of appearance in the cardiac lymph, we may develop a model of interstitial structure. In our studies both the large and small molecules appeared in the cardiac lymph very quickly. Interestingly, the large molecule appears in greater concentration than the smaller molecule early in the collection process. This indicates that the myocardial interstitium is acting like a chromatography column and supports the existence of free fluid channels.

Molecular and biochemical properties

The extracellular matrix (ECM) of the heart is a network composed of primarily collagen that functions in the structural support of the heart and allows the myocardium to contract as a single unit. Collagen is produced by the cardiac fibroblasts. The myocardium contains primarily type-I and type-III fibrillar collagens [21]. Type-I collagen is the most abundant collagen, comprising approximately 85% of the total collagen in the heart [22]. Collagen I is very strong; its tensile strength is greater than that of steel. Therefore, a small increase in type-I collagen can greatly increase the stiffness of the myocardium. Type-III collagen comprises approximately 11% of the total collagen in the normal heart [22]. Collagen types I and III form fibrils which surround and support groups of myocytes or myofibres. These fibrillar collagens also connect individual myocytes to one another [22]. Fibronectin, the major non-collagenous protein in the ECM, may also be produced by the cardiac fibroblasts [23].

The properties of ECM change in many diseases. In a post mortem histological study of hearts from hypertensive patients compared with normal patients, an increased accumulation of connective tissue around blood vessels and in the myocardial interstitium surrounding myocytes was observed [24]. Myocytes in fibrotic areas appeared smaller or atrophied compared with myocytes from non-fibrotic areas of the ventricles of hypertensive patients [24]. In a rat model of left ventricular hypertrophy, an increase in mRNA levels for collagen types I and III was detected after aortic banding [25,26]. This increase in collagen mRNA was also correlated with an increase in collagen protein [25,26]. An increase in collagen content was also reported in an experimental model of pulmonary artery hypertension. In this model, an increase in collagen was observed both in the overloaded right ventricle and in the left ventricle which experienced a normal haemodynamic load [16]. Changes in the ECM can affect many properties of the heart. An increase in collagen can alter the passive properties of the heart such as chamber stiffness and also the active properties of the heart such as contractility through direct effects on the myocytes. Fibronectin may play a role in connecting myocytes to the collagen matrix in the heart and may therefore also have an impact on myocardial chamber stiffness [27]. It is important to note that turnover, both deposition and degradation, of interstitial components may be involved in remodelling. It is clear that although the ECM changes in various diseases, the mechanisms are unknown.

There is evidence that a mechanical signal may be involved in the initiation of ECM remodelling. Carver and his co-workers reported an increase in collagen type-III expression in cardiac fibroblasts in response to mechanical stimulation [28]. Stretch of cultured cardiac cells also causes an induction of the immediate-early gene sequence similar to that associated with the hypertrophic response *in vivo* [29]. However, the mechanism by which a mechanical signal may be transduced into a change in cardiac gene expression is not clear. Sadoshima and co-workers examined the role of several possible mechanotransducers in the development of cardiac hypertrophy [30]. They concluded that stretch-activated action channels, microtubules, and microfilaments are not involved in the transduction of a mechanical signal for hypertrophy [30].

Other experimental evidence points to a humoral signal for ECM remodelling in hypertension. Interstitial fibrosis has been demonstrated in both the left and right ventricles in arterial hypertension even though the right ventricle is not subjected to an increased load [31]. Therefore, a signal other than a mechanical signal may be involved. Since angiotensin stimulates collagen production in a cardiac fibroblast cell culture model, it has been proposed as the hormonal signal for ECM remodelling [32]. In one set of experiments, three rat models of arterial hypertension with various levels of angiotensin II (A-II) and aldosterone (ALDO) were used to investigate the role of angiotensin in ECM remodelling [31]. In the first model, the renovascular hypertension model, A-II and ALDO levels are both elevated. In the infrarenal aortic banding model, A-II and ALDO levels are normal. In the third model, ALDO was infused into the rats so ALDO levels were elevated and A-II levels were suppressed. Although left ventricular hypertrophy occurred in all three models, interstitial fibrosis only occurred in the renovascular hypertension model and the ALDO infusion model [31]. The investigators concluded from these experiments that A-II and/or ALDO cause interstitial fibrosis in arterial hypertension [31]. However, ALDO levels were elevated in both arterial hypertension models in which interstitial fibrosis occurred and A-II levels were actually decreased in one model of hypertension in which fibrosis occurred.

There is some additional evidence that is not consistent with the proposed A-II hormonal signal for interstitial fibrosis. In pulmonary hypertension, right ventricular hypertrophy occurs. There is very little change in systemic blood pressure in pulmonary hypertension; consequently, the renin–angiotensin–aldosterone system should not be activated. However, as in arterial hypertension, an increased collagen content has been reported in both the left and the right ventricles in pulmonary hypertension [16,33,34]. Furthermore, most patients with essential arterial hypertension who develop interstitial fibrosis of the heart have renin levels below normal and only about 17% have renin levels above normal [35].

Another postulated mechanism for inducing interstitial fibrosis does not involve a humoral factor. Myocardial interstitial oedema may be involved in the development of interstitial fibrosis during hypertension. Fibrosis is usually associated with interstitial oedema in other tissues. Chronic pulmonary oedema and systemic lymphoedema are associated with pulmonary fibrosis and interstitial fibrosis respectively [36]. Although it is not clear how oedema causes fibrosis, increased interstitial volume causes an increase in interstitial pressure which may act as a signal to induce collagen deposition. Support for the involvement of oedema in the development of interstitial fibrosis comes from experiments in pulmonary artery hypertension in dogs. When pulmonary artery hypertension is induced in dogs by banding the pulmonary artery, left ventricular interstitial oedema develops and left ventricular collagen content is increased [16]. In addition, preliminary data suggest that there is an increase in mRNA for collagen type I in the left ventricle of rats after pulmonary artery banding [37]. Oedema develops relatively early in pulmonary hypertension and may therefore act as a signal to induce myocardial interstitial fibrosis [38].

A combination of mechanical signals and hormonal signals is probably responsible for the induction and maintenance of fibrosis during hypertension. In a set of experiments by Hammond et al., left ventricular hypertrophy was induced by aortic banding in dogs [39]. Then an extract was taken from the hypertrophied left ventricle and used to perfuse a normal heart. They observed an increase in total translational activity of RNA, indicating hypertrophy induction [39]. In a similar set of experiments in a cardiac cell culture system, non-stretched cardiac cells were treated with 'stretch-conditioned medium' from cells that were stretched to induce hypertrophy [40]. Changes in gene expression similar to that seen in the stretched cells were observed in the unstretched culture [40]. From these experiments one can conclude that some factor is released from the cardiac cells due to a mechanical stimulus, perhaps increased interstitial pressure or an increase in stretch due to oedema, and this factor induces cardiac interstitial remodelling.

Another interstitial component, glycosaminoglycan (GAG), performs a number of functions in the cardiac interstitium. Hyaluronan comprises the largest fraction of GAGs in cardiac tissue and has been the most extensively studied. It is found in relatively high tissue concentrations in the heart compared with other organs. Possible functions for cardiac hyaluronan include fluid balance regulation and lubrication. The latter function is supported by histochemical studies that demonstrate intense staining in the tissue surrounding the cardiac muscle fibres [41,42]. Hyaluronan is also found in high concentrations in the periarteriolar tissue and there appears to be more hyaluronan in the atria than the ventricles.

Because of its water-binding properties, hyaluronan may play a role in the accumulation of myocardial oedema. Investigators have demonstrated a relationship between increased hyaluronan and interstitial myocardial oedema in several experimental models. Hällgren et al. studied the effect of cardiac transplantation and found that surgery results in an increase both in cardiac water content and in hyaluronan concentration and that both were minimized in syngeneic (identical) transplants [43]. In transplants between different strains of rats, transplantation oedema progressed over several days accompanied by increases in hyaluronan. Immunohistochemical analysis confirmed interstitial hyaluronan accumulation [43]. In another model of inflammation, Waldenström *et al.* demonstrated an increase in myocardial hyaluronan concentration in mice in whom viral myocarditis was induced [44].

The impact of hyaluronan accumulation following myocardial infarction on patient outcome has received considerable interest. Myocardial ischaemia and infarction result in interstitial oedema and hyaluronan accumulation [45]. Myocardial oedema may worsen patient outcomes by increasing oxygen diffusion distances, increasing heart work, or compromising microvascular flow. Hyaluronidase administration has been shown to decrease mortality following myocardial infarction in patients [46]. Thus, degradation of hyaluronan probably results in mobilization of oedema fluid. This may occur due to either the loss of the water-binding effect of hyaluronan or decreased interstitial resistance to fluid flow. This latter mechanism is supported by increased cardiac lymph flow rates observed following hyaluronidase administration [47].

We have studied myocardial lymphatic hyaluronan flux under control and experimental conditions. Our preliminary data suggest that daily myocardial hyaluronan turnover is about 1% and doubles when microvascular filtration increases. As in other tissues, not all of myocardial hyaluronan is freely available for lymphatic removal and these turnover values may underestimate the activity of that hyaluronan involved with interstitial fluid regulation.

GAGs have been shown to increase in the heart following various manipulations to induce arterial hypertension. Lipke and Couchman used an aortic coarctation rat model to demonstrate increased cardiac GAG production [48]. However, although several functions have been attributed to GAGs, the physiological significance of this change in the heart is unknown.

Myocardial lymphatics

The mammalian heart has a dense network of lymphatic capillaries which drain myocardial interstitial fluid from the subendocardium to the subepicardium via intramyocardial channels. The subepicardial plexus drains into the subepicardial collecting trunks forming left and right coronary lymphatics which, eventually, terminate in the 'principal' cardiac lymphatic. The 'principal' cardiac lymphatic reaches the cardiac lymph node located in the connective tissue between the innominate artery and superior vena cava. Lymph collected for studies of the myocardial interstitium or lymphatics should be collected prenodally to eliminate changes which occur when lymph passes through a node [49]. From the cardiac lymph node, several lymphatics ascend to the thoracic duct and finally empty into the central venous circulation at the level of the left subclavian vein. Since myocardial interstitial fluid primarily exits the heart via the lymphatics, which then enter the central venous circulation; any lymphatic blockage or increase in central venous pressure can result in excess fluid accumulation within the myocardial interstitium [16]. It is important to note the existence of many valves within the myocardial lymphatics which maintain unidirectional flow [50,51].

Myocardial lymph flow rates

Drinker *et al.*, in 1940, were the first to cannulate a cardiac lymphatic in order to determine myocardial lymph flow rate [52]. Subsequently, several other investigators measured cardiac lymph flow rates in normal hearts, which were substantially higher than Drinker's values (Table 1). Most likely, Drinker *et al.* did not cannulate the principal cardiac lymphatic, thus measuring only a fraction of total cardiac lymph flow. In a recent study, we estimated the amount of cardiac lymph being drained through the principal cardiac lymphatic to be approximately 85% of total myocardial lymph and we calculated a total myocardial lymph flow rate of 5.0 ± 2.2 ml/h under control conditions [53].

There are several factors which can affect myocardial lymph flow rate. Short periods of generalized hypoxia, coronary artery occlusion, as well as saline infusion, have been shown to increase cardiac lymph flow [54–58]. Coronary sinus pressure and concomitant myocardial microvascular pressure elevation have been demonstrated to raise cardiac lymph flow rates significantly [17,59,60]. Laine demonstrated that chronic arterial hypertension in dogs caused myocardial oedema which was associated with a significant myocardial lymph flow rate increase compared with normotensive controls [61]. We also recently demonstrated that acute arterial hypertension is directly related to cardiac lymph flow increases [62]. In another study from our laboratory, we demonstrated that myocardial oedema caused by cardiopulmonary bypass and cardioplegic arrest was associated with significantly increased myocardial lymph flow [53]. Furthermore, we showed that myocardial lymph flow rate decreased substantially during ventricular fibrillation

Table 1	Reference	*n*	Body weight (kg)	Lymph flow rate (ml/h)
	Drinker et al., 1940 [52]	10	12.0±2.0	0.8±0.5
	Miller et al., 1964 [63]	13	17.7±3.4	3.1±1.6
	Uhley et al., 1969 [64]	6	15.0–30.0	2.3±1.1
	Leeds et al., 1970 [59]	20	16.7 (10.4–20.4)	1.2±0.6
	Ullal, 1972 [65]	15	n.a.	3.3 (2.5–4.0)
	Feola and Glick, 1975 [55]	12	16.0–24.0	2.1±0.3
	Fjeld et al., 1976 [56]	9	15.0–22.0	2.7 (0.8–4.8)
	Michael et al., 1979 [58]	14	n.a.	0.5–5.6
	Laine and Granger, 1985 [17]	18	>17.0	7.0±2.7
	Laine, 1988 [61]	7	>17.0	3.1±2.1
	Laine and Allen, 1991 [16]	8	>15.0	3.1±2.1
	Mehlhorn et al., 1995 [53]	9	28.4±3.6	4.2±1.9

Normal values [mean S.D. (range)] for myocardial lymph flow rate in dogs

Abbreviations: n, *number of dogs;* n.a., *not available.*

on normothermic cardiopulmonary bypass. In the absence of any myocardial activity in the arrested, plegic heart, lymph flow rate approaches zero.

Myocardial lymph driving pressure

The rhythmic contraction and relaxation of the heart has been hypothesized to be the 'motor' for myocardial lymph propulsion [50]. Thus, we speculated that the pressure in the myocardial lymphatics is mainly created by ventricular contraction. To evaluate this theory, we measured myocardial lymph driving pressures in normal beating hearts, as well as in the absence of organized contraction during ventricular fibrillation and in the arrested heart on cardiopulmonary bypass [53]. We found a linear relationship between myocardial lymph flow rate and lymph driving pressure. Neither uncoordinated myocardial contraction (ventricular fibrillation) nor the formation of oedema during cardio-plegic arrest appeared to increase either lymph driving pressure or lymph flow rate significantly. Myocardial oedema was associated with an increase in both lymphatic driving pressure and flow rate only when sinus rhythm resumed. Thus, we concluded that organized myocardial contraction is the major factor generating myocardial lymph driving pressure and consequently myocardial lymph flow rate.

Another factor affecting myocardial lymph driving pressure appears to be arterial blood pressure. In their original publication, Drinker *et al.* briefly mentioned that myocardial lymph pressure was 15.5 cmH$_2$O at a mean blood pressure of 112 mmHg and rose to 18.6 cmH$_2$O after an adrenaline injection [52]. Recently, we found that myocardial lymph driving pressure increased by 0.15 mmHg for each 1 mmHg increase in arterial blood pressure [62]. This suggests that hypertensive arterial pressures are transmitted to the myocardial micro-vascular exchange vessels leading to increased myocardial microvascular fluid filtration, increased myocardial lymph flow and, possibly, myo-cardial oedema formation [61].

Myocardial lymphatic resistance

The only data regarding myocardial lymphatic resistance determination have been published by Laine *et al.* [57]. Using myocardial lymph flow rate versus outflow pressure relationships, they showed that myocardial lymph flow rate decreased linearly with increases in outflow pressure. Thus, they calculated a myocardial lymphatic resistance of between 0.88 and 1.6 cmH$_2$O/min per μl under baseline conditions in dogs. After volume infusion, the myocardial lymphatic resistance decreased to between 0.15 and 0.08 cmH$_2$O/min per μl [57]. It may be speculated that myocardial lymphatic resistance decreases as myocardial lymph flow rate increases, thus acting as a safety mechanism to improve lymph drainage from the myocardial interstitium before substantial myocardial oedema can occur. However, at high myocardial microvascular filtration rates, the capability of further lymphatic resistance decreases may be exhausted, and myocardial oedema may develop. Certainly, further studies are necessary to understand the role of myocardial lymphatic function in myocardial fluid balance.

We have attempted to provide some insight into the clinical and basic importance of the myocardial interstitium and lymphatics in maintaining normal cardiac function. New techniques and experimental protocols to evaluate the dynamic properties of the interstitium and lymphatics are needed. Cardiac motion, lymphatic cannulation techniques, maintenance of chronic myocardial lymphatic cannulae, as well as various standards for evaluation of cardiac function, have made studying the myocardial interstitium and lymphatics both challenging and rewarding.

References

1. Davis, K., Rohn, D., Warters, D., Dreyer, J., Adams, D., Laine, G. and Allen, S. (1993) Myocardial edema compromises left ventricular function following cardiopulmonary bypass. *FASEB J.* 7, A562
2. Foglia, R., Lazar, H., Steed, D., Follette, D., Manganaro, A., Deland, E. and Buckberg, G. (1978) Iatrogenic myocardial edema with crystalloid primes: effects on left ventricular compliance, performance, and perfusion. *Surg. Forum* 29, 312–315
3. Weng, Z., Nicolosi, A., Detwiler, P., Hsu, D., Schierman, S., Goldstein, A. and Spotnitz, H. (1992) Effects of crystalloid, blood, and University of Wisconsin perfusates on weight, water content, and left ventricular compliance in an edema-prone, isolated porcine heart model. *J. Thorac. Cardiovasc. Surg.* 103, 504–513
4. Davis, K., Stewart, R., Warters, D., Laine, G. and Allen, S. (1993) Pulmonary hypertension and left ventricular function. *FASEB J.* 7, A882
5. Hosenpud, J., Douglas, J., Cobanoglu, M., Floten, H., Conner, R. and Starr, A. (1987) Serial echocardiographic findings early after heart transplantation: evidence for reversible right ventricular dysfunction and myocardial edema. *Transplant* 6, 343–347
6. Lund, G., Morin, R., Olivari, M. and Ring, W. (1988) Serial myocardial T_2 relaxation time measurements in normal subjects and heart transplant recipients. *J. Heart Transplant* 7, 274–279
7. Gotloib, L., Shostak, A., Galdi, P., Jaichenki, J. and Fudin, R. (1992) Loss of microvascular negative charges accompanied by interstitial edema in septic rats' heart. *Circ. Shock* 36, 45–56
8. Yankopoulos, N., Davis, J., Cotlove, E. and Trapasso, M. (with surgical assistance of Casper, A.) (1960) Mechanism of myocardial edema in dogs with chronic congestive heart failure. *Am. J. Physiol.* 199, 603–608
9. Chandraratna, P., Bardley, W., Kortman, K., Minagoe, S., Delvicario, M. and Rahimtoola, S. (1987) Detection of acute myocarditis using nuclear magnetic resonance imaging. *Am. J. Med.* 83, 1144–1146
10. Carlson, R., Aisen, A. and Buda, A. (1992) Effect of reduction in myocardial edema on myocardial blood flow and ventricular function after coronary reperfusion. *Am. J. Physiol.* 262, H641–H648
11. Garcia-Dorado, D., Theroux, P., Munoz, R., Alonso, J., Elizaga, J., Fernandez-Aviles, F., Botas, J., Solares, J., Soriano, J. and Duran, J. (1992) Favorable effects of hyperosmotic reperfusion on myocardial edema and infarct size. *Am. J. Physiol.* 262, H17–H22
12. Kahles, H., Mezger, V., Hellige, G., Spieckermann, P. and Bretschneider, H. (1982) The influence of myocardial edema formation on the energy consumption of the heart during aerobiosis and hypoxia. *Basic Res. Cardiol.* 77, 158–169
13. Laine, G.A. and Allen, S.J. (1992) Increased cardiac energy consumption accompanies myocardial interstitial edema. *FASEB J.* 6, A2038
14. Allen, S., Drake, R., Laine, G. and Gabel, J. (1991) Effect of thoracic duct drainage on hydrostatic pulmonary edema and pleural effusion in the sheep. *J. Appl. Physiol.* 71, 314–316
15. Laine, G.A. and Allen, S.J. (1991) Edema of the heart decreases left ventricular diastolic compliance. *FASEB J.* 5, A1753
16. Laine, G.A. and Allen, S.J. (1991) Left ventricular myocardial edema: lymph flow, interstitial fibrosis, and cardiac function. *Circ. Res.* 68, 1713–1721
17. Laine, G.A. and Granger, H.J. (1985) Microvascular, interstitial, and lymphatic interactions in the normal heart. *Am. J. Physiol.* 249, H834–H842
18. Laine, G. (1990) Physicochemical properties of the myocardial interstitial matrix. *FASEB J.* 4, A1258
19. Marmarou, A., Poll, W., Shulman, K. and Bhagavan, H. (1978) A simple gravimetric technique for measurement of cerebral edema. *J. Neurosurg.* 49, 530–537
20. Laine, G. (1990) Microvascular permeability and interstitial matrix changes in the heart following chronic venous hypertension. *FASEB J.* 4, A590
21. Medugorac, I. (1982) Characterization of intramuscular collagen in mammalian left ventricle. *Basic Res. Cardiol.* 77, 589–598
22. Medugorac, I. and Jacob, R. (1983) Characterization of left ventricular collagen in the rat. *Cardiovasc. Res.* 17, 15–21
23. Mamuya, W.S. and Brecher, P. (1992) Fibronectin expression in the normal and hypertrophic rat heart. *J. Clin. Invest.* 89, 392–401
24. Pearlman, E.S., Weber, K.T., Janicki, J.S., Pietra, G. and Fishman, A.P. (1982) Muscle fiber orientation and connective tissue content in the hypertrophied human heart. *Lab. Invest.* 46, 158–164

25. Eleftheriades, E.G., Durand, J.-B., Ferguson, A.G., Englemann, G.L., Jones, S.B. and Samarel, A.M. (1993) Regulation of procollagen metabolism in the pressure-overloaded rat heart. *J. Clin. Invest.* **91**, 1113–1122

26. Villarreal, F.J. and Dillman, W.H. (1992) Cardiac hypertrophy-induced changes in mRNA levels for TGF-β1, fibronectin, and collagen. *Am. J. Physiol.* **262**, H1861–H1866

27. Ahumada, G.G. and Saffitz, J.E. (1984) Fibronectin in rat heart: a link between cardiac myocytes and collagen. *J. Histochem. Cytochem.* **32**, 383–388

28. Carver, W., Nagpal, M.L., Nachtigal, M., Borg, T.K. and Terracio, L. (1991) Collagen expression in mechanically stimulated cardiac fibroblasts. *Circ. Res.* **69**, 116–122

29. Sadoshima, J.-I., Jahn, L., Takahashi, T., Kulik, T.J. and Izumo, S. (1992) Molecular characterization of the stretch-induced adaptation of cultured cardiac cells. *J. Biol. Chem.* **267**, 10551–10560

30. Sadoshima, J.-I., Takahashi, T., Jahn, L. and Izumo, S. (1992) Roles of mechano-sensitive ion channels, cytoskeleton, and contractile activity in stretch-induced immediate-early gene expression and hypertrophy in cardiac myocytes. *Proc. Natl. Acad. Sci. U.S.A.* **89**, 9905–9909

31. Brilla, C.G., Pick, R., Tan, L.B., Janicki, J.S. and Weber, K.T. (1990) Remodeling of the rat right and left ventricles in experimental hypertension. *Circ. Res.* **67**, 1355–1364

32. Brilla, C.G., Zhou, G. and Weber, K.T. (1992) Angiotensin II and collagen synthesis in cultured adult rat cardiac fibroblasts. *J. Hypertens.* **10** (Suppl. 4), S125

33. Buccino, R.A., Harris, E., Spann, J.F. and Sonnenblick, E.H. (1969) Response of myocardial connective tissue to development of experimental hypertrophy. *Am. J. Physiol.* **216**, 425–428

34. Kohama, A., Tanouchi, J., Hori, M., Kitabatake, A. and Kamada, T. (1990) Pathologic involvement of the left ventricle in chronic cor pulmonale. *Chest* **98**, 794–800

35. Laragh, J.H. (1992) Role of renin secretion and kidney function in hypertension and attendant heart attack and stroke. *Clin. Exp. Hyper. Theory Practice* **A14**, 285–305

36. Szidon, J.P. (1989) Pathophysiology of the congested lung. *Cardiol. Clinics* **7**, 39–48

37. Davis, K., Mehlhorn, U., Laine, G.A. and Allen, S.J. (1994) Left ventricular remodeling and myocardial edema in pulmonary artery hypertension. *FASEB J.* **8**, A795

38. Davis, K.L., Mehlhorn, U., Laine, G.A. and Allen, S.J. (1995) Myocardial edema, left ventricular function and pulmonary hypertension. *J. Appl. Physiol.* **78**, 132–137.

39. Hammond, G.L., Wieben, E. and Markert, C.L. (1979) Molecular signals for initiating protein synthesis in organ hypertrophy. *Proc. Natl. Acad. Sci. U.S.A.* **76**, 2455–2459

40. Sadoshima, J.-I. and Izumo, S. (1993) Mechanical stretch rapidly activates multiple signal transduction pathways in cardiac myocytes: potential involvement of an autocrine/paracrine mechanism. *EMBO J.* **12**, 1681–1682

41. Hellström, S., Tengblad, A., Johansson, C., Hedlund, U. and Axelsson, E. (1990) An improved technique for hyaluronan histochemistry using microwave irradiation. *Histochem. J.* **22**, 677–682

42. Laurent, C., Johnson-Wells, G., Hellström, S., Engström-Laurent, A. and Wells, A. (1991) Localization of hyaluronan in various muscular tissues. A morphological study in the rat. *Cell Tissue Res.* **263**, 201–205

43. Hällgren, R., Gerdin, B., Tengblad, A. and Tufveson, G. (1990) Accumulation of hyaluronan (hyaluronic acid) in myocardial interstitial tissue parallels development of transplantation edema in heart allografts in rats. *J. Clin. Invest.* **85**, 668–673

44. Waldenström, A., Fohlman, J., Ilbäck, N., Ronquist, G., Hällgren, R. and Gerdin, B. (1993) Coxsackie B3 myocarditis induces a decrease in energy charge and accumulation of hyaluronan in the mouse heart. *Eur. J. Clin. Invest.* **23**, 277–282

45. Waldenström, A., Martinussen, H.J., Gerdin, B. and Hällgren, R. (1991) Accumulation of hyaluronan and tissue edema in experimental myocardial infarction. *J. Clin. Invest.* **88**, 1622–1628

46. Roberts, R., Braunwald, E. and Muller, J.E. (1988) Effect of hyaluronidase on mortality and morbidity in patients with early peaking of plasma creatinine kinase MB and non-transmural ischaemia. *Br. Heart J.* **60**, 290–298

47. Taira, A., Uehara, K., Fukuda, S., Takenaka, K. and Koga, M. (1990) Active drainage of cardiac lymph in relation to reduction in size of myocardial infarction: an experimental study. *Angiology* **42**, 1029–1036

48. Lipke, D. and Couchman, J. (1991) Increased proteoglycan synthesis by the cardiovascular system of coarctation hypertensive rats. *J. Cell Physiol.* **147**, 479–486

49. Adair, T., Moffatt, D., Paulsen, A. and Guyton, A. (1982) Quantitation of changes in lymph protein concentration during lymph node transit. *Am. J. Physiol.* **243**, H351–H359

50. Miller, A.J. (1982) *Lymphatics of the Heart.* Raven Press, New York

51. Patek, P.R. (1939) The morphology of the lymphatics of the mammalian heart. *Am. J. Anat.* **64**, 203–249

52. Drinker, C.K., Field Warren, M., Maurer, F.W. and McCarrell, J.D. (1940) The flow, pressure, and composition of cardiac lymph. *Am. J. Physiol.* **130**, 43–55

53. Mehlhorn, U., Davis, K.L., Burke, E.J., Adams, D., Laine, G.A. and Allen, S.J. (1995) Impact of cardiopulmonary bypass and cardioplegic arrest on myocardial lymphatic function. *Am. J. Physiol.* **268**, 178–183

54. Dobbs, W.A. (1974) The flow of lymph to the cardiac node following saline infusion in the dog. *Microvasc. Res.* **8**, 14–19

55. Feola, M. and Glick, G. (1975) Cardiac lymph flow and composition in acute myocardial ischemia in dogs. *Am. J. Physiol.* **229**, 44–48

56. Fjeld, N.B., Kluge, T.H., Stokke, K.T. and Skrede, S. (1976) The effect of generalized hypoxia

upon flow and composition of cardiac lymph in the dog. *Eur. J. Clin. Invest.* **6**, 255–259

57. Laine, G.A., Allen, S.J., Katz, J., Gabel, J.C. and Drake, R.E. (1987) Outflow pressure reduces lymph flow rate from various tissues. *Microvasc. Res.* **33**, 135–142

58. Michael, L.H., Lewis, R.M., Brandon, T.A. and Entman, M.L. (1979) Cardiac lymph flow in conscious dogs. *Am. J. Physiol.* **237**, H311–H317

59. Leeds, S.E., Uhley, H.N., Sampson, J.J. and Friedman, M. (1970) The cardiac lymphatics after ligation of the coronary sinus. *Proc. Soc. Exp. Biol. Med.* **135**, 59–62

60. Miller, A.J., Pick, R. and Johnson, P.J. (1972) The rates of formation of cardiac lymph and pericardial fluid after the production of myocardial venous congestion in dogs. *Lymphology* **5**, 156–160

61. Laine, G.A. (1988) Microvascular changes in the heart during chronic arterial hypertension. *Circ. Res.* **62**, 953–960

62. Mehlhorn, U., Davis, K.L., Laine, G.A. and Allen, S.J. (1994) Myocardial microvascular filtration is directly related to arterial blood pressure in anesthetized dogs. *FASEB J.* **8**, A1050

63. Miller, A.J., Ellis, A. and Katz, A.J. (1964) Cardiac lymph: flow rates and composition in dogs. *Am. J. Physiol.* **206**, 63–66

64. Uhley, H.N., Leeds, S.E., Sampson, J.J. and Friedman, M. (1969) The cardiac lymphatics in experimental chronic congestive heart failure. *Proc. Soc. Exp. Biol. Med.* **131**, 379–381

65. Ullal, S.R. (1972) Cardiac lymph and lymphatics. *Ann. R. College Surg. Engl.* **51**, 282–298

20

Integration of capillary, interstitial and lymphatic function in the pleural space

Daniela Negrini
Istituto di Fisiologia Umana, Università degli Studi, Milano, Italy

Introduction

The pleural space may be considered as an enlarged tissue space whose free liquid volume largely exceeds that of the solid elements, mainly consisting of a complex mesh of microvilli of the mesothelial cells. Traditionally, interest in the pleural space was mainly focused on mechanical coupling between lung and chest wall and little attention was paid to a quantitative evaluation of the mechanisms controlling pleural fluid turnover. As a matter of fact, the pleural space represents an invaluable experimental model to study the integration between capillary, interstitial and lymphatic functions with the least invasive techniques.

Historical background

The ability of the serous spaces to remove fluid and particulates at high flow rate was already known in 1799 [1]. In 1863 Recklinghausen revealed the existence of the Kampfmeier foci, as well as of the mesothelial stomata, on the peritoneal surface of the diaphragm [2]; furthermore, he demonstrated that mesothelial cells are flat and very similar to the capillary endothelial cells in which he identified the presence of fenestrae. In 1866 Dybkowsky [3] acknowledged Recklinghausen's findings on serosal lymphatics and put forward the suggestion that respiratory movements would enhance lymphatic drainage through stomata. A controversy on the mechanisms of serosal fluid and solute turnover arose in 1895, when Heidenhain proposed that fluid leaves the peritoneal space mainly through absorption into the blood capillaries [4]. At about the same time the pioneering studies of Sir Ernest Starling [5,6] showed that: (1) osmotic gradients are important to sustain fluid exchanges across mesothelial membranes and (2) after "the establishment of osmotic equilibrium...the absorption of fluid from the pleural cavity is extremely slow, so that it might perhaps be affected by the lymphatics alone" [6]. Furthermore, Leathes and Starling introduced the important concept that the mesothelia act as size-selective barriers for solute exchange [7]. In 1901, Hertzler denied the existence of lymphatic stomata and endothelial fenestrae claiming that Recklinghausen's anatomical findings only resulted from technical artifacts [8]. In 1927, Florey pointed to the importance of rhythmic contraction of the large collecting lymphatics to propel lymph [9,10].

The existence of lymphatic stomata in the serous spaces remained controversial until 1937 [11,12] and was finally confirmed by scanning and transmission electron microscopy performed by Wang [13].

Based on the Starling osmotic hypothesis, in 1923 Neergard reasoned that the negative pleural liquid pressure could result from fluid reabsorption through the visceral pleura because plasma colloid osmotic pressure largely exceeds the hydraulic pressure in the pulmonary capillaries [14]; according to this hypothesis, which neglected any role of pleural lymphatics, the main route of pleural fluid drainage would be through the pulmonary capillaries.

In 1972, Agostoni [15], further developing Neergard's hypothesis, made an estimate of transpleural pressure gradients in dogs based on the balance between hydraulic and colloid-osmotic pressures, thereby assuming that pleural membranes are perfectly impermeable to proteins. He calculated a filtration pressure gradient of 10 cmH$_2$O through the parietal pleura and an absorption pressure gradient of 14 cmH$_2$O through the visceral pleura: the higher gradient through the visceral pleura would force fluid absorption to attain a minimum volume of pleural fluid and a tight fitting between lung and chest wall. This view remained substantially unchanged up to 1986 [16]; as such, it overlooked the role of parietal extrapleural and pulmonary interstitial spaces and failed to consider the size-selective properties of pleural membranes (as first formulated by Starling). Pleural lymphatics were considered a pathway for removal of cells, particles and probably protein in physiological conditions, and as an emergency route for fluid drainage in case of pleural effusion.

Therefore, up to the 1980s, many questions on (1) the perm-selectivity of the mesothelia in physiological conditions, (2) the mechanism setting pleural liquid pressure and (3) the relative role of Starling-dependent and lymphatic flows in the turnover of the pleural fluid in physiological conditions and with pleural effusions, were still unanswered.

This chapter intends to focus on these three main aspects of pleural space physiology, dealing primarily with solute and water transport between pleural compartments and with lymphatic drainage. It will purposefully neglect: (a) the mechanical lung–chest wall coupling [17]; (b) the lubrication between sliding pleurae [18–20]; (c) the intra-pleural flows [21–28] and recirculation of pleural fluid [29]; and (d) the control of pleural fluid turnover [30].

General features of the pleural space

The main function of pleural fluid is to guarantee a close apposition of lung and chest wall, allowing frictionless sliding of visceral and parietal pleurae during respiratory movements. The pleural fluid displays some specific features: (a) its volume is very small (from 0.4 to 2.5 ml per kg of body weight from both pleural spaces, depending upon the species considered [31,32]), so that only a thin layer of fluid separates the opposing pleurae, evaluated by different methods, pleural liquid thickness averages about 10–20 μm [13,20,33]; (b) its hydraulic pressure is subatmospheric in physiological conditions; therefore, the pleural cavity may be considered as a relatively dehydrated interstitium; (c) its total protein concentration is low compared with other interstitial spaces, ranging between 1 and 2.5 g/dl and decreasing with increasing mammal size [31,32]; (d) it contains surfactant phospholipids that act as boundary lubricants [18,19]; (e) its viscosity is essentially equal to that of water; (f) its ionic content is similar to that of other extracellular fluids and plasma [34]; and (g) it contains about 2200–2400 cells per mm^3, including defoliated mesothelial cells, monocytes and lymphocytes [31].

Anatomy of the pleural space

The pleural space, as are all serous cavities, is derived from the embryological development of the primitive coelomatic body space. Figure 1 shows the morpho-functional arrangement of pleural structures; the pleural cavity is delimited by the parietal and visceral mesothelia covering the inner thoracic cavity and the lung respectively.

The maximum thickness of a mesothelial body cell is about 4 μm [35]. The Golgi apparatus and the rough endoplasmic reticulum are barely developed and few mitochondria are dispersed in a scant cytoplasm; adjacent cells are connected by tight junctions on the luminal side, and by desmosomes on the basal portion of the intercellular junction [13,35,36]. These features are common to mesothelia and vascular and lymphatic endothelia [13].

Mesothelial cells are covered by 1–3 μm-long microvilli, whose density varies from 2 to 30 per μm^2 [35,37]. High concentrations of glycoproteins and hyaluronic acid are trapped by microvilli on the most mobile lung caudal surface [13,37]. The cells, particularly the cuboidal ones [13], contain the enzymic chains for production and assembly of macromolecules (such as collagens I, III and IV) of the subpleural interstitial space, produced at a rate similar to that of the interstitial fibroblasts [36,38]; mesothelial cells also synthesize elastin, laminin, fibronectin, glycoproteins and proteoglycans [36,39]. Oxidative and glycolytic metabolisms are low in cultured mesothelial cells [40].

The mesothelia lie on a continuous basal lamina connected to the subpleural interstitium; the latter extends up to the alveolar and septal pulmonary interstitial space on the visceral side and to the endothoracic fascia on the parietal side. In mammals with thin pleurae [41], such as dogs, rabbits and cats, the thickness of the parietal subpleural interstitium (about 20 μm [42]) is fairly similar to that of the visceral side, whereas in mammals with thick pleurae such as sheep, pigs, horses and human beings, the parietal interstitium is about four times thinner than the visceral one [37,43,44].

In all mammalian species, blood supply to the parietal pleura is provided by a systemic microvascular network; the visceral pleural microvasculature derives from the pulmonary circulation in mammals with thin pleurae and from branching of the systemic bronchial artery in mammals with thick pleurae. The average distance between mesothelial cells and the subpleural microvascular network is from two to five times smaller in the parietal than in the visceral pleura [43,44].

Figure 1

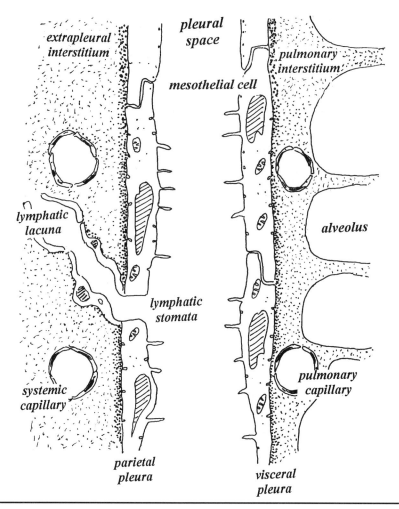

*extrapleural
interstitium*

*pleural
space*

*pulmonary
interstitium*

mesothelial cell

*lymphatic
lacuna*

alveolus

*lymphatic
stomata*

*systemic
capillary*

*pulmonary
capillary*

*parietal
pleura*

*visceral
pleura*

Morpho-functional arrangement of the pleural structures

Pleural lymphatic system

The visceral pleural lymphatic plexus runs parallel to the mesothelium with no connection between the lymphatic lumen and the pleural space [44]. Conversely, the parietal pleura, as well as the parietal peritoneum, is supplied by a peculiar network of lymphatics [45–50], characterized by the existence of the so-called 'stomata' (Figure 2a), which establish a direct patent link between the pleural cavity and an extensive mesh of submesothelial lymphatic lacunae (Figure 2b) [13,50,51]. The latter consists of wide lymphatic vessels running parallel to the mesothelium from which they are separated by a thin stratum of submesothelial interstitial space [13,50,51]; stomata are delimited by edges of adjacent mesothelial cells at the points where they make contact with the endothelium of the lymphatic lacunae.

Stomata may be either isolated, grouped in clusters [49], or organized to form a cribriform membrane made of a net-like arrange-

Figure 2

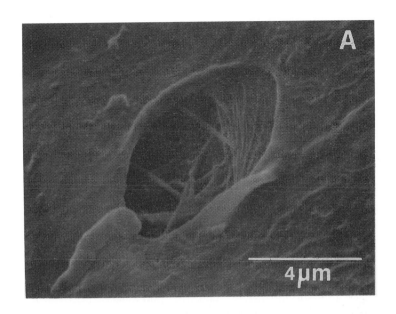

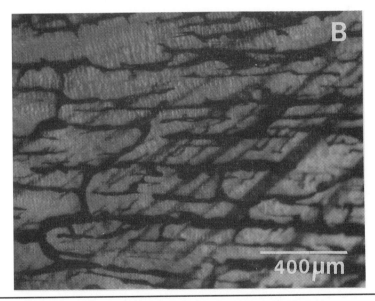

Scanning electron microscopic image (A) of pleural stomata on the tendinous portion of the diaphragm and (B) a microscopic image of this area to show the network of lymphatic lacunae

ment of collagen fibres irregularly covering the roof of the underlying lacunae [13]. Their density ranges from 100/cm^2 on the intercostal surface to 8000/cm^2 on the diaphragm, which also displays the highest stoma/lacuna ratio [48,49]. At the end-expiratory lung volume, the average stoma diameter is about 1.3 μm, ranging from less than 1 μm for stomata grouped into clusters up to 40 μm for the widest isolated ones;

their surface area (about 0.7 μm^2 [49]) may increase up to threefold during inspiration [52].

The cytoplasm of the endothelial cells delimiting the lumen of the lacunae contains actin filaments [50], suggesting that the very initial portion of the pleural lymphatics may actively contract; furthermore, the endothelium of lacunae may differentiate to form unidirectional flap-like valves [13,47,53].

Transpleural water and solute flows

An effort has been made in recent years to quantify transpleural solute and water fluxes [see eqns. (1) and (3)] in spontaneously breathing mammals. Figure 3 shows, as an example, the lung surface viewed through the intact parietal pleura exposed after removal of the intercostal muscles [54]; this preparation allowed us to measure, through the micropuncture technique, the hydraulic pressure in the extrapleural parietal interstitium [55], the pleural space [55], the subpleural pulmonary interstitium [54,56] and the pulmonary microvasculature [57]. A new technique was also devised to measure solute and water permeability of parietal mesothelium *in situ* [58].

Permeability characteristics of the pleural mesothelia
Studies on specimens of parietal and visceral mesothelia stripped off the underlying tissues [59,60] in sheep and dogs would suggest that the

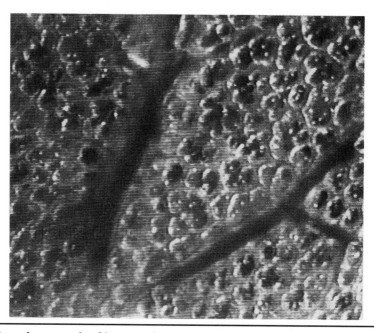

Microphotograph of lung surface viewed through the intact parietal pleura exposed by removal of the intercostal muscles

mesothelia behave as 'non-selective' barriers to water and solutes as large as proteins. Similar conclusions were drawn from experiments aimed at measuring transpleural fluxes in lungs enclosed in an artificial pleural space [61–64]. However, since normal pleural fluid turnover rate is rather slow, these results are not compatible with the physiological evidence that pleural fluid protein concentration is very low. Hence, to measure the mesothelial permeability coefficients in spontaneously breathing mammals under physiological conditions, we devised a new method [58,65,66] which enabled us to determine transpleural fluxes by driving pleural fluid, down a known pressure gradient, from the pleural space into a capsule glued to the exposed parietal pleura.

Solute permeability coefficients were determined for proteins of different molecular mass (albumin, 68 000 Da; lactate dehydrogenase, 140 000 Da and α_2-macroglobulins, 625 000 Da) injected into the pleural space. Permselectivity, pore size and distribution were determined through an analysis previously applied to pulmonary and systemic endothelium [67–70].

Membrane selectivity can be derived from the permeability coefficients to water and to solutes of different size. The coefficients considered in the present analysis are: (1) the reflection coefficient of the membrane with respect to a given solute (σ_d); (2) the solute permeability coefficient (P) and (3) the hydraulic conductivity (L_p).

Transpleural protein flux (J_s) is described by the equation:

$$J_s = J_v (1 - \sigma_d) C_{pl} + PS (C_{pl} - C_c) \frac{x}{e^x - 1} \tag{1}$$

where J_v is the transpleural liquid flux; σ_d is the mesothelial pleural solvent drag reflection coefficient for the protein considered; C_{pl} is the pleural liquid protein concentration; P is the permeability coefficient of mesothelium with respect to a given protein; S is the pleural surface area through which exchange takes place; C_c is the protein concentration of capsular fluid; x is the Peclect number, equal to $J_v(1-\sigma_d)/PS$, a factor accounting for the ratio between convective and diffusional protein fluxes. The first term on the right-hand side of eqn. (1) quantifies protein movements due to convective phenomena through the membrane pores, whereas the second one is the diffusive component depending upon uneven distribution of solute across the membrane. As such, the equation can hardly be solved experimentally, since it is not possible to determine all the parameters simultaneously. However, by imposing high transpleural pressure gradients (~ 30 cmH$_2$O), the diffusive component tends to be nullified when $x/(e^x - 1)$ approaches zero and J_s becomes purely convective so that $J_s = J_v(1-\sigma_d)C_{pl}$. Since J_s, J_v and C_{pl} are known, σ_d for a given protein can be calculated as:

$$\sigma_d = 1 - \frac{C_c}{C_{pl}} \tag{2}$$

The parietal pleura hydraulic conductivity, L_p, can be obtained from the Starling equation for fluid fluxes:

$$J_v = L_p \cdot S\left[(P_{liq} - P_c) - \sigma_d(\pi_{liq} - \pi_c)\right] \tag{3}$$

solved for: $L_p = J_v / \{S[(P_{liq} - P_c) - \sigma_d(\pi_{liq} - \pi_c)]\}$, where P_{liq}, P_c, π_{liq} and π_c are the experimentally measured hydraulic and colloid-osmotic pressures in the pleural and capsular fluid. Colloid-osmotic pressures could also be derived from the experimental regression: $\pi = 4.64C + 0.0027C^2$, where C is total protein concentration in g/dl [71].

Knowledge of σ_d allowed us to determine the equivalent pore radius, r_p, of the parietal pleura; indeed, from hydrodynamic theory of solute drag [18], σ_d relates to the ratio between solute and equivalent pore radius ($\alpha = r_s/r_p$) according to the relationship given in eqn. (4):

$$1 - \sigma = 1 - \frac{16}{3}\alpha^2 + \frac{20}{3}\alpha^3 + \frac{7}{3}\alpha^4 \tag{4}$$

Solution of the above equation allowed us to model protein transport as occurring through two separate populations of pores: large pores allow transit of molecules of 140 000–625 000 Da ($r_p = 157$–223 Å), whereas small pores grant movement of molecules about the size of albumins ($r_p = 83$–90 Å).

Considering pores arranged as parallel cylinders crossing the pleura, the total surface area provided by each pore population is given by:

$$A_p = \frac{L_p 8\eta S \Delta X}{r_p^2} \tag{5}$$

where η is pleural fluid viscosity (assumed to be equal to that of water), S is membrane surface area and ΔX is the thickness of the parietal pleura. Dividing A_p by the area of a single pore yields the number of small and large pores for unit membrane surface area.

The protein permeability coefficients due to large and small pores were determined by solving the relationship:

$$P = \frac{A_p}{S\Delta X} \cdot D_p \phi \tag{6}$$

where D_p is the diffusion coefficient of the protein considered and $\phi = (1 - \alpha)^2$ is the solute partition coefficient depending upon the exclusion of the protein at the pore walls.

The permeability coefficients and pore size and distribution for the parietal pleura in spontaneously breathing rabbits are summarized in Table 1. L_p values ranged from 1.22 to 1.36 μl·h^{-1}·cmH$_2$O^{-1}·cm^{-2} in spontaneously breathing dogs [65,66], and were fourfold higher in isolated portions of the chest wall [58]. σ_d was lower compared with rabbits, being 0.3 for albumin and 0.5 for lactate dehydrogenase [66]. The average total P value in the isolated dog chest preparation was 1×10^{-5} cm/s, higher than that obtained in spontaneously breathing rabbits.

Parameter	Small pores	Large pores	Total	Table 1
L_p ($\mu l \cdot h^{-1} \cdot cmH_2O^{-1} \cdot cm^{-2}$)	1.6; *1.7*	0.58; *0.4*	2.18 ± 1.54	
σ_d (albumin)			0.44 ± 0.2	
σ_d (LDH)			0.84 ± 0.1	
σ_d (α_2-macroglobulin)			0.93 ± 0.05	
Equivalent pore radius (Å)	83; *90*	157; *223*		
Total pore area (cm^2)	0.115; *0.11*	0.012; *0.004*		
Pore number ($10^{-9} \cdot cm^{-2}$)	53; *43*	1.5; *0.26*		
P (albumin) ($10^6 \cdot cm \cdot s^{-1}$)	1.14; *1.06*	0.21; *0.08*	1.35; *1.14*	
P (LDH)	0.23; *0.76*	0.089; *0.065*	0.32; *0.83*	
P (α_2-macroglobulin)	0.007; *0.43*	0.026; *0.01*	0.33; *0.53*	

Hydraulic permeability (L_p), protein reflection coefficient (σ_d), solute permeability coefficient (P) and other parameters describing the permselectivity properties of the parietal pleura

The outcome of the analysis varies according to the solutes radii assumed. Estimates are based on solute radii derived from diffusion coefficients [albumin, 35 Å; lactate dehydrogenase (LDH), 56 Å; α_2-macroglobulin, 89 Å], or from gel filtration (numbers in italics) (albumin, 37 Å; LDH, 42 Å; α_2-macroglobulin, 108 Å).

In the species studied, a low pleural σ_d was associated with a low P. This means that transpleural protein movements take place through populations of relatively large pores that provide little restriction to proteins, but which are few in number (about one-tenth compared with the continuous capillary endothelium [72]) per unit surface area. Accordingly, sieving of plasma proteins through the parietal pleura is as high as that through the continuous capillaries.

The L_p value indicates that the permeability to water is also low, being of the same order of magnitude as that estimated for the endothelium of lung and muscle continuous capillaries, normally considered among the least permeable capillaries of the entire circulatory system [72,73]. These conclusions are at variance with those reached through experimental approaches more distant from physiological conditions, like the isolated stripped pleurae (parietal and visceral) or the artificial pleural space. The most reasonable explanation for such a discrepancy is that the pleural mesothelium is an extremely delicate membrane that can be easily damaged by direct manipulation.

The restriction offered by the parietal pleura to protein movements explains why pleural liquid protein concentration is low (1 g/dl [31,32,71]) and actually lower than the extrapleural interstitial protein concentration (2.5 g/dl [71,74]).

Starling balance of pressures at pleural level

The micropuncture technique enabled us to measure the hydraulic pressure in the pulmonary microvasculature on the lung surface [75]; from the pressure profile shown in Figure 4(a), in intact *in situ* rabbit lung under zone-3 conditions the pulmonary capillary pressure averages 10 cmH$_2$O. These microvascular pressure values differ from those gathered in: (i) open-chest rabbits with lung expanded at an alveolar pressure of 7 cmH$_2$O (zone-2 condition) [76]; (ii) isolated perfused dog lungs maintained in zone-3 condition [77]; and (iii) double occlusion technique in artificially perfused and ventilated dog lungs [78]. This variability may be at least partially due to experimental preparation; indeed, for example, setting left atrial pressure at values higher than physiological ones [77,78] necessarily affects the pressure in all the uphill microvascular segments. Futhermore, the degree of interstitial oedema induced by lung lobe isolation and perfusion might also affect the microvascular pressure distribution [79]. Figure 4(b) shows the percentage pressure drop in the pulmonary circulation corresponding to segmental flow resistance: micropuncture data indicate that about 55% of total pulmonary resistances are encountered in the microvascular district from 60–40 μm arterioles to 30 μm venules; conversely, double

Figure 4

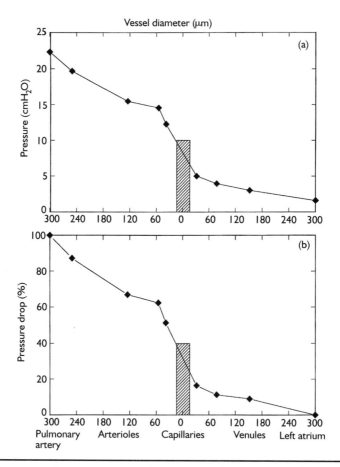

(a) Microvascular pressure profile in the pulmonary circulation in *in situ* rabbit lung and (b) percentage pressure drop across the various vascular segments

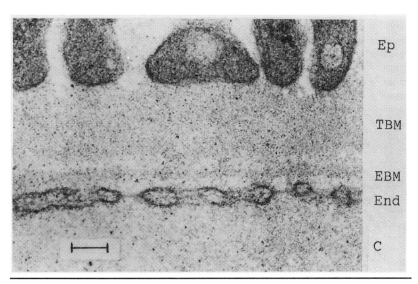

Figure 4

Narrow cortical interstitium between capillary (C) and proximal tubular epithelium (Ep)

Abbreviations: TBM and EBM, tubular and endothelial basement membranes; End, fenestrated capillary endothelium. Bar = 100 nm.

include perivascular interstitium and medulla. A much lower value, about 5%, was obtained for extravascular space on the basis of an albumin blood-to-lymph transit time of 30–40 min [14,15]. While this method excludes the medulla (see below), the distribution space for inulin may well exceed that of albumin.

We have recently made an attempt to determine medullary interstitial volume by measuring the distribution space for aprotinin [16]. Aprotinin is a basic polypeptide (M_r 6500) which is filtered in the glomeruli but completely reabsorbed by the proximal tubules. This means that aprotinin will enter the medulla only through the vasa recta, while no aprotinin reaches the loops of Henle and collecting ducts. In hydropenic rats the average aprotinin distribution space (arterial plasma equivalent space) in the inner medulla was 57%. With a simultaneous albumin space of 23% we arrive at an extravascular space of 34%. This is clearly higher than the anatomical estimates cited above, possibly reflecting enrichment of the positively charged aprotinin in the inner medullary interstitium.

Renal lymphatics and lymph flow

Lymphatics are found along all intrarenal arteries, extending into the loose interstitium around the interlobular arteries and at least in part along the afferent arterioles. The best studies also agree that there are no lymphatics in the medulla, while there are still different opinions about their existence in the cortical labyrinth, i.e. between the tubules in the cortex. While O'Morchoe and co-workers (e.g. [17]) describe intertubular lymphatics in rats and hamsters, but not in rabbits, Kriz [18] has found no such vessels in the rat, but has stressed that there is free communication from the wide cortical interstitia to the loose connective tissue surrounding the interlobular arteries. Anyhow, there is evidence that the renal lymph in part derives from tubular reabsorbate and, if this is so, the anatomical disagreement may not be functionally important.

A more provocative question is: do the renal lymphatics serve any transport function beyond presenting immunological signals through lymph-borne cells? While lymph flow per gram of kidney is high compared with that of many other tissues (e.g. in the rat kidney $0.5-5 \, \mu l \cdot min^{-1} \cdot g^{-1}$), it is less than 1% of the amount of fluid delivered to the interstitium by tubular reabsorption. However, is not removal of plasma protein which is found in lymph at a concentration of about one-third of that in plasma a necessary function?

We do not believe that we have the answer: the medulla has a higher microvascular surface area per gram of tissue than cortex, and uptake of horseradish peroxidase ($r = 25$ Å) and ferritin ($r = 55$ Å) after intravenous or intra-aortic infusion [4,19] makes it highly unlikely that the vasa recta should be impermeable to plasma proteins. Nevertheless, the medulla is doing well without lymph drainage and labelled albumin deposited in the interstitium is rapidly drained off by blood flow in the vasa recta (v.i.). Moreover, renal lymphoedema remains to be described, and attempts to block all renal lymph vessels have apparently not given any consistent picture of their functional importance.

Fluid transport through the cortical interstitium

In a 1 g rat kidney 1 ml of fluid is filtered from glomerular plasma every minute. From the tubular lumina practically all this fluid is reabsorbed through an osmotic pressure created by active tubular cell transport of low-M_r solutes. From the interstitium the fluid is taken up by the peritubular capillaries and vasa recta. In the case of the cortex, there is good evidence that in this step the driving force is the colloid osmotic pressure of peritubular plasma proteins, being concentrated by filtration in the glomeruli. However, direct measurements of all Starling forces are not available because the narrow interstitial spaces between the renal tubules are not accessible even with fine micropipettes. Instead we have to rely on renal lymph for estimating protein concentration and colloid osmotic pressure, and measurement of pressure in implanted porous capsules [20] or by fine polyethylene tubes inserted in the thin atubular subcapsular layer [21]. While interstitial fluid communication has been demonstrated within the cortex, pressure gradients can hardly be excluded. Peritubular capillary pressure is measured by direct micropuncture on the kidney surface and plasma colloid osmotic pressure is calculated from arterial plasma protein concentration and the glomerular filtration fraction.

The most complete data, obtained by Larson *et al.* [22], are visualized in Figure 5, showing a net driving force of 15.4 mmHg — as integrated over the whole capillary length. This is similar to the net

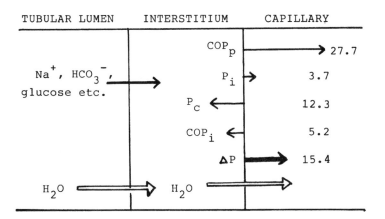

Figure 5

Driving forces for fluid uptake by cortical peritubular capillaries in the normal rat kidney
Abbreviations: COP_p and COP_i, colloid osmotic pressures in plasma and interstitial fluid respectively; P_c and P_i, hydrostatic pressures in plasma and interstitial fluid. Net driving pressure, 15.4 mmHg, integrated along the whole length of the capillary. Based on data from Larson et al. [13]. Reproduced from Aukland et al. [9] with permission from the American Physiological Society.

filtration pressure in glomeruli, indicating that the two sets of capillaries have about the same filtration coefficient per gram of kidney.

While this seems straightforward, under some experimental conditions these 'Starling forces' are clearly not sufficient: Pinter and co-workers (for summary, see [15]) have shown that in old rats lymph protein concentration may exceed that of plasma. However, the capillary absorption will go on in spite of little or no colloid osmotic driving force. Moreover, several groups have shown that reabsorption will go on in the isolated kidneys perfused with colloid-free solutions (for references, see [9]). However, nobody seems to have asked the intriguing question: what can replace plasma colloid osmotic pressure as the driving force for capillary fluid intake? The problem could be somewhat reduced by an increase of the capillary filtration coefficient and by reduction of interstitial fluid protein and colloid osmotic pressure. However, in order to establish a net absorption pressure there seems to be no other solution than the build-up of an interstitial pressure exceeding the capillary pressure by 5–10 mmHg. While this has never been measured, it is well established that the subcapsular pressure rises during saline expansion with lowered plasma protein concentration [22].

The conclusion that a hydrostatic pressure gradient from the interstitium to the peritubular capillary lumen can take over the role of plasma oncotic pressure has two interesting consequences. First, it might prevent entrance of macromolecules from the plasma to the interstitium and, secondly, it requires some mechanism to prevent collapse of the capillaries.

Uptake of ferritin from capillary plasma

Plasma proteins are assumed to enter the interstitium by diffusion through a small number of large pores in the capillary wall. The protein reflection coefficient across these pores is so low that the oncotic gradient is insufficient to counteract the capillary–interstitial hydrostatic pressure gradient. As shown schematically in Figure 6, fluid flow in the large pores may even be directed from plasma to interstitium [23]. Under protein-free perfusion, however, the higher hydrostatic pressure in the interstitium should create fluid absorption in the wide pores also, tending to oppose protein transport from plasma to interstitium.

In order to test this hypothesis we perfused rat kidneys with either 5% or 0.1% bovine serum albumin, adding ferritin for periods of 3–30 min before fixation and electron microscopy. Uptake of ferritin was found in both narrow and wide interstitium in all rats perfused with 5% albumin, whereas only two out of five kidneys perfused with 0.1% albumin showed some uptake. While the semi-quantitative estimates shown in Table 1 do not provide statistically significant differences, the results fit well with the hypothesis of reversal of the transcapillary hydrostatic pressure gradient and flow direction in the large pores during 'protein-free' perfusion. This will clearly contribute to removal of plasma protein from the interstitium.

Figure 6

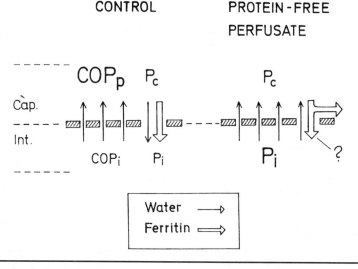

Hypothesis for interstitial uptake of ferritin from peritubular capillaries

Left-hand panel: the normally higher colloid osmotic pressure of plasma (COP_p) than that of interstitial fluid (COP_i) absorbs fluid through small pores impermeable to plasma proteins, but not through large permeable pores. In the latter, fluid flows into the interstitium because hydrostatic pressure in the capillary (P_c) exceeds that of the interstitium (P_i), and thereby adds to diffusive transport of the large ferritin molecules. Right-hand panel: during protein-free perfusion the hydrostatic pressure gradient and fluid direction in the large pores is reversed and will now tend to oppose diffusion of ferritin into the interstitium.

BSA, 50 g/l	BSA, 1 g/l	Table 1
+++*	++	
+++	+	
+++	0	
++	0	
	0	

Interstitial uptake of ferritin in nine rat kidneys perfused with bovine serum albumin (50 or 1 g/l)
Semi-quantitative estimate of interstitial ferritin concentration, +++ corresponding to about one-third of plasma concentration. Observations by Aukland et al. [9].

Compression of the peritubular capillaries?

The glomerular filtration rate and fractional tubular reabsorption is usually considerably reduced during protein-free perfusion. Nevertheless, a rough estimate assuming unaltered capillary hydraulic conductivity indicates that the hydrostatic pressure in the interstitium must exceed that in the peritubular capillaries by 5–10 mmHg in order to take care of the tubular reabsorbate.

If, however, the hydraulic conductivity is reduced by a factor of 2–3, as estimated by Larson et al. [22] after saline expansion (10% of body weight), a pressure gradient of 2–4 mmHg might be sufficient. The latter estimate depends strongly on the assumption that the pressure measured in the atubular layer under the renal capsule is equal to the interstitial pressure between the tubules. Especially at high pressure, fluid leakage along the subcapsular catheter might easily give too low a pressure, leading to an overestimate of the filtration coefficient. Moreover, intrarenal extravascular pressure gradients are not excluded. Anyhow, it seems *a priori* unlikely that the 25–100 nm-thick and densely fenestrated endothelial cells should *per se* have enough rigidity to withstand this compressive force. However, if collapse did occur, cessation or a great reduction of blood flow would immediately reduce the pressure gradient in precapillary vessels, increase capillary pressure and distend the capillary, but now with a luminal pressure that would stop fluid reabsorption. Continued fluid delivery from the tubules would increase interstitial pressure even more, capillary pressure would in turn increase, and the outcome of these escalating pressures would probably be a self-strangulation as in a compartment syndrome, with cessation or a great reduction of blood flow.

Clearly, the surroundings of the capillaries must in some way prevent collapse. In the areas where the peritubular capillary is closely apposed to the tubules through the thin interstitium, it seems likely that fibrils between the tubular and capillary basement membranes would prevent expansion of the interstitium. This fits well with the finding of equal width of the narrow interstitium during perfusion with or without protein [9]. One might in fact just as well envisage the transport as a direct filtration from the basolateral tubular infoldings into the capillary lumen. However, this easy way out clearly does not apply to the wide interstitium, which probably receives about two-thirds of the reabsorbed fluid. Here we must assume that the sustentacular cells with their attachments to tubular and capillary basement membranes, as well as the interstitial fibrils, will contribute to prevention of expansion of the interstitium and keeping the capillaries open. Such tethering is consistent with the finding of unchanged interstitial fluid volume during saline infusion and a subcapsular pressure increased from 3.7 to 12 mmHg [13].

At this point it may be pertinent to emphasize that the normal driving force for peritubular fluid uptake in the renal cortex is the osmotic pressure of the plasma proteins and not a hydrostatic pressure gradient. However, as discussed in a recent review [9], automatic adjustment of interstitial pressure may provide an efficient and extremely rapid buffering of any change in tubular fluid reabsorption or plasma colloid osmotic pressure.

Fluid and protein reabsorption by the vasa recta

The fluid reabsorbed from the collecting ducts in the concentrating process is generally assumed to be drained off through the vasa recta. However, the transcapillary Starling forces in the medulla are even less accessible than in the cortex. The most comprehensive experimental and model studies have been performed by R.L. Jamison and T.L. Pallone and their respective co-workers (for references see [24–26]).

On the basis of (i) the finding that NaCl gradients in the ascending limb of the vasa recta do not contribute appreciably to water uptake [25,26], (ii) measured values for vasa recta plasma hydrostatic and oncotic pressures, and (iii) an assumed 'reasonable' value for interstitial pressure, they concluded that the interstitial protein concentration and oncotic pressure must be low. This is consistent with the findings that protein tracers do gain access to the interstitium, but in spite of a large anatomical interstitial space [8] and a large distribution volume for aprotinin [16], several studies have failed to measure any extravascular albumin distribution space in the papilla, while some studies suggest appreciable amounts of extravascular albumin in the inner medulla [27–29]. Now, if protein diffuses out from the vasa recta down a large concentration gradient, how can the interstitial concentration be kept low? Or, to rephrase the question, how is albumin removed from the interstitium in the absence of lymph drainage? Recent unpublished studies in our laboratory showed that ^{125}I-albumin delivered to the papillary interstitium at an infusion rate of 5 nl/min was rapidly drained off by renal venous blood, while less than 0.5% appeared in renal lymph. Moreover, injection of Evans Blue–albumin gave no visual evidence for interstitial transport towards the cortex. Thus it appears that albumin has to enter the vasa recta by bulk flow through pores large enough to admit albumin molecules. Since neither oncotic nor hydrostatic interstitial pressures are known, some speculations on the driving force may be excusable.

(1) A high interstitial pressure, exceeding capillary pressure, might easily build up by fluid absorption from the collecting ducts,

driven by a large small-solute osmotic pressure gradient. The recent finding by McPhee and Michel [30] that the vasa recta can withstand an interstitial to lumen pressure gradient of $+3$ mmHg, possibly assisted by the stellate interstitial cells, indicates that the hypothesis should not be *a priori* rejected, even if it implies an interstitial pressure of at least 10 mmHg compared with the 3–4 mmHg measured in the cortex.

(2) Alternatively, and maybe more likely, the high plasma oncotic pressure might cause bulk flow through large pores, carrying with it protein from the interstitium [31]. In the general circulation this 'bootstrap mechanism' [32] has the disadvantage that the protein concentration in the reabsorbate will always be lower than that of interstitial fluid. Accordingly, it will tend to increase interstitial protein concentrations and therefore has to be assisted by lymph drainage. In the renal medulla, which contains no lymph vessels, this drawback may well be compensated by the diluting effect of protein-free fluid delivered from the collecting ducts. In fact, in order to maintain some protein concentration in the medullary interstitium one may even have to postulate periodic diffusional loss through the large-pore system, for instance caused by variation in interstitial pressure induced by pelvic contraction [33], or by diffusion through extra large pores with a low reflection coefficient.

Concluding remarks

While the architecture and composition of the renal interstitium seem well described, quantitative data on *in vivo* spaces and pressures are still uncertain or incomplete. The first step in the reabsorption of glomerular filtrate, from the tubular lumen to the interstitium, has been studied by a large number of investigators, in principle agreeing that fluid is driven by a small-solute osmotic pressure gradient, created by active tubular transport mechanisms. The last transport step, capillary fluid uptake from the interstitium, has received less attention, and is less accessible for study, especially in the medulla where the nature of the driving force is still unresolved. Obviously, the kind of speculations presented above do not solve any problems, but might hopefully stimulate interest and experimental attacks.

References

1. Kaissling, B. and LeHir, M. (1994) Characterization and distribution of interstitial cell types in the renal cortex of rats. *Kidney Int.* **45**, 709–720
2. Takahashi-Iwanaga, H. (1991) The three-dimensional cytoarchitecture of the interstitial tissue in the rat kidney. *Cell. Tissue Res.* **264**, 269–281
3. Lemley, K.V. and Kriz, W. (1991) Anatomy of the renal interstitium. *Kidney Int.* **39**, 370–381
4. Langer, K.H. (1975) Niereninterstitium: Feinstrukturen und Kapillarpermeabilität I-III. *Cytobiologie* **10**, 161–216
5. Desjardins, M. and Bendayan, M. (1989) Heterogenous distribution of type IV collagen, entactin, heparan sulfate proteoglycan, and laminin among renal basement membranes as demonstrated by quantitative immunocytochemistry. *J. Histochem. Cytochem.* **37**, 885–897
6. Öjteg, G. and Wolgast, M. (1993) Charge density of renal interstitium. *Acta Physiol. Scand.* **147**, 297–303
7. Pedersen, J.C., Persson, A.E.G. and Maunsbach, A.B. (1980) Ultrastructure and quantitative characterization of the cortical interstitium in the rat kidney. In *Functional Ultrastructure of the Kidney* (Maunsbach, A.B., Steen Olsen, T. and Christensen, E.I., eds.), pp. 443–456, Academic Press, London

8. Pfaller, W. (1982) Structure function correlation on rat kidney. *Adv. Anat. Embryol. Cell. Biol.* **70**, 1–106
9. Aukland, K., Bogusky, R.T. and Renkin, E.M. (1994) Renal cortical interstitium and fluid absorption by peritubular capillaries. *Am. J. Physiol.* **266**, F175–F184
10. Kriz, W. and Napiwotzky, P. (1979) Structural and functional aspects of the renal interstitium. *Contr. Nephrol.* **16**, 104–108
11. Knepper, M.A., Danielson, R.A., Saidel, G.M. and Post, R.S. (1977) Quantitative analysis of renal medullary anatomy in rats and rabbits. *Kidney Int.* **12**, 313–323
12. Gärtner, K. (1966) Das Volumen der interstitiellen Flüssigkeit der Niere bei énderungen ihres hämodynamischen Widerstandes; Untersuchungen an Kaninchen. *Pflügers Arch.* **292**, 1–12
13. Larson, M., Sjöquist, M. and Wolgast, M. (1984) Renal interstitial volume of the rat kidney. *Acta Physiol. Scand.* **120**, 297–304
14. Bell, D.R., Pinter, G.G. and Wilson, P.D. (1978) Albumin permeability of the peritubular capillaries in rat renal cortex. *J. Physiol. (London)* **279**, 621–640
15. Pinter, G.G. (1988) Renal lymph: vital for the kidney and valuable for the physiologist. *News Physiol. Sci.* **3**, 189–193
16. Hestholm, F., Tenstad, O. and Aukland, K. (1993) Extracellular space in the inner renal medulla. *Acta Physiol. Scand.* **149**, 30A
17. Niiro, G.K., Jarosz, H.M., O'Morchoe, P.J. and O'Morchoe, C.C.C. (1986) The renal cortical lymphatic system in the rat, hamster and rabbit. *Am. J. Anat.* **177**, 21–34
18. Kriz, W. (1987) A periarterial pathway for intrarenal distribution of renin. *Kidney Int.* **31** (Suppl. 20), S51–S56
19. Venkatachalam, M.A. and Karnowsky, M.J. (1972) Extravascular protein in the kidney. An ultrastructural study of its relation to renal peritubular capillary permeability using protein tracers. *Lab. Invest.* **27**, 435–444
20. Ott, C.E., Navar, L.G. and Guyton, A.C. (1971) Pressures in static and dynamic states from capsules implanted in the kidney. *Am. J. Physiol.* **221**, 394–400
21. Wunderlich, P., Persson, E., Schnermann, J., Ulfendahl, H. and Wolgast, M. (1971) Hydrostatic pressure in the subcapsular interstitial space of rat and dog kidneys. *Pflügers Arch.* **328**, 307–319
22. Larson, M., Hermansson, K. and Wolgast, M. (1983) Hydraulic permeability of the peritubular and glomerular capillary membranes in the rat kidney. *Acta Physiol. Scand.* **117**, 251–261
23. Wolgast, M. (1985) Renal interstitium and lymphatics. In *The Kidney: Physiology and Pathophysiology* (Seldin, D.W. and Giebisch, G., eds.), vol. 1, pp. 497–517, Raven Press, New York
24. Pallone, T.L., Morgenthaler, T.I. and Deen, W.M. (1984) Analysis of microvascular water and solute exchanges in the renal medulla. *Am. J. Physiol.* **247**, F303–F315
25. Pallone, T.L. (1991) Transport of sodium chloride and water in rat ascending vasa recta. *Am. J. Physiol.* **261**, F519–F525
26. Pallone, T.L., Yagil, Y. and Jamison, R.L. (1989) Effect of small-solute gradients on transcapillary fluid movement in renal inner medulla. *Am. J. Physiol.* **257**, F547–F553
27. Pinter, G.G. (1967) Distribution of chylomicrons and albumin in dog kidney. *J. Physiol. (London)* **192**, 761–772
28. Rasmussen, S.N. and Iversen, P. (1976) The extravascular pool of albumin in the non-diuretic rat kidney estimated by means of radioactive tracers and quantitative immunochemistry. *Pflügers Arch.* **363**, 239–244
29. Rasmussen, S.N. (1978) Red cell and plasma volume flows to the inner medulla of the rat kidney. *Pflügers Arch.* **373**, 153–159
30. McPhee, P.J. and Michel, C.C. (1992) Microvascular closing pressures in the renal medulla of anesthetized rats and in the mesentery of pithed frogs. *Int. J. Microcirc. Clin. Exp.* **2** (Suppl. 1), S78
31. Casley-Smith, J.R. (1975) A theoretical support for the transport of macromolecules by osmotic flow across a leaky membrane against a concentration gradient. *Microvasc. Res.* **9**, 43–48
32. Perl, W. (1975) Convection and permeation of albumin between plasma and interstitium. *Microvasc. Res.* **10**, 83–94
33. Schmidt-Nielsen, B. and Graves, B. (1982) Changes in fluid compartments in hamster renal papilla due to peristalsis in the pelvic wall. *Kidney Int.* **22**, 613–625

Physiology and biophysics of synovial extracellular matrix-capillary system

J.R. Levick* and J.N. McDonald
Department of Physiology, St George's Hospital Medical School,
London SW17 0RE, U.K.

Overview

The synovial joint (Figure 1) is an organ in which extracellular matrix attains particular functional importance, because it not only determines the properties of articular cartilage (see Chapter 5 by Maroudas *et al.*) but also the permeability of the synovial lining, which is responsible for the formation and absorption of synovial fluid. Synovial fluid is vital to joint function, both as a source of nutrition for the avascular articular cartilage and as a lubricant during joint motion, and the fluid is continually being absorbed and replaced by the joint lining.

The synovial lining (synovium) is about 20 μm thick (rabbit knee) to 60 μm (human knee), and the three key elements of synovium involved in fluid turnover are shown in Figure 1. They are the synovial capillary, the synovial interstitium and the lymphatic drainage system.

Capillaries

The thin synovial lining contains a row of capillaries about 5 μm (rabbit knee) to 30 μm (human knee) beneath the surface. Capillary density is high (700–800 mm^{-2} section in rabbit, 240 mm^{-2} in human knee [1]) and many of the capillary profiles bear patches of fenestrations. These 50 nm-diameter, membrane-spanned windows through the endothelium are regions of high permeability to water and small solutes [2], though not to plasma proteins [3]. Fenestrations are generally located on the half of the capillary facing the joint cavity, and along with the high capillary density and superficial location they represent structural adaptations for synovial fluid formation. Synovial fluid is formed primarily by passive ultrafiltration of plasma across the fenestral membranes, driven by a net imbalance in the 'Starling pressures' acting across the membrane. The Starling pressure imbalance is the pressure drop from plasma to synovial interstitium minus the difference in effective colloidal osmotic pressure (COP) across the capillary wall, which is due to the unequal concentration of plasma protein on the two sides. The influence of capillary pressure, plasma COP and intra-articular pressure (IAP) on net trans-synovial flow have all been studied by direct experiment and reviewed previously [4,5]. The influence of intra-articular colloids, however, has only recently been reported and is the main theme of this chapter.

---

*To whom correspondence should be addressed.

Figure 1

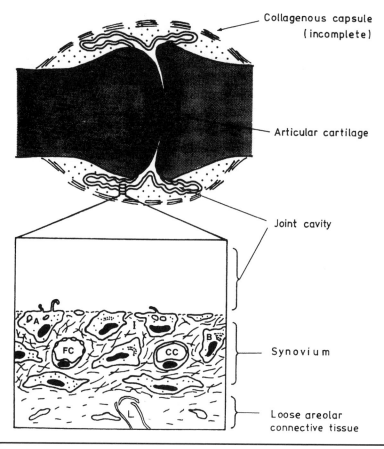

Collagenous capsule (incomplete)

Articular cartilage

Joint cavity

Synovium

Loose areolar connective tissue

Sketch of saggital section through a synovial joint, with synovium enlarged to show lining A cells (macrophages) and B cells (fibroblast-like), naked interstitium at the surface (I), fenestrated and continuous capillary profiles (FC, CC), and subsynovial initial lymphatic vessel (L)

Plasma ultrafiltrate is the raw material for synovial fluid formation and accounts for most of its constituents, but to it the synovial lining cells then add the glycosaminoglycan hyaluronan and smaller amounts of the glycoprotein lubricin by active secretion, to produce the final viscous, lubricating, synovial fluid [6].

Synovial interstitium

The pathway into the joint cavity from the outer surface of the capillary, and from the joint cavity to lymphatic vessels in the subsynovium, is an intercellular one several micrometres wide passing between a discontinuous layer of cell bodies and processes (Figure 2). The lining cells comprise macrophage-like A cells and fibroblast-like B cells [6]. The interstitial pathway contains a complex fibrous matrix in open contact with intra-articular fluid (see Figures 2 and 15). The matrix comprises type-I, III and V collagen fibrils, type-VI microfibrils, hyaluronan, chondroitin and heparan sulphate proteoglycans (including

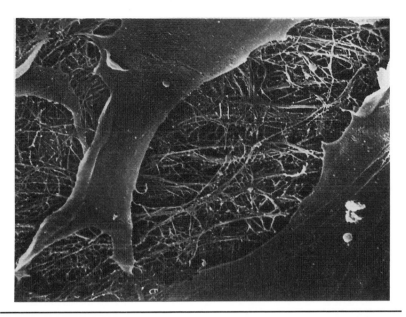

Figure 2

Scanning electron micrograph of the synovial surface in rabbit knee, showing two cell processes and intervening fibrous interstitium in direct contact with synovial fluid
Scale bar = 2 μm.

decorin and biglycan) and glycoproteins such as fibronectin. The hydraulic conductivity of the matrix has been estimated from pressure–flow relations and morphometric data, and appears to be low, in the order of $10^{-11}\,\mathrm{cm^4 \cdot s^{-1} \cdot dyn^{-1}}$ [7,8]. The low conductivity presumably helps to reduce the rate of escape of the vital intra-articular fluid when joint pressure is raised, for example during acute flexion of a joint.

Synovial lymphatic system
A plexus of lymphatic end-vessels is found in the subsynovium close to the border with the synovium, and this drains away fluid and macromolecules escaping from the joint cavity [9,10]. The subsynovium itself comprises loose areolar tissue over substantial areas of the joint, and fatty or fibrous tissue in other regions. Areolar subsynovium connects with surrounding connective-tissue planes and, like areolar tissue elsewhere (see Chapter 11 by Guyton), is thought to act as a highly compliant, low-pressure, quasi-infinite sink for fluid when fluid is driven into it, as in the experiments described later.

Effect of joint motion
A major factor affecting net flow across the synovial interstitium, besides the capillary blood pressure and plasma COP, is the pressure of the intra-articular fluid. This opposes capillary filtration by raising pericapillary interstitial pressure, and it also directly promotes interstitial flow from joint cavity to subsynovium. Movement of a joint has a marked effect on synovial fluid pressure, as Figure 3 shows, and is

Figure 3

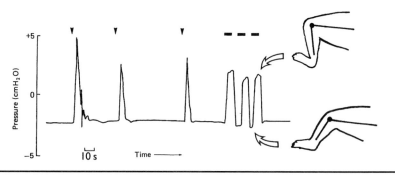

Effect of joint angle on intra-articular pressure (IAP) in the normal knee of a lightly anaesthetized rabbit
Commencing with the joint in extension (subatmospheric IAP), flexion raised IAP above atmospheric pressure. Arrowheads indicate active flexion reflex to heel pinch. Bars indicate passive flexion from 110° to 75°. Much higher pressures, 25 cmH₂O or more, are generated by flexion in the presence of joint effusions.

therefore an important factor in fluid exchange. Flexion of a normal joint, either actively or passively, can raise IAP to several cmH$_2$O above atmospheric pressure, whereas in extension IAP is a few cmH$_2$O subatmospheric. At subatmospheric pressures, net flow is often into the joint cavity, and at higher pressures net flow is out of the cavity in non-inflamed joints [4,5].

Effect of intra-articular albumin on trans-synovial flow

It has long been known that raising IAP increases the rate of seepage of fluid out of the joint cavity through the lining's interstitium, and that the pressure–flow relationship grows steeper at pathological joint pressures due to a fall in synovial hydraulic resistance (see [11] and Figures 13 and 14 later). Only recently, however, has there been any systematic investigation of how macromolecules in synovial fluid affect trans-synovial flow. The principal intra-articular macromolecules are albumin, the most abundant plasma protein in synovial fluid (normal concentration 40–45% of that in plasma), responsible for most of the COP of synovial fluid; and hyaluronan (around $3 \, g \cdot l^{-1}$), which dominates the viscosity of synovial fluid. Albumin is a virtually ubiquitous component of interstitial fluid throughout the body, and its effect on interstitial flow is therefore of general interest; yet there has been remarkably little direct experimental study of albumin's local effect on the process of interstitial flow. The synovial joint, whose cavity is in open contact with a defined area of interstitium, offers a possibly unique opportunity to study this experimentally.

Albumin has two physiologically important effects on the physical properties of a solution; it raises the solution's COP, and it also raises the solution's viscosity modestly, both relationships being curvilinear. To study how these changes affect interstitial fluid kinetics, two cannulae were inserted into the joint cavity of the rabbit knee under anaesthesia — one to record IAP, and the other to infuse albumin solution and thereby manipulate synovial interstitial fluid composition. The height of the open, gravity-fed infusion reservoir controlled IAP, and an in-line drop counter recorded the rate of absorption of the infusate. Flows were measured in the steady state and a small correction was applied for viscous creep of the cavity walls. The absorbed fluid passes mostly into the subsynovium by a process of interstitial flow, but transcapillary flow is involved too, as will emerge. In experiments like that in Figure 4, albumin solutions of various concentrations were infused alternately with Krebs solution for 15 min or more, the joint space being flushed out three times with each fresh infusate. Because there was some variation in control flow (zero albumin), the trans-synovial flow of albumin solution was expressed as a fraction of that of Krebs solution interpolated to the same point in time (Figure 4; 'fractional flow').

   The effect of albumin on fractional flow is plotted as a function of the relative fluidity of the intra-articular liquid in Figure 5. Fluidity (ψ) is the reciprocal of viscosity (η), and the reason for choosing this form of plot relates to Darcy's law; that is for flow ($\dot{Q}$) through a rigid macroscopic porous medium (e.g. gravel):

$$\dot{Q} = \kappa\,(\mathrm{d}P/\mathrm{d}x)\,(A/\eta) = \psi\kappa A\,(\mathrm{d}P/\mathrm{d}x) \tag{1}$$

where κ is specific hydraulic conductivity. It can be seen that, when the flow of a solution is divided by that of solvent, the fractional flow equals relative fluidity, provided that the pressure gradient, $\mathrm{d}P/\mathrm{d}x$, and bed

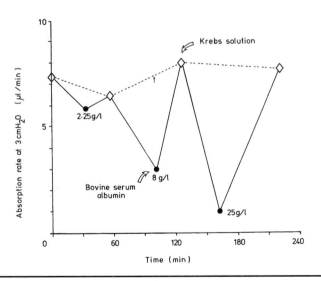

Figure 4

Effect of infused albumin on steady-state net trans-synovial flow (fluid absorption rate) in the rabbit knee
Infusions of albumin solution (●) and Krebs solution (◇) were alternated, the joint cavity being flushed three times upon changing infusates. The small arrow shows how the control value was interpolated.

Figure 5

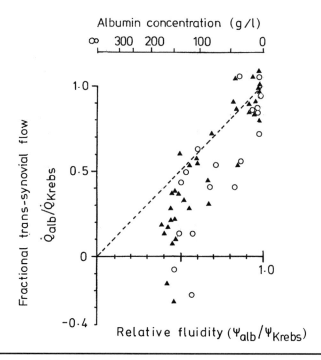

Albumin concentration (g/l)

Trans-synovial flow of albumin solution, expressed as a fraction of control flow of Krebs solution ($\dot{Q}_{alb}/\dot{Q}_{Krebs}$), plotted as a function of the intra-articular relative fluidity ψ_{alb}/ψ_{Krebs} measured on aspirates $\bigcirc$, *IAP = 3 cmH$_2$O (five joints);* $\blacktriangle$, *IAP = 6 cmH$_2$O (five joints). The broken line of the slope depicts Darcy's law for flow through a macroscopic porous medium or tube, where flow is linearly proportional to fluidity. Reproduced from [17] with permission.*

area, *A*, are constant. The line of equality in Figure 5 thus serves as a guide as to whether the results are simply obeying Darcy's law. This is evidently not the case. At a constant IAP of 3 or 6 cmH$_2$O, the reduction in net trans-synovial flow by albumin *in vivo* greatly exceeded the reduction in the permeating liquid's fluidity; indeed, at very high concentrations net flow even reversed direction to net filtration into the cavity. The deviation below the Darcy line was due to enhancement of capillary filtration by the interstitial fluid's COP (Starling's principle), the increased filtration then partially or wholly counteracting interstitial drainage from the joint cavity. This explanation was confirmed by experiments *post mortem*, but before describing these, two other illuminating features *in vivo* must be considered.

Is the pericapillary interstitial COP the same as that of bulk interstitium?

The first of the features just referred to is that the reduction in net trans-synovial outflow by intra-articular albumin was less marked than might be predicted from the known effect of intravascular albumin on trans-synovial flow [12]; if one were to assume that the pericapillary albumin concentration in the present experiments was the same as in the joint cavity 5 μm away, a steeper effect than that observed would be expected. This led us to consider the possibility that albumin concentration in the immediate pericapillary space might be less than in the joint cavity in these experiments. This was supported by modelling studies (see below) and is of significance in that it is often assumed that interstitial fluid sampled some distance from the capillary wall represents the composition of the fluid immediately around the porous regions of a capillary. This point is returned to later.

Evidence for simultaneous bidirectional flow across the lining

The second interesting feature, referred to earlier, was that when joint fluid was aspirated for analysis after 15 min of continuous infusion (the latter always preceded by a triple flush), its albumin concentration was found to be lower than that being infused (Figure 6). Moreover, the higher the infused concentration, the greater was the fractional intra-articular dilution. Also, the lower the IAP and hence net outflow, the greater was the dilution. These features lead us to postulate that an internal circulation of fluid might be occurring, along the lines shown in the inset to Figure 6. Pericapillary albumin, acting osmotically, should increase the rate of capillary ultrafiltration into the joint cavity, leading to intra-articular dilution. At the same time a net outflow could occur if outflow through the interstitial pathway parallel to and some distance from the capillary were greater in magnitude than the capillary filtration rate. For this explanation to work, however, albumin would have to diffuse continuously against the filtration stream in order to reach the pericapillary region and sustain an enhanced capillary filtration rate. The question arises, is this feasible, taking into account the local albumin diffusion coefficient and the size of the opposing local fluid velocities? To answer this question, a transport model was developed.

Interaction of interstitial albumin and the filtration stream

To address the above issue quantitatively, a two-dimensional mathematical model for trans-synovial flow was constructed, based on a detailed morphometric study of synovial structure. The structure of the lining, with its row of capillaries just below the surface (Figure 7, top), lends itself to modelling, although anatomical heterogeneity was perforce neglected. A basic repeating unit, a half-capillary with an orientated fenestral cluster and a neighbouring tissue domain, formed the core of the model (Figure 7, middle). Estimates of key parameters such as capillary wall conductance and interstitial hydraulic resistance were available from previous work. The tissue was subdivided into tiny cubic elements of tissue, and the solute flux across each face was calculated using the non-linear equation of Patlak et al. [13], which combines convective and diffusional solute transport. Each minute cube of

Figure 6

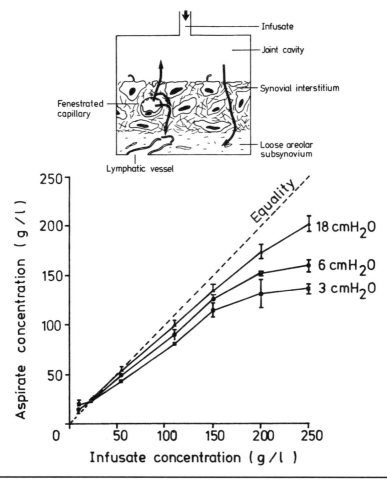

Albumin concentration in a joint cavity of the rabbit knee after continuous infusion for 15 min preceded by a triple flush, plotted as a function of infused concentration (mean ± S.E.M.)
Results at three different IAPs are shown. Inset shows a proposed explanation based on net trans-synovial flux comprising two oppositely directed flows. Adapted from [28].

interstitial matrix was treated as a leaky porous membrane with a finite concentration and pressure drop across it, and a local hydraulic resistance, partial albumin exclusion, albumin reflection coefficient, and restriction to diffusion. All of these material properties were related to glycosaminoglycan concentration, using random-fibre matrix theory (Table 1). An important difference from other interstitial transport models was the incorporation of an interstitial reflection coefficient to albumin (based on the degree of steric exclusion and hence on matrix concentration). This affected not only solute flux but also interstitial water flow, because a small effective interstitial osmotic pressure then resulted from any local difference in interstitial albumin concentration. The effect of albumin on interstitial fluid viscosity was also modelled

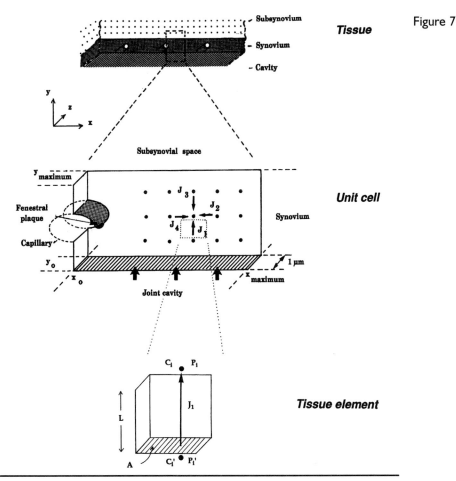

Figure 7

Tissue

Unit cell

Tissue element

Two-dimensional model upon which net flux calculations were based
*Note that the orientation is inverted compared with Figures 1 and 6 to make
the y-axis positive. Synovial lining in situ (top) was subdivided into identical unit
cells (middle), and the unit cell was further subdivided into tiny blocks
(bottom). Abbreviations: J, flux of water or albumin in given direction; P_i and C_i,
interstitial pressure and protein concentration respectively at defined point; A
and L, surface area and length of each tiny tissue element. Reproduced from [8]
with permission.*

(see later), as was discrete (localized) capillary hydraulic permeability.
The common modelling assumption of uniform permeation of water
across the capillary perimeter was shown to result in significant errors, at
least for this tissue.

The model solutions made several useful contributions.

(i) Modelling support for simultaneous bidirectional flow across the lining

An example of the solution for a certain set of boundary conditions is
shown in Figure 8. Over the synovial surface as a whole, a net outflow

Table 1

Property	Key biophysical relations*	References/assumptions
Hydraulic conductance	$k_i = \kappa_i/\eta_i L$ ($\kappa = 1.6 \times 10^{-18} \cdot \theta^{-2.3}$)	[30]
	$K_{AV} = \exp[-(\theta/r_f^2)(r_f + r_s)]$	[20,31]
	($\phi = K_{AV}/e^{-\theta}$)	
Reflection coefficient	$\sigma_i = (1 - \phi)^2$	[29,31]
Effective viscosity	$\eta_i = f(\eta_{bulk}, \phi, r_s)$	[23]; particle-in-tube method
Water flow	$J_v = k_i(\Delta P_i - \sigma_i \Delta \pi_i)$	[32]
Restricted diffusion	$D_{res} = D \cdot \exp[-(\theta/r_f^2)^{0.5}(r_f + r_s)]$	[33]
Albumin transport by diffusion and convection	$J_s = f(\Delta C_i, Pec)$ where $Pec = J_v(1 - \sigma_i)/M_i A$	Non-linear transport; [13]

Biophysical aspects of interstitial transport

The properties of the extracellular matrix are governed primarily by the concentration of interstitial biopolymers, especially glycosaminoglycan, whose volume fraction is θ. Key to symbols: A, area; C, concentration; D_{res}, restricted diffusion coefficient within matrix; J, transport rate; K_{AV}, fraction of extrafibrillar water space available to solute; k, hydraulic conductance of unit area of material; L, length of path; M, diffusional permeability; Pec, Peclet number; r, radius of solute or bipolymer chain; ΔP_i, pressure difference across a small element of tissue; θ, volume fraction occupied by a component; ϕ, solute partition coefficient in extrafibrillar space; η, viscosity; κ, specific hydraulic conductivity of a material; π, colloid osmotic pressure due to plasma protein (oncotic pressure); σ, osmotic reflection coefficient. Subscripts: f, fibre (molecular chain); i, interstitium; s, solute; v, volume.

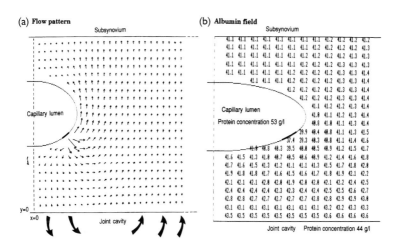

Figure 8

Predicted bidirectional pattern of flow across a synovial interface with joint cavity (a) and corresponding interstitial albumin concentrations (b; x-axis expanded for clarity)

Boundary conditions: IAP, 6 cmH$_2$O; subsynovial pressure, atmospheric; intra-articular albumin concentration, 44 g·l^{-1}; capillary pressure = plasma COP. (a) Thin arrows are flow vectors; flow into cavity 0.2 μl·min^{-1}, flow out of cavity 10.7 μl·min^{-1}, capillary filtration fraction 0.044. Larger inflow/outflow ratios occur upon raising intra-articular albumin concentration or lowering IAP. (b) Numbers represent concentrations in available, non-excluded interstitial water. Note the substantial dilution immediately around the filtering fenestral plaque (thickened line). Over the capillary, albumin is diffusing out of the cavity against the inward filtration stream. Reproduced from [8] with permission.

due to flow through interstitium distant from the capillary was predicted; but in addition there was a smaller local inflow through the interstitium immediately over the capillaries, caused by capillary filtration, and this gave rise to intra-articular dilution. It was shown that the experimental observations on intra-articular dilution could be explained quantitatively in this way (see Figure 9b). The bidirectional interstitial flow pattern is thought to be functionally important, because it provides a mechanism by which synovial fluid can turn over even in a stationary joint where IAP is not varying, provided that the joint angle is such that IAP is greater than subsynovial pressure.

(ii) Modelling support for perifenestral reduction of interstitial COP

Because most of the hydraulic permeability of the capillary is concentrated into very small, geometrically discrete areas (the fenestral plaques here; intercellular junctions in continuous capillaries), the velocity of the filtration stream at these points is orders of magnitude higher than if water escaped at a uniform rate around the entire perimeter of the capillary. The high water velocity at the pore exits tends to wash protein molecules away from the exits, reducing the local concentration of interstitial plasma protein around the exits from the fenestral small-pore system (Figure 8b). Perifenestral protein concentration is maintained at a certain fraction of that in the bulk phase by diffusion against the ultrafiltration stream, down the locally steepened concentration gradient. As a result of the standing pericapillary concentration gradient, a given intra-articular concentration of albumin has less effect on capillary filtration rate than does intracapillary albumin, as noted earlier.

In the experimental situation being modelled here, the main source of interstitial albumin was the intra-articular cavity and infusion line, an obviously unnatural situation. The question arises whether perifenestral gradients of similar nature might occur under normal conditions. To answer this, we must consider the normal route(s) by which plasma protein enters the interstitium. The fenestral membrane itself has a high protein reflection coefficient (0.8 for albumin, [3]) and it is generally accepted that much of the extravascular plasma protein, especially the larger species, enters the interstitium via the capillary large-pore system [14]. There is controversy as to whether the large-pore system comprises a vesicular transport system and/or continuous large apertures, but it is sufficient to note here that in either event much protein enters the interstitium at regions spatially separate and removed from the site of fenestral filtration. It follows therefore that perifenestral gradients along the lines shown in Figure 8 may also occur under normal conditions. Thus, mean interstitial COP measured a few micrometres from the capillary wall can under some circumstances mis-estimate the COP around the capillary small-pore system, where COP matters most from the point of view of Starling balance. It is thus possible that the substantial 'buffering' of fluid filtration by changes in bulk interstitial COP, described in Chapter 4 by A.E. Taylor and co-workers and Chapter 11 by Guyton, may even be underestimates of the magnitude of osmotic buffering, especially in fenestrated tissues. The above findings also lead one to conclude that mathematical models that assume a uniform capillary hydraulic permeability, and therefore falsely low fluid velocities at the small pore, require cautious interpretation.

Experimental results for intra-articular dilution and for the effect of albumin on fractional flow are compared with model predictions in Figure 9. The set of model curves covers various alternative scenarios concerning heterogeneity of interstitial glycosaminoglycan and capillary distribution. The predictions broadly follow the data, which themselves show considerable scatter.

Interstitial glycosaminoglycan concentration and resistance

The above model predictions are based on an average concentration of around 14 mg of molecular fibre (glycosaminoglycan, proteoglycan and glycoprotein) per ml of extrafibrillar space i.e. space between collagen fibrils. This matrix concentration was deduced from experimental estimates of synovial hydraulic resistance [8,15] and gave an appropriate predicted control flow. Recently, attempts have been made to analyse the tiny (milligram) quantities of synovium present in a rabbit knee by quantitative biochemical methods. The combined concentration of chondroitin sulphate, heparan sulphate and hyaluronan in control

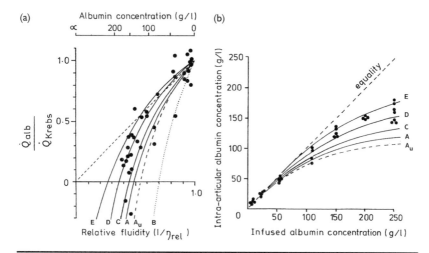

Figure 9

Comparison of experimental data (points) and model predictions (curves)

(a) Fractional trans-synovial flow versus relative fluidity at 6 cmH$_2$O (as in Figure 5, triangles). (b) Steady-state dilution of infusate (as in Figure 6, 6 cmH$_2$O). Model curves: A, uniform interstitial matrix of conductivity 60 μm^2·min^{-1}·cmH$_2$O^{-1} (10^{-11} cm^4·s^{-1}·dyn^{-1}) and extrafibrillar fibre concentration 14 mg·ml^{-1}; A$_u$, as for A but capillary permeability assumed to be uniformly distributed around its perimeter; B, as for A but conductivity reduced to one-fifth by doubling interstitial matrix concentration; C, effect of heterogeneity of matrix concentration along x axis, with lower conductivity around capillary but same overall tissue conductance, otherwise as A; D, as for C but unit cell length doubled along x axis to incorporate capillary profile heterogeneity, that is alternating fenestrated and continuous capillaries; E, as for D but lower estimate of fenestral hydraulic conductivity. Reproduced from [8] with permission.

synovium from the rabbit knee was found to be approximately 4 mg per ml of extrafibrillar space (recalculated from [16]). There thus exists a substantial material deficit of around 10 mg·ml^{-1}. This must be due, at least in part, to the presence of materials not assayed, such as fibronectin and the core protein of proteoglycan, which are known to be present from qualitative immunohistochemical work. The reconciliation of bio-chemical composition and physiologically estimated hydraulic resistance is thus incomplete at present.

Interstitial flow studied in the absence of capillary filtration; viscosity anomalies

Experimental evidence that the deviation below the Darcy line in Figure 5 is caused by capillary filtration was obtained by killing the animal to abolish capillary filtration. In Figure 10(a), which is again a plot of fractional flow versus intra-articular fluidity in the presence of albumin,

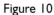

Figure 10

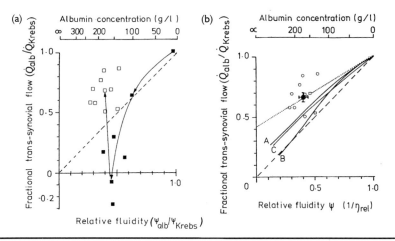

Effect of interstitial albumin on fractional interstitial flow in the absence of a functional microcirculation

For explanation of axes, see Figure 5 and text. (a) Effect of albumin first in vivo (■) and then post mortem (□) at 3–6 cmH₂O IAP. Arrowed lines join up a sequence of results in a single joint. Results post mortem lie above the Darcy line of equality (broken line). (b) Model predictions for interstitial flow post mortem (solid curves) based on anomalous viscosity and a finite interstitial reflection coefficient (0.09, curve A). Labels A and B are as for Figure 9; C, matrix concentration halved to 7 mg·ml⁻¹. ● with S.E.M. bars is mean of data post mortem and dotted line through it is predicted effect of apparent viscosity if reflection coefficient were zero; see text for further explanation. Reproduced from [8] and [17] with permission.

the filled squares represent results *in vivo*. Upon killing the animal, the low net outflows in the presence of albumin rose to much higher values, indicating that net outflows below the Darcy line had been caused by capillary filtration.

Surprisingly, however, interstitial flows *post mortem* lay above the Darcy line, rather than around it. Although certain experimental factors might have exaggerated this deviation, as discussed in [17], the results also fit with the view that the viscosity of the interstitial fluid was less than that of the feeding, bulk phase, i.e. intra-articular fluid. There is a fundamental theoretical reason why this should be so, and it stems from the well-known ability of interstitial glycosaminoglycans to exclude albumin from part of the water space [18,19]. As Figure 11 shows, a glycosaminoglycan chain creates an annular space into which the centre of mass of a large globular solute cannot penetrate due to steric exclusion, whereas the much smaller water molecules freely access the space. The greater the glycosaminoglycan concentration, the greater is the excluded volume fraction [18,20]. If the interstitial pressure gradient drives a flow of water through the albumin-excluded space, as well as driving a flow of albumin solution through the albumin-available space, then the effective overall fluidity will be a flow-weighted average of the relative fluidity of water (1) and the albumin solution in the non-excluded space (<1). The result will be an effective interstitial fluidity

Figure 11

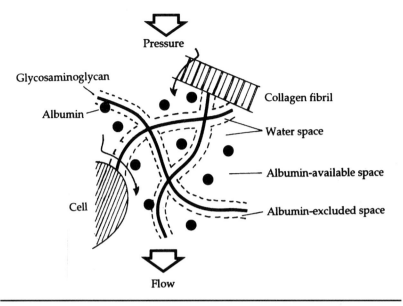

Sketch of extracellular, extrafibrillar space illustrating the difference in space available to water and to the centre of a globular macromolecular solute

that is greater (closer to 1) than that of the feeding phase, as in the results *post mortem* in Figure 10. The effect is obscured *in vivo* by large, COP-induced changes in capillary filtration, except perhaps at low albumin concentrations.

Because fluid close to the molecular chain moves less quickly than that in the centre of the 'channel' (the effect of shear [21]) a large macromolecule confined by exclusion to the central stream can be expected to have a faster transit time than a smaller solute that also travels in the slower marginal stream. This might explain the gel-chromatography effect observed in interstial transport studies, where large macromolecules have shorter transit times than small molecules, without recourse to the ill-defined 'free-fluid channels' postulated by some reviewers.

Protein exclusion and effective interstitial fluid viscosity

No formalism based on first principles appears to exist for the anomalous viscosity of a solution of macromolecules flowing through a partially excluding matrix; indeed, the issue has usually been ignored in models of interstitial flow. A simple, first-approximation treatment is proposed, therefore, based on an analogy with the anomalous viscosity of a particulate suspension flowing down a narrow tube, where there is likewise marginal steric exclusion. The Fahreus–Lindquist effect, in which decreasing tube diameter causes an apparent decrease in blood viscosity, is an example familiar to most physiologists [22]. In the present context, flow between cylindrical fibres exhibits Poiseuille-like laminar patterns [21] and the channel can be likened to an inside-out tube in that the fluid is wrapped around and shearing radially against a cylindrical solid, whereas in a tube the cylinder is wrapped around the fluid. Whitmore [23] considered the exclusion of suspended particles at the solid–fluid interface in a tube, and showed that the anomalous viscosity of a suspension of particles (radius r) flowing down a narrow tube of radius R_{tube} is described by:

$$1/\eta_{apparent} = 1 - \{(R_{core}/R_{tube})^4 [1 - (1/\eta_{core})]\} \tag{2}$$

where $\eta_{apparent}$ and η_{core} are the apparent relative viscosity and the bulk viscosity of the liquid in the non-excluded core respectively; solvent relative viscosity is 1; and the radius of the non-excluded region, R_{core}, is $R_{tube} - 0.735r$. To apply this formalism to a glycosaminoglycan matrix it is necessary to define an equivalent tube radius for the irregular channels between molecular fibres. This can been done by calculating the tube radius that produces the same fractional steric exclusion of the particle (i.e. albumin molecule here) as does the matrix.

The model curves in Figure 10(b) show the result of this approach. The predicted relationship does indeed deviate above Darcy's line but not as much as the mean observation. The reason is that there is a linked effect of exclusion on the interstitial reflection coefficient as well as fluidity. The predicted effective interstitial fluidity *per se* is high, as shown by the broken line well above the Darcy line in Figure 10(b). However, concomitant interstitial molecular sieving of albumin sets up small interstitial osmotic gradients according to the model, and these reduce the flow and so displace the model prediction down towards the Darcy line. It is concluded that the issues of interstitial reflection coefficients to macromolecules, interstitial molecular sieving and interstitial effective viscosity are far from well understood and require further investigation, both experimentally and theoretically.

Hyaluronan and trans-synovial flow

As stated in the introductory overview, the other major macromolecule that governs the physical properties of synovial fluid is the giant, non-sulphated glycosaminoglycan, hyaluronan ($M_r > 10^6$). The normal concentration of hyaluronan in synovial fluid is around $3\ g\cdot l^{-1}$ and its properties contrast sharply with those of albumin (Figure 12). The osmotic pressure of hyaluronan *per se* is slight compared with that of albumin (although hyaluronan does amplify the COP of synovial fluid by excluding intra-articular plasma protein from part of the water space), whereas hyaluronan's non-Newtonian viscosity is very high indeed. Studies on the effect of hyaluronan on trans-synovial flow are still in their infancy but striking effects are emerging, as shown in Figure 13. Here, the protocol was different from that of Figure 4; instead of holding IAP fixed and varying the intra-articular solute concentration, a single concentration was infused (3 or $6\ g\cdot l^{-1}$ hyaluronan) and IAP was raised in steps at 15–20 min intervals to define a pressure–flow

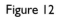

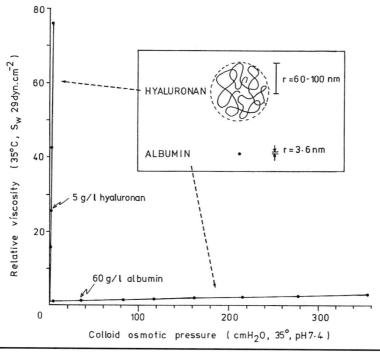

Figure 12

Comparison of effect of albumin on osmotic pressure and viscosity with that of hyaluronan

Points represent increasing concentrations. Molecular dimensions are compared in the inset, roughly to scale. Abbreviations: r, molecular radius; S_w, wall shear stress at which viscosity recorded (J.R. Levick and J.N. McDonald, unpublished work).

relationship. The control curve using Krebs solution shows the well-known increase in slope with pressure, indicating a fall in hydraulic resistance [11]. This is partly due to stretching of the lining with pressure [24] and partly due to dilution of the synovial ECM [16]. Albumin reduces absorption rate *in vivo* at any given pressure but does not alter the basic shape of the relation. The relation in the presence of hyaluronan, however, is fundamentally different in shape. At low IAPs, flows were reduced by hyaluronan (to one- to two-thirds of control), but the reduction was remarkably modest when compared with the huge reduction in bulk fluidity (to between one-tenth and one-sixteenth of control) induced by hyaluronan [25]. At higher IAPs, trans-synovial flow in the presence of hyaluronan fell increasingly below the control curve, until eventually the trans-synovial flow began to plateau. Indeed, in several joints, including that used in Figure 13, raising IAP actually resulted in a slight fall in the steady-state absorption rate. A reduction in steady-state flow upon raising IAP is suggestive of an increasing resistance to flow. To illustrate this, the pressure required to drive unit flow across the synovial lining is plotted as a function of IAP in Figure 14: if one assumes that subsynovial pressure did not change substantially over the experiment (there are grounds for such an assumption), Figure

Figure 13

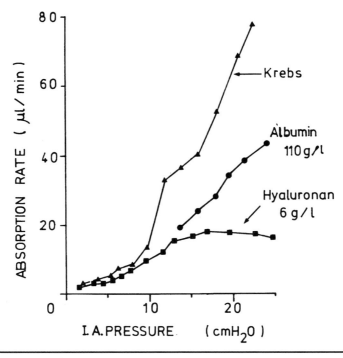

Relationship between IAP and net trans-synovial flow out of a joint cavity (absorption) for Krebs solution, albumin solution and hyaluronan solution in three individual rabbit knees

14 represents a plot of hydraulic resistance versus IAP. With Krebs solution as the infusate, the resistance parameter decreased with an increase in IAP, as has been recognized for some time. But when hyaluronan was present, the resistance parameter increased with pressure.

Hyaluronan molecular filtercakes

A very similar phenomenon was reported *in vitro* by Parker and Winlove [26]. When hyaluronan solution was driven through a Millipore membrane with pores as wide as 0.45 μm, the membrane resistance increased. This was caused by the formation of a hyaluronan filtercake or 'concentration polarization layer' at the surface; the hydrated, mutually overlapping molecular domains of the vast hyaluronan molecules were too large to pass easily though the pores, so they accumulated just upstream. The accumulated hyaluronan chains offer a high resistance to the passage of water [27]. Since the equivalent tube radius within synovial ECM is ≪0.45 μm [8,15] it is to be expected that a hyaluronan filtercake should likewise form at the synovial surface (Figure 15). Preliminary studies using non-specific staining of the synovial surface for polyanionic material by Ruthenium Red supports this, in so far as electron micrographs reveal an accumulation of Ruthenium Red-positive

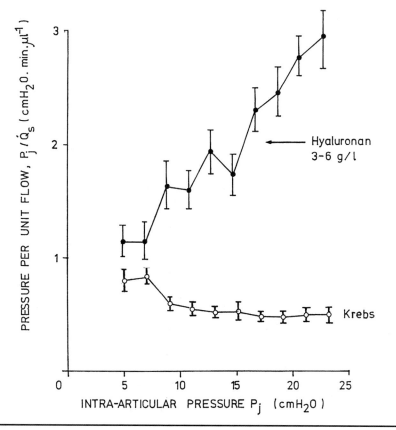

Figure 14

Resistance of synovial lining, as indicated by IAP required to drive unit trans-synovial flow, in the presence and absence of hyaluronan, plotted as a function of IAP
Points are means with S.E.M. bars for 10 joints.

material just within the superficial interstitium and at the surface after infusion of hyaluronan solution [25].

Whatever the mechanism, hyaluronan has a major effect on the hydraulic resistance of the joint cavity lining. This may be functionally important; by acting as a 'dynamic waterproofing', hyaluronan may help the synovial lining to retain the vital synovial fluid during periods of joint flexion and raised IAP.

Summary

(1) Discrete sites of capillary hydraulic permeability (fenestral plaques here) produce highly localized 'divergent jet' patterns of ultrafiltration (cf. diffuse water passage). As a result of the relatively high local fluid velocities, functionally significant gradients of interstitial COP can exist around fenestral exits over a micrometre or so. This attenuates the effect

Figure 15

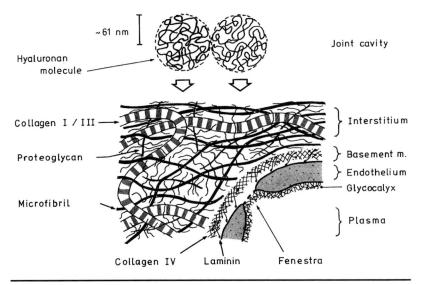

Sketch showing composition of pathway between joint cavity and
plasma, comprising three distinct fibrous matrices in series —
synovial interstitium, capillary basement membrane and endothelial
glycocalyx
*The voluminous hyaluronan molecules of synovial fluid are thought to permeate
the lining less freely than water, leading to an accumulation of hyaluronan at
the interface when IAP is raised.*

of the bulk (measurable) interstitial COP on capillary fluid exchange and
should be considered in fluid-exchange models.

(2) Effective interstitial fluid viscosity is probably modified
(reduced) by steric exclusion of plasma protein from part of the
water-conducting space.

(3) At certain IAPs and albumin concentrations, a bidirectional
flow pattern can develop across that synovial surface, providing a
mechanism for synovial fluid turnover even when a joint is static.

(4) Hyaluronan raises the outflow resistance of the lining in a
flow-dependent fashion, and this may help conserve synovial fluid and
lubricant when IAP is raised.

References

1. Stevens, C.R., Blake, D.R., Merry, P., Revell, P.A. and Levick, J.R. (1991) A comparative study by morphometry of the microvasculature in normal and rheumatoid synovium. *Arthritis Rheum.* **34**, 1508–1513
2. Levick, J.R. and Smaje, L.H. (1987) An analysis of the permeability of a fenestra. *Microvasc. Res.* **33**, 233–256
3. Knight, A.D., Levick, J.R. and McDonald, J.N. (1988) Relation between trans-synovial flow and plasma colloid osmotic pressure, with an estimation of the albumin reflection coefficient in the rabbit knee. *Q. J. Exp. Physiol.* **73**, 47–66
4. Levick, J.R. (1984) Blood flow and mass transport in synovial joints. In *Handbook of Physiology, Section 2 , The Cardiovascular System, vol. IV, The Microcirculation* (Renkin, E.M. and Michel, C.C., eds.), pp. 917–947, Am. Physiol. Soc., Bethesda, MD
5. Levick, J.R. (1987) Synovial fluid and trans-synovial flow in stationary and moving joints. In *Joint Loading: Biology and Health of Articular Structures* (Helminen, H., Kiviranta, I., Tammi, M.,

Saamaren, A.M., Paukonnen, K. and Jurvelin, J., eds.), pp. 149–186, Wright and Sons, Bristol

6.   Henderson, B. and Edwards, J.C.W. (1987) *The Synovial Lining*, Chapman and Hall, London

7.   Levick, J.R. (1991) A two-dimensional morphometry-based model of interstitial and transcapillary flow in rabbit synovium. *Exp. Physiol.* **76**, 905–921

8.   Levick, J.R. (1994) An analysis of the interaction between extravascular plasma protein, interstitial flow and capillary filtration; application to synovium. *Microvasc. Res.* **47**, 90–125

9.   Simkin, P.A. and Benedict, R.S. (1990) Iodide and albumin kinetics in normal canine wrists and knees. *Arthritis Rheum.* **33**, 73–79

10. Jensen, L.T., Henriksen, J.H., Olesen, H.P., Risteli, J. and Lorenzen, I. (1993) Lymphatic clearance of synovial fluid in conscious pigs; the aminoterminal propeptide of type III procollagen. *Eur. J. Clin. Invest.* **23**, 778–784

11. Edlund, T. (1949) Studies on the absorption of colloids and fluid from rabbit knee joints. *Acta Physiol. Scand.* **18** (Suppl. 62), 1–108

12. Levick, J.R. and Knight, A.D. (1988) Interaction of plasma colloid osmotic pressure and joint fluid pressure across the endothelium-synovium layer; significance of extravascular resistance. *Microvasc. Res.* **35**, 109–121

13. Patlak, C.S., Goldstein, D.A. and Hoffman, J.F. (1963) The flow of solute and solvent across a two-membrane system. *J. Theor. Biol.* **5**, 426–442

14. Rippe, B. and Haraldsson, B. (1994) Transport of macromolecules across microvascular walls: the two-pore theory. *Physiol. Rev.* **74**, 163–219

15. Levick, J.R. (1987) Flow through interstitium and other fibrous matrices. *Q. J. Exp. Physiol.* **72**, 409–438

16. Mason, R.M., Price, F.M. and Levick, J.R. (1994) A quantitative investigation of the glycosaminoglycans of the synovium. *Trans. Orthop. Res. Soc.* **19**, 403

17. Levick, J.R. and McDonald, J.N. (1994) Viscous and osmotically mediated changes of interstitial flow induced by extravascular albumin in synovium. *Microvasc. Res.* **47**, 68–89

18. Ogston, A.G. (1958) The spaces in a uniformly random suspension of fibres. *Trans. Faraday Soc.* **54**, 1754–1757

19. Aukland, K. and Reed, R.K. (1993) Interstitial-lymphatic mechanisms in the control of extracellular fluid volume. *Physiol. Rev.* **73**, 1–78

20. Ogston, A.G. (1970) On the interaction of solute molecules with porous networks. *J. Phys. Chem.* **74**, 668–669

21. Happel, J. and Brenner, H. (1965) *Low Reynolds Number Hydrodynamics*, pp. 392–404, Prentice-Hall, Englewood Cliffs, NJ

22. Goldsmith, H.L., Cokelet, G.R. and Gaehtgens, P. (1989) Robin Fahreus; evolution of his concepts in cardiovascular physiology. *Am. J. Physiol.* **257**, H1005–H1015

23. Whitmore, R.L. (1968) *Rheology of the Circulation*. Pergamon Press, Oxford

24. Levick, J.R. and McDonald, J.N. (1989) Ultrastructure of transport pathways in stressed synovium of the knee in anaesthetized rabbits. *J. Physiol. (London)* **419**, 493–508

25. McDonald, J.N. and Levick, J.R. (1994) Hyaluronan reduces fluid escape rate from joints disparately from its effect on fluidity. *Exp. Physiol.* **79**, 103–106

26. Parker, K.H. and Winlove, C.P. (1984) The macromolecular basis of the hydraulic conductivity of the arterial wall. *Biorheology* **21**, 181–196

27. Johnson, M., Kamm, R., Ethier, C.R. and Pedley, T. (1987) Scaling laws and the effect of concentration polarization on the permeability of hyaluronic acid. *Physicochem. Hydrodynamics* **9**, 427–441

28. McDonald, J.N. and Levick, J.R. (1992) Evidence for simultaneous bidirectional fluid flux across synovial lining in knee joints of anaesthetized rabbits. *Exp. Physiol.* **77**, 513–515

29. Anderson, J.L. and Malone, D.M. (1974) Mechanism of osmotic flow in porous membranes. *Biophys. J.* **14**, 957–982

30. Comper, W.D. and Zamparo, O. (1989) Hydraulic conductivity of polymer matrices. *Biophys. Chem.* **34**, 127–135

31. Curry, F.E. (1984) Mechanics and thermodynamics of transcapillary exchange. In *Handbook of Physiology, Section 2, The Cardiovascular System, vol. IV, The Microcirculation* (Renkin, E.M. and Michel, C.C., eds.), pp. 309–374, Am. Physiol. Soc., Bethesda, MD

32. Kedem, O. and Katchalsky, A. (1958) Thermodynamic analysis of the permeability of biological membranes to non-electrolytes. *Biochim. Biophys. Acta* **27**, 229–245

33. Ogston, A.G., Preston, B.N. and Wells, J.D. (1973) On the transport of compact particles through solutions of chain polymers. *Proc. R. Soc. Ser. A* **333**, 297–316

Accumulation of hyaluronan, 8
Action potential, 221–227
Active tubular transport, 311
Acute inflammation, 92
Adhesion receptor, 29
Adrenergic nerve, 206
Afferent lymph, 247
Afferent lymphatics, 237
Aggrecan
  carbohydrate structure, 14
  cell synthesis, 74
  composition in matrix, 67
  hydrodynamic volume, 23
  physiological function, 138
  protein structure, 14, 16
  rheological property, 23
  schematic representation, 139
  viscoelastic property, 24
Aggregate, 15
Albumin, 317, 324
Allograft, 251
Amiloride, 294
Anaphylaxis, 93
Annulus fibrosus, 70
Anomalous viscosity, 327
ANP (see Atrial natriuretic
  peptide)
Arachidonic acid metabolite, 186
Articular cartilage, 14, 55, 67
ATP, 215
Atrial natriuretic peptide, 262, 263

Basement membrane, 302
Bidirectional flow, 319
Binding
  of calcium to elastin, 157
  of elastin to lipid, 138
  of proteoglycan, 147
Biosynthesis of hyaluronan, 5
Blood lymphocyte, 247
Blood volume expansion, 261
Bovine lymphatics, 206
Burn injury, 91

C48/80, 93
Ca^{2+}-activated K^+ channel, 233
Ca^{2+}-activated Cl^- channel, 231

Cable, 230
Calcium , 157
Cannulation, 212
Capillary
  coefficient for volume filtration,
    177
  filtration coefficient, 307
  network, 126
  pressure, 173, 259
  protein leakage, 178
Carbohydrate composition of
  proteoglycan, 21
Cardiac function, 271
Carrageenan, 93
Cartilage
  compressive property, 55, 59
  two-compartment model, 56
  degeneration, 71, 78
  electromechanics, 76
Cartilaginous tissue, 55
Catecholamine, 186
Cell-surface glycosaminoglycan,
  147
Cellular lifespan, 252, 253
Cellular turnover, 252
Cerebral ischaemic response, 185
Chain–chain interaction, 10
Chemical reactivity, 157
Cholinergic nerve, 206
Chondrocyte, 73
Chondroitin sulphate, 21, 22, 138
Chronically implanted perforated
  capsule 86
Clinical use of hyaluronan, 8
Coefficient for volume filtration,
  177
Collagen, 55, 67, 103, 122, 137,
  274
  classification, 148
  composition in extracellular
    matrix, 67, 137
  constitutive model of network,
    60
  contribution to hydraulic
    conductivity, 103
  electrical property, 153
  fibre network, 55, 137

in distributed model, 122
interaction, 151
interaction with fibroblast, 34
mechanical property, 149
physicochemical property, 137
production by cardiac fibroblast,
274
synthesis, 152
Colloid osmotic pressure, 306,
307, 313, 315, 318, 324
Compaction, 107
Compartmental model, 120–122
Compliance, 89, 121
Composite medium, 110
Compressive property of cartilage,
55, 59
Compressive stress, 55, 60
Concentration, 167
Conduit network, 112
Constitutive model of collagen
network, 60
Continuity equation, 111
Contraction frequency, 194
Contractility, 294
Control mechanism, 296
Convection, 130, 134
Convective hindrance, 122
Convective transport, 258
COP (see Colloid osmotic
pressure)
Cortex, 239
Creep, 55, 62
Creeping flow, 102, 105
Critical probability, 115
Current-generated stress, 77
Cut segment, 234
Cyclic AMP, 95
Cyclic loading, 73

Darcy equation, 60
Darcy's law, 62, 101, 128
Debye–Brinkman equation, 101
Decorin, 139
Deformation of matrix, 60
Desensitization, 185
Dextran anaphylaxis, 93
Diffusion, 134

Diffusive transport, 258
Diffusivity, 122, 144, 145
Distension, 231
Distributed model, 120, 122
Distribution of solute, 144
Distribution, 290
Drag force, 104
Drag theory, 105

ECF (see Extracellular fluid)
EDRF (see Endothelium-derived
relaxing factor)
Effective fluid chemical potential,
128
Efferent lymphatics, 239
Ejection fraction, 194
EJP (see Excitatory junction
potential)
Elasticity, 156
Elastic tension, 58
Elastin
biochemistry, 153
calcium binding, 157
chemical reactivity, 157
composition in extracellular
matrix, 137
elasticity, 156
in distributed model, 122
lipid binding, 158
mechanical property, 154
molecular basis of elasticity, 156
network structure and
permeability, 158
organization, 154
physicochemical property, 137
structure, 155
synthesis, 154
Electrical activity, 207
Electrical property, 153
Electrically coupled cell, 234
Electrokinetic effect, 76
Electromechanical spectroscopy,
78
Electromechanics, 76
Electrophysiology, 221
Elemental volume, 106
Endothelial cell, 187, 245, 248, 309

Endothelial factor, 50
Endothelial fenestra, 303
Endothelium-derived relaxing
    factor, 186
Endotoxin, 183
Energy dissipation, 109
Equivalent hydraulic radius, 104
Excitatory junction potential, 208
Excluding property, 58, 103, 128
Exclusion chromatography, 146
Expression of integrin, 30
Extracellular electrical recording,
    222
Extracellular fluid, 169, 255
Extracellular matrix, 2, 137
Extracellular pH, 74
Extracellular space, 303
Extravasation of plasma protein,
    258
Extravascular space, 305

Facilitation, 209
FCD (see Fixed charge density)
Femoral head cartilage, 62
Ferritin, 308
Fibre matrix theory, 104
Fibroblast, 274
Fibroblast–collagen interaction, 34
Fibrosis, 271
Filtration coefficient, 42
Filtration pressure, 42
Fixed charge density, 55, 62, 80
Flow cytometry, 252
Flow resistance, 103
Fluid exchange, 120
Fluid flow, 57
Fluid mechanics, 101
Fluid permeability, 69
Fluid transport, 122, 128
Focal adhesion, 31
Free fluid channel, 273

G1 domain, 16–18
G2 domain, 16–18
G3 domain, 20
GAG (see Glycosaminoglycan)
Gel-chromatography effect, 327

Geometrical model, 62
Globular domain, 16–21
Glycocalyx, 111
Glycosaminoglycan, 57, 103, 122,
    138, 145, 276
Granulomatous lesion, 252
Guanethidine, 214

Haemorrhage, 217
Heart disease, 271
Heterogeneity, 57, 103, 106, 122
Heteroporous membrane, 258
Homing, 250
Horse lymph node, 238
Humoral regulation, 185
Hyaladherin, 7
Hyaluronan
    accumulation, 8
    biosynthesis, 5
    cell synthesis, 74
    chain length, 15
    clinical use, 8
    concentration in synovial fluid,
        328
    effect on hydraulic conductivity,
        103
    filtercake, 330
    function, 276
    in model tissue, 128
    interaction with globular
        domain, 138
    oligosaccharide, 10
    serum level, 7
    turnover, 6
Hydration, 58, 103, 138
Hydraulic conductivity, 101, 102,
    122, 134, 141, 142, 289
Hydraulic permeability, 55, 59
Hydraulic resistance, 324, 330
Hydrodynamic volume, 23
Hydrogen peroxide, 195
Hydrostatic pressure, 71, 132
Hypersensitivity, 251
Hypoproteinaemic rat, 97
Hypovolaemia, 185

IFNγ (see Interferon γ)

IGD (see Interglobular domain)
IGF-I (see Insulin-like growth factor I)
IL-I (see Interleukin I)
Immunological memory, 253
Incompressible fluid, 109
Inflammation, 92–94, 192
Inositol trisphosphate, 231
Insulin-like growth factor I, 72
Integrin, 29–36, 95
Interaction, 151
Interfacial property, 147
Interferon γ, 248
Interglobular domain, 19
Interleukin I, 72
Interstitial compliance, 89
Interstitial flow pattern, 323
Interstitial fluid
  accumulation, 271
  dynamics, 172
  flux, 128
  physical condition, 167
  pressure, 85, 167, 216, 264
  protein concentration, 167
  transport, 101, 128
  viscosity, 320
  volume, 167, 216, 264
Interstitial matrix, 271
Interstitial pathway, 314
Interstitial pressure, 35, 307
Interstitial reflection coefficient, 320
Interstitial space, 124
Interstitial transport, 119
Interstitium, 1, 101, 128, 271
Intervertebral disc, 67
Intra-articular albumin, 316
Intra-articular dilution, 319
Intrafibrillar space, 56
Intravital microscopy, 193
Inward rectifier, 233
Ionic dependence, 226
IP$_3$ (see Inositol trisphosphate)
ISF (see Interstitial fluid)

Joint motion, 315

K$^+$ channel, 226
Keratan sulphate, 21, 138
Kinetics, 250
Kozeny–Carman equation, 104
Krogh cylinder, 127

Large lymphatic vessel, 232
Length scale, 105
Link protein, 25, 74
Lipid binding, 158
Lubrication, 284
Lumbar disc, 71
Lymph
  flow, 167, 176, 211, 266
  node, 237, 246, 247
  propulsion, 266
  pump, 181, 185, 192
  pump flow index, 194
  vessel, 176
Lymphangion, 181, 221, 230
Lymphatic contractility, 294
Lymphatic contraction frequency, 194
Lymphatic contraction propagation, 194, 197
Lymphatic diastole, 193
Lymphatic ejection fraction, 194
Lymphatic electrical activity, 207
Lymphatic endothelial cell, 187, 248
Lymphatic exchange, 129
Lymphatic filling, 49
Lymphatic flow, 295
Lymphatic innervation, 205
Lymphatic safety factor, 42
Lymphatic smooth muscle, 221
Lymphatic stroke volume, 194
Lymphatic system
  contractile activity, 181
  in fluid homoeostasis, 191
  pumping capability, 49, 212
Lymphatic systole, 193
Lymphatic vessel, 237
Lymphatics, 124, 169, 213
Lymphocyte circulation, 245–253
Lymphocyte tracking, 249

Macromolecular exclusion, 264
Mass balance, 129
Mast cell, 96
Mathematical modelling, 119, 171
Matrix, 1–3, 55, 60
Mechanical property, 137, 149, 154
Medulla, 239
Membrane potential, 224
α, β-Methylene ATP, 213, 215
Mesothelial cell, 283
Micropuncture technique, 87, 288
Microvascular district, 292
Microvascular endothelial barrier, 49
Microvascular exchange, 119
Microvascular permeability, 260, 273
Microvillus, 285
Monocyte, 248
Myocardial interstitial compliance, 273
Myocardial interstitial pressure, 273
Myocardial interstitium, 271
Myocardial lymph flow, 271
Myocardial lymphatics, 273

Navier–Stokes equation, 102, 111
Negative feedback control system, 170
Network model, 101, 112
Neurogenic inflammation, 94
Niflumic acid, 232
Nitric oxide, 186
Non-enzymic glycosylation, 152
Noradrenaline, 215, 228
Noradrenergic innervation, 213
Nucleus pulposus, 70

Oedema, 43, 90, 122, 169, 170, 185, 271
Oedema-dependent lymphatic factor, 48
Oedema safety factor, 44
Organization of matrix, 3
Osmolality, 75

Osmotic pressure, 42, 55, 70, 143, 311
Osmotic reflection coefficient, 273
Outflow pressure, 182
Oxyhaemoglobin, 186

Pacemaking, 226–228, 232–235
Partition of extracellular fluid volume, 256
Percolation network, 116
Percolation theory, 115, 116
Pericapillary interstitial colloid osmotic pressure, 318
Pericardial effusion, 273
Pericellular coat, 8
Periodicity, 112
Permeability, 47, 55, 59, 69, 138
Permeability coefficient, 289
Permselectivity, 284
Physicochemical property, 137
Physiological regulatory mechanism, 259
Pig lymph node, 241
Plasma protein
   colloid osmotic pressure, 306
   concentration, 175
   extravasation, 258
   transport, 128
   turnover, 255
Plasma volume expansion, 261
Plasminogen activator, 248
Pleural lymphatic flow, 295
Pleural space, 283
Polyelectrolyte property, 141
Polymyxin B, 93
Polysaccharide, 3
Pore, 57, 104, 290, 323
Pore exit, 323
Porosity, 102
Postnodal mesenteric vessel, 182
Prenodal duct, 182
Pressure–flow relationship, 183, 328
Pressure sensitivity, 184
Pressure at pleural level, 291
Protein
   diffusivity, 122

-excluded volume, 273
-free perfusion, 308
leakage, 178
osmotic pressure, 42
Proteoglycan, 21, 55, 67, 103,
  137–148, 302
Pump flow index, 194
Pumping capability, 49
Purinergic transmission, 215

Random-fibre matrix theory, 320
Reabsorption, 134, 310
Reactive oxygen metabolite, 192
Reflection coefficient, 46, 128, 320
Regulation of integrin activity, 32
Remodelling, 138, 275
Renal allograft, 251
Renal cortex, 301
Renal interstitium, 301
Renal medulla, 311
Reserpine, 215
Resistance to lymph flow, 176
Reynolds number, 102
Rheological property, 23, 140

Scale, 106
Sensitivity analysis, 110
Sensory C-fibre, 97
Serum hyaluronan, 7
Sheep, 213, 238, 245
Short cable, 230
Simulation, 131
Small chamber, 234
Smooth-muscle neuromuscular
  junction, 209
Solute
  diffusivity, 144
  distribution, 144
  exchange, 120
  permeability coefficient, 289
Splanchnic nerve, 212
Spontaneous transient
  depolarization, 228–233
Starling balance of pressures at
  pleural level 291
Starling's hypothesis, 42, 257
Starling's law, 121

Static loading, 73
STD (see Spontaneous transient
  depolarization)
Stokes equation, 111
Stoma, 286
Streaming potential, 74
Stroke volume, 194
Subcapsular sinus, 238
Superoxide anion, 195
Superoxide dismutase, 195
Supramolecular structure, 15
Suramin, 215
Swelling, 55, 127
Swelling pressure, 58
Sympathetic chain, 211
Synovial joint, 67, 313
Synthesis of elastin, 154
Systems analysis, 119

Tension, 55, 58
TGF-β (see Transforming growth
  factor β)
Thoracic duct, 277
Tissue fluid hydrostatic pressure,
  42
Tissue functional unit, 127
TNF-α (see Tumour necrosis
  factor α)
Tortuosity, 104, 122
Tortuous fluid pathway, 122
Tracking, 249
Transforming growth factor β, 72
Trans-synovial flow, 317, 319, 320
Transcapillary fluid flux, 133
Transcapillary pressure gradient,
  85
Transmural pressure, 182
Transpleural fluid, 293
Transvascular fluid filtration, 41
Tumour necrosis factor α, 72, 248
Turnover
  cell, 252, 253
  hyaluronan, 6
  plasma protein, 255
Two-compartment model of
  cartilage, 56